Bion, Rickman, Foulkes and the Northfield Experiments

Community, Culture and Change
(formerly Therapeutic Communities)

Series editors: Rex Haigh and Jan Lees

Community, Culture and Change encompasses a wide range of ideas and theoretical models related to communities and cultures as a whole, embracing key Therapeutic Community concepts such as collective responsibility, citizenship and empowerment, as well as multidisciplinary ways of working and the social origins of distress. The ways in which our social and therapeutic worlds are changing is illustrated by the innovative and creative work described in these books.

Community Culutre and Change 5

Bion, Rickman, Foulkes and the Northfield Experiments
Advancing on a Different Front

Tom Harrison

Foreword by Bob Hinshelwood

Jessica Kingsley Publishers
London and Philadelphia

The quotation on page 24 is from *Flight to Arras* by Antoine de Saint-Exupéry and is reproduced by kind permission of Penguin.
The quotation on page 182 is from *War Poems and Others* by Wilfred Owen and is reproduced by kind permission of Chatto and Windus Ltd.

First published in the United Kingdom in 2000
by Jessica Kingsley Publishers
116 Pentonville Road
London N1 9JB, UK
and
400 Market Street, Suite 400
Philadelphia, PA 19106, USA

www.jkp.com

Copyright © Tom Harrison 2000
Foreword copyright © Bob Hinshelwood 2000
Printed digitally since 2009

Library of Congress Cataloging in Publication Data
Harrison, Tom, 1947–
    Bion, Rickman, Foulkes and the Northfield experiments: advancing on a different front / Tom Harrison
        p.   cm.
    Includes bibliographical references and index.
    ISBN 1-85302-837-1 (pb. : alk. paper)
        1. Group psychotherapy--History. 2. Military psychiatry--History.
I. Title.
RC488.H37   1999
616.89'152'09--dc21   99-39959
                                                                            CIP

British Library Cataloguing in Publication Data

A CIP catalogue record for this book is available from the British Library

ISBN 978 1 85302 837 3

Contents

Dedication

To all those soldiers who fought on 'a different front'
at Northfield Military Hospital

Foreword

The legend of Northfield is one of those myths of creation. Everyone who works in group psychotherapy, the therapeutic community, art therapy, therapeutic social clubs or a number of other related fields knows where their origins were. Northfield Military Hospital in the early 1940s was populated by Olympian psychiatrists and psychotherapists. We can treasure this fabled past, and know that we are the descendants of gods. But now Tom Harrison has been to Mount Olympus and has come back with more than just traveller's tales. He has brought back a full and vibrant account of the place, the ideas and the persons in all their brilliance and failings.

This book is a kind of biography of an institution, born in 1943 and lasting, as institutions often do, only a few years. Nevertheless it had a full life. In the midst of war, it represented the triumph of hope and initiative. Its life is marked by the clash of desperate originality with the forces of conservatism. Ultimately perhaps the outcome was a draw; but not without the demonstration of immense experiment and thought. As is well known, there was not just one Northfield experiment, but two. And in themselves they generated a good deal of friction between them, and it seems between those players within the hospital who represented the separate experiments. The hopes of one side and then of the other fluctuated and the life of this institution can be seen to be as organic as the life of any individual person. The fortunes of Northfield were short-lived but glittering, and totally dependent on the fluctuations of the war. Then, you the reader, will feel a sadness as we come to 1946 and the hospital declined into dirty dereliction as it faced closure; it is a sadness reminiscent of the closing chapter of an actual biography with the death of its subject.

Within the hospital is a galaxy of names that were subsequently to become stars – Wilfred Bion, Michael Foulkes, Tom Main, Harold Bridger, Joshua Bierer, Pat de Maré, and, in this account, above all John Rickman. Harrison finds amongst these and the many others, his friends, colleagues and foes, just as anyone living there must have done. The author has in fact worked, and thus professionally inhabited, the buildings at Hollymoor

Hospital in South Birmingham, which housed Northfield, and he has met more than the ghosts of his predecessors. He has used the surviving texts to resurrect the life of this old community; and he has interviewed some of the ageing participants, or their relatives, as well as inmates.

None of the main contributors to the Northfield experiments had a reputation before their drafting to the hospital. How is it, one wonders, that so many came from this army hospital to flourish afterwards in so many directions? Was it that the army was merely fortunate in gaining such a supply of brilliant people which the navy and airforce lacked – or was it something about Northfield that instilled so many of them with a lasting creative stimulus? My own preferred guess is that it was the latter – no-one could go through such an involvement, and come out unscathed. Northfield occurred at a national moment of collective need and, for people rising to that challenge, mostly at the beginnings of their careers, a sense of achievement, perhaps even of achieving the impossible, must have stayed with them as a springboard for their own personal careers.

One gets a sense of Bion's irascible impatience with authority, Rickman's Quaker inner stillness, Foulkes' rather frantic ambitiousness, Main's overbearing but eloquent anxiousness, all combining as a community of real people. Those arriving at Northfield with more experience provided some degree of a stabilising influence, but at the same time acted as agents provocateurs with imaginative ideas for the newer generation to take up and run with. The greatest of these was John Rickman. His actual role at Northfield seems to be not clear, because he was also, it seems, at a great many other army experiments in social psychology and psychiatry all over the country. He was a close background figure for Bion in all his troubled experiences in army psychiatry. There seemed to be a guru quality about Rickman, a prodding inspiration rather than an administrator or an academic writer. That quality of direct inspiration of others leaves a quiet record, and Tom Harrison clearly wants to rescue his hero, and rehabilitate him to the centre of this psychiatric pantheon. All of us readers will have our particular heroes, but I for one am persuaded to take Rickman a lot more seriously than I had hitherto.

Despite its wave upon wave of enthusiastic initiatives that swept the institution, Northfield was perhaps the first and prototype self-reflective institution. Central to its purpose was a constant questioning of the proper way to perform the task of treating soldiers who break down. Perhaps this constant questioning and reflection is due to the actual impossibility of the job. Do you serve the army and return men to a death in the front line? Or do you serve the patients and repair their health? In wartime the good of the army and the good of the patient pull in diametric opposition. Though many of its inmates returned to administrative and supportive roles, it is to the credit of Northfield that it seemed continually to worry away at this contradiction across which it was straddled, and did not settle on some stale and easy pretence about its task.

Although Northfield did not theorise itself as a reflective institution, in the way, say that Main later described the 'culture of enquiry', nevertheless it simply did keep on enquiring about its role and is methods. From this came the therapeutic community, or more precisely, one could say that the energy and enquiry at Northfield brands it as a genuine therapeutic community before they knew what one was. This book is in effect a full-scale description of a therapeutic community as a going concern; and at the same time, Tom Harrison implies, a description of how a psychiatric institution today should be functioning. It is of great interest that the origins of the therapeutic community were in rehabilitation work with casualties of war and later, after the war, in the rehabilitation of the inmates of the long-stay psychotic patients in the countries mental hospitals. Somehow, we need to go back to our roots and recognise that such rehabilitation jobs still need to be done, and they need to be done humanely. They need to be done with an eye on the subjective quality of those in our charge, that is to say, we need to match their self-reflective capacities with a self-reflective institution.

One of the strengths of this account is that it contextualises the thinking that was done in Northfield, in the period of the 1930s when social psychology was at its height. Mostly when psychology commenced at the beginning of this century it arose from an amalgam of doctors interested in mental illness and philosophers interested in the philosophy of mind. Such an unlikely marriage created our interesting profession of psychologists. However there was a third strand which arose from political thinking. Following the French revolution in 1789, the nineteenth century had remained very anxious about the turmoil of crowds and masses who could behave, collectively, in primitive ways which contrasted drastically with the notions, held by the middle classes, of civilised people. Political descriptions of crowd behaviour, more or less objective, gradually came to be graced with the title of 'social psychology' after 1900. This was a European anxiety, but it mingled with the American study of work conditions in factories which would maximise output. Together, the notion of social psychology mushroomed in its political and egonomic variants. So in wartime, when group morale was a higher priority than individual health, it was natural to seek psychological ideas in that prevailing climate. This was the context of Northfield, and one which is covered interestingly in this book.

Northfield did not happen in a vacuum, nor did its star performers do so without each other. It was a living experience and not a designed environment, and it had the pell-mell inconsistencies and flaws, as well as the vibrancy, of any ordinary institution. Its contradictions and confusions are the reality of the rough edges of life. Who wants a myth of this wonderful place, when the reality is so much more fascinating, and touches exquisitely on those nerves that worry about the contradictions in our present institutions?

Bob Hinshelwood
October 1999

Acknowledgements

This book has taken some fifteen years to research and write. During that time I have received support, help, advice and information from a number of people. I will endeavour to acknowledge them all; but I apologise in advance for any failure to recognise a particular contribution.

In embarking on such an enterprise, the people one lives with have to tolerate an obsession. They must cope with one's rushing off at a few hours' notice to interview someone, holidays devoted to one's writing, conversations larded with references to events fifty years ago, strangers coming to the door requiring hospitality and then being closeted in discussion for hours on end, weekends taken up with meetings and sporadic mood disturbances occassioned by successes or disappointments. This is not easy. Writing a book tends to a solitary occupation excluding those around you, and my family – particularly Jane – have tolerated all this with great forebearance and love, for which I thank them.

A number of people have been enthusiastic supporters, contributing encouragement as well as practical help. First among these is Craig Fees of the Planned Environment Therapy Trust Archive, who, with his patience over my amateurish recording techniques, knowledge, considerate enthusiasm for the project and expertise, has been a pillar on which I have leant many times. I am also grateful to David Clarke, who as a trainee psychiatrist working with me, stimulated me to actually embark on the voyage for real and brought his expertise in writing papers to our first tentative publication on Northfield. One graduate of Northfield itself has consistently put up with enquiries, letters and bursts of enthusiastic reporting on progress; he has also provided essential background material. This is Professor Laurence Bradbury, whose friendship I value deeply. Others who have given me support and advice include Malcolm Pines, Bob Hinshelwood, Ian Lowery, the late Dr Stephen MacKeith for setting me straight on Forward Psychiatry, Ben Shepherd for helping to clear the way and Eric Rayner.

Others have helped in organising and recording interviews. Alistair Wilson was kind enough to enlist my help in his excellent documentary for Radio 4, 'War in the Head', which gave me access to a number of participants. Sally Lindsay of Blakeway Productions Ltd was also kind enough to give me similar assistance during her production of 'Shell Shock' for Channel 4. Craig Fees, David Clarke, Ian Lowery and Jane Willey too have helped in this part of the enterprise.

Two archives in particular have yielded especially valuable material: the Wellcome Contemporary Medical Archives and those of the British Psycho-Analytic Society. I would like to thank the archivists at both for their invaluable assistance. Pearl King from the latter facility was also kind enough to make available other materials concerning John Rickman, and also to give me some of her time in an interview about her memories and knowledge of the relevant period in psycho-analysis. Her articles have proved invaluable.

Many people were interviewed. All spoke openly and all gave information that has proved essential: in addition, many gave documents and photographs. These are: Mrs Lucy Baruch, Mrs Francesca Bion, Dr Julian Bion, the late Mrs Parthenope Bion, Mrs Bird, Professor Laurence Bradbury, Mr Harold Bridger, Mr K. Charlton, Mrs June Clayton, Mr R. Curtis, Doctor Pat de Maré, the late Dr Millicant Dewar, Mr J. Eden, the late Mr Sam Gaskin, Mrs Irene Gaskin, Mrs May Goble, the late Dr H.E. Haas, Mr S. Harvey, Mrs Lilian Hewitt, Mr E. Howell, Mrs B. Hughes, the late Dr Charles Lewsen, Dr Ronald Markillie, the late Dr Tom Main, Mr D. Morgan, Mr W. Perry, Mr E. Rawson-Lax, Mr and Mrs J. Ross, Mrs B. Sargent, Mr G. Siddall, Mr Skinner, Mr G. Smith, Mr C. Walsh, Mr Peter Wiggall and Mr G. Young.

I have also been in correspondance with others who have sent me their memories, and memorabilia. Thank you, therefore, to: Professor William Abse, the Reverend R.C.H. Corbin, Dr Susannah Davidson, Dr Eric Cunningham Dax, Dr Thomas Freeman, Dr Jennifer Johns and Mrs Denise Leigh.

I have a particular debt to acknowledge to Mr Vernon Scannell, who has kept me in touch with the emotional pain of what happened in Northfield. His poem 'Compulsory Mourning' is compulsory reading for anyone who is interested in the events there (Ambit, 1992). I only wish I could directly thank his colleague, the late Mr Rayner Heppenstall, for the insights and descriptions given in his book *The Lesser Infortune*, which unfortunately is out of print.

Finally, three of my secretaries have consistently supported the enterprise, fielding telephone calls, showing unfeigned interest and gently nudging me back into the present day when duty called.

CHAPTER 1

The Psychological Offensive

DECODING THE SPHINX: BION, RICKMAN AND THE FIRST NORTHFIELD EXPERIMENT

Whilst General Montgomery was on the offensive in North Africa, military psychiatrists advanced into enemy territory in England. In one year of the Second World War they broke through twice. During 1942, Sigmund Foulkes elucidated the concept of group transference (Foulkes and Lewis 1944). Over the winter of 1942 to 1943, Wilfred Bion and John Rickman penetrated even further in what has come to be known as 'the First Northfield Experiment'. The front they opened up in the conflict against neurosis has been a centre of operations ever since.

Like 'two vast and trunkless legs of stone', a pair of terse articles, 'Intra-group tensions in therapy: their study as the task of the group' (Bion and Rickman 1943) and 'The leaderless group project' (Bion 1946) abide as records of these events. These remain as a reminder of a lost world from which few artifacts remain. One or two other expositions elaborate on this sketchy picture, but all descriptions of the First Northfield Experiment have had to rely primarily on their account, often quoting significant amounts of it verbatim (Trist 1985; Bridger 1990a; Bléandonu 1994).

Eric Trist pointed out that their ideas, as contained in Bion's work *Experiences in Groups* (Bion 1961), were 'no more than the first etchings for a theory', and that 'no one has so far appeared to continue the work of decoding the sphinx' (Trist 1985). This metaphor refers to Bion's perception of the conundrum of his leadership within the therapeutic group: 'the enigmatic, brooding, and questioning sphinx from whom disaster emanates' (Bion 1961, p.162). The reconstruction given here provides some further clues to help solve the riddle.

The circumstances of working in a military hospital with conscripted soldiers led to specific conditions which have not subsequently been replicated in British group therapy. These conditions forced particular modes of operation, particularly the concatenation of group therapy and functional activity, which has rarely been repeated since.

By reviewing this early work, and in particular its relationship with earlier theory, it is possible to view Bion's later writing in a new light. The influence of Rickman, often remarked upon but rarely explored, offers an entirely novel vantage point. Whilst the latter never fully developed a theory of his own, his writings contain the seeds of many of his colleague's insights.

Process, leadership and social obligations: A threefold strategy

The First Northfield Experiment, although curtailed abruptly and unable to establish any permanent gain, is the pivotal event of this book. It established the principles upon which subsequent workers built. Bion and Rickman identified the core issues that had to be faced, and shifted therapeutic thinking from individual treatment with its limited horizons to enabling men to survive the relationships and responsibilities of fighting in a war. By sundering the traditional doctor/patient relationship and reconfiguring the task as one of mutual endeavour they engaged the men in the process of recovery. The issue of illness became secondary. The task was to re-establish the individual as someone who could operate effectively in a social environment, carrying out their responsibilities and sharing comradeship.

Three crucial aspects underlay this: understanding the group process, elucidating concepts of leadership and acknowledging the social obligations of therapists.

Group process

Fundamental to Bion and Rickman's way of working was that they enabled the dynamics of a group to reveal themselves rather than dictating the direction the group should take. This is a commonplace now, but they pioneered it in practice. Sigmund Foulkes, who also claimed this distinction, probably introduced the concept; but at this time he would open a session with a mini-tutorial, apparently unaware of the fact that as the leader he was already determining its course. Rickman observed one of his sessions and was shocked to find that he opened it by announcing: 'I want you to look on me as you would the doctor in a white coat and not as someone in uniform' (Bridger 1985). Another therapist at Northfield Military Hospital announced to his patients that it was possible to 'say what you like here, for within these four walls we are not in the army!' (quoted in Rickman 1945).

This undermined the necessity for the group members to deal with the reality of the 'here and now', particularly in a time of war when the aim was to provide the army with as many effective soldiers as possible – a task which was not always the same as treating symptoms.

Bion and Rickman recognised that the power of the group lay not in the uncovering of past material through mass individual therapy but in the explicit resolution of intra-group dynamics, exploring the 'here and now' experience of the participants. Through this, the individual was able to explore the impact of his behaviour on others and modify his relationships in real time. This was both an intellectual, discursive task and a practical exercise in group living. The men in the training wing under Bion decided upon their own activities, and were then encouraged to look at the consequences of their decisions. Fundamentally, it was expected that once the soldiers had a say in what was happening to them they would begin to take charge of their lives. This was no libertarian democracy, but an opportunity for them to face up to their responsibilities.

These concepts had their antecedents in the work of the Americans, Trigant Burrows and J.L. Moreno; but neither had amalgamated them with the still-emerging ideas of object relations theory or applied them to a complete institution. The concepts were entirely new to British practice.

Leading by wandering about: Concepts of command

Turning the headlong flight of men who had lost all confidence, all sense of belonging, and who wished only to run to a mythical 'home', required leadership. It could take one of three courses: punishment, treatment or the methods that Rickman and Bion attempted. The first approach was tried and tested, but singularly ineffectual. The second avoided the problem altogether by identifying problematic behaviour as illness. The last required a complete reconceptualisation of how effective command could be re-established. Bion and Rickman argued that only when the men considered themselves as valuable and effective partners in the enterprise would they begin to rally.

Leadership was a central concern, not only in their own practice, but also in its relationship to morale. As we shall see, they were both involved in officer selection. They had to ensure these men's competence in maintaining the aggression of those under their command towards the enemy, whilst retaining friendship and support for their colleagues. The selection procedures were modified, particularly by Bion, to enable the observer to identify whether the candidate actually performed, as well as spoke, like a potential leader.

Whilst at Northfield Bion and Rickman deliberated on how leadership was expressed most effectively. Rickman openly discussed issues of rank in his group sessions on the ward (Bion and Rickman 1943). Bion's technique of walking around the unit and discussing progress with the soldiers prefigured the observations of the management guru Tom Peters on 'Management by Wandering About' (Peters and Austin 1985).

The wider social content

Military necessity painfully exposed the social responsibilities of psychiatrists. Soon after the war was over Ahrenfeldt complained of the tendency to forget this :

> One of the most serious deficiencies on the part of psychiatry as a whole was its emphasis on the individual, almost as an isolated unit independent of group dynamics, and its relative neglect of 'social psychiatry.'

He recognised that individuals should not be treated in isolation and 'society' should not be considered in the abstract. The two are inextricably interrelated and interdependent (Ahrenfeldt 1968). This reflected the confluence of a number of streams of social theory and experimentation: psychoanalysis, the American social psychology of Slavson, Moreno and Lewin, the British schools of thought of Trotter, McDougall and Rivers, and the practical experience of the Peckham and Hawkspur Experiments. These will be elaborated on later; here it is important to recognise that much thinking at this time emphasised the intimate and dynamic interrelationship of the person and their social environment, and the impossibility of individuals living in isolation from one another.

Bion and Rickman were aware of the ramifications of their work for the community at large, particularly as it related to the army. For instance, they emphasised that the task of the therapy was to enable as many men as possible return to military service in one role or another. This might well be at the expense of a full recovery. It was better to return an experienced soldier to his unit to function effectively for six months than to treat him fully and then discharge him from the army. Main emphasised this when he castigated his colleagues at Northfield for being 'treaters' (1984).

Bion and Rickman, however, failed to take into account the macro-environment of the hospital, leading to the premature demise of the experiment. This issue was taken up more explicitly in the later work of Foulkes, Main and Bridger in the Second Northfield Experiment.

Perhaps this last issue, the interrelationship of social systems, is the most significant contribution to present day psychiatry, which is commonly preoccupied with individual patient care, often to the exclusion of the family, and has relatively little concern for the responsibilities of both the individual and the professionals to the wider society. There is evidence that this is changing, particularly with treatment being increasingly carried out in people's own homes. The story of the First Northfield Experiment could provide a significant contribution to how this might progress, particularly with regards to these wider social obligations.

THE SECOND NORTHFIELD EXPERIMENT

It is surprising that after the apparent debacle of the First Northfield Experiment, which ended six weeks after it had begun, another attempt was not only sanctioned by the British Army but received active support from the Establishment.

In this second and more substantial bridgehead into enemy territory, Sigmund Foulkes, Tom Main, Laurence Bradbury and Harold Bridger resurveyed the ground and exploited it rather differently. They were only partially aware of their predecessors' foray into the field and consequently they tackled the foe with different tactics. It was with Bridger's arrival that the lessons of the first reconnaissance began to be understood. The whole hospital, including the commanding officer, had to be part of the enterprise. This was never achieved entirely, but the attempt proved fascinating. Again the men were placed in the position of re-evaluating their experience and taking responsibility for their actions rather than blaming everyone and everything else. On this occasion the creativity and enterprise released was reflected in magazines, mutual aid groups, concerts, contributions to children's hospitals and, finally, international recognition in the form of a visit by a very eminent American delegation. The ferment spread wider than previously and involved a much broader group of psychiatrists, many of whom continued as group therapists for the rest of their lives.

In the background was John Rickman, visiting, writing, constantly aware of what was going on and supporting the most active participants. His contributions, whilst intermittent and brief, reinforced the original concepts that he and Bion had hammered out earlier. Always considerate, thoughtful and self-deprecating, his visit in 1945 was welcomed by Tom Main as being as effective as a bomb in clearing a slum (Main 1945).

Neither of the two expeditions were successful in establishing a bridgehead that could sustain a full-blooded assault, but they prepare the ground for others to follow in the future.

ARTEFACTS AND CONTEXT: THE METHOD OF EXCAVATION

Some readers may feel that too much of this book is taken up by early social psychology and military history rather than the events themselves.

As in an archaeological exploration, the task is not only to find artefacts, but also to place them into their historical and cultural context in order to understand their purpose and importance. They in turn amplify the understanding of the society that produced them. The few shards of evidence available from the Northfield Experiments can only really be understood in the context of contemporary socio-psychological theories and the practice of military psychiatry during the Second World War. Foulkes' recollections of his mentor Kurt Goldstein come to mind here. This neurologist believed in a holistic approach to his patients, setting them and their symptoms into a social and psychological context. He understood that this method allowed one to gain a more complete picture of the issues and resulted in a better formulation of the problem and plan of treatment (Foulkes 1936).

The section following this introduction outlines the development of psychoanalysis and conceptualisations of group behaviour during the first part of the twentieth century. These developments were integral to both Bion and Rickman's experience and training before joining the army; indeed, they had had direct contact with with many of the main theorists, either as pupils or colleagues. Both British and American schools of social psychology were influential, the most significant and direct contribution stemming from the work of Kurt Lewin on an early version of systems theory. Psychoanalysis was at the heart of all their thinking, and the contemporary 'Controversial Discussions' held at the British Psycho-Analytic Society were followed closely by both.

It comes as a shock to modern practitioners to realise how profound an influence psychiatrists and psychologists had on the organisation of the British Army between 1941 and 1945. They pioneered, on a practical level, the implementation of insights gained from the social psychology theory described above. The two main protagonists of this book were central to this process, and the story of their involvement is essential background to an account of their activities in the hospital. Two particular aspects are detailed: the evolution and practice of the War Office Selection Boards (WOSBs) and the development of psychiatric rehabilitation services.

On examination of these two streams of theory and practice it becomes clear that the Northfield Experiments did not emerge from a vacuum. There were clear antecedents, and this goes some way towards explaining how, after the failure of the First Experiment, the Second was able to take place. The setting itself also influenced their course. This included the nature of the hospital itself, the patients and the staff. In describing these, some of the conflicting aims and methods of treatment are elucidated, thus giving an idea of the barriers that Bion and Rickman faced when setting up their experiment.

The six weeks' drama of the First Experiment has been described before. The reconstructions have gained immeasurably from the first-hand accounts of people who were there at the time as well as archived records. Published accounts provide a framework, but are not always clearly expressed. The terseness of Bion's writing has in certain instances hidden what it sought to reveal. This is particularly true for later readers who are unaccustomed to some of the language. The contemporary social psychology and psychoanalysis discussed in the early chapters of this book should go some way towards overcoming this difficulty.

The ideas of Bion and Rickman are best evaluated through examination of their practical implementation. The Second Northfield Experiment provides an obvious opportunity to do this. Here the conditions imposed by the exigencies of war were virtually identical to those imposed during the first; but the edifice had to be rebuilt, often without awareness of its predecessor. Rickman acted as the intermediary, corresponding with many of the participants and on occasion visiting. As a result the architecture changed, with accretions of many varied styles being tacked on. There is more evidence relating to this second experiment. Others have explored it in some depth, although they have not always agreed with one another on details.

The final chapter attempts to review the outcomes of the Northfield Experiments. This is both an account of effects on the individuals involved and also a highly selective and personal view of the longer-term consequences. This will allow for a degree of speculation that is deliberately avoided in the rest of the book.

To follow through fully the holistic approach expounded earlier it would be relevant to explore the economic, political and social environment. A complete and definitive systems analysis would require this. The difficulty with this is that the relationship of this particular sequence of events is too dissociated from the macro-environment for direct connections between cause and effect to be demonstrable. There was evidently some interaction that enabled explorations of the group approach recurred so frequently during the 1930s and 1940s. It was almost certainly interwoven with the flourishing of idealistic left-wing politics among intellectuals of the time. However, it is beyond the scope of this book to explore these relationships, and it is also unlikely that any associations so drawn could be anything more than highly conjectural.

COMRADES IN ARMS: BION, RICKMAN
AND THEIR COLLEAGUES

At the outset, one issue may appear incongruous to many readers. Usually, most of the credit for the Northfield Experiment goes to Wilfred Bion, and John Rickman figures only in the small print. Here they are paired together as equally significant collaborators. There is a lot of evidence that demonstrates that they had a close relationship at this point in their lives and shared interests in many issues. From 1938 to 1939 Bion had been in psychoanalysis with Rickman. They both wrote papers on air raids and shared similar ideas about military psychiatric rehabilitation, and the first paper on the Northfield Experiments was co-authored. Rickman's deference concerning his own contributions was remarked upon by Bion himself (Payne 1957, pp.12–13). Bléandonu suggests that Rickman's analysis of Bion laid the foundations for further work with Melanie Klein, and that Rickman's interpretations 'fanned the embers dormant in the ashes of the past' rather than playing intellectual games, as had been Bion's experience of analysis previously (Bléandonu 1994). The importance of the analysis was emphasised by Eric Trist, who pointed out that subsequently Bion married and began to demonstrate his 'immense powers of insight and intellect' (1985, p.3). Tom Main emphasised that 'a lot of what Bion says is borrowed direct from Rickman, at that period' (1984).

As the research for this book progressed, the importance of Rickman's role became increasingly evident. He had been considering the con-sequences of Melanie Klein's work on social situations long before war broke out. Papers and lectures given by Rickman in the 1930s are probably the first public application of object relations theory to groups and social psychology (1938a). He organised international conferences of psychiatrists during the first part of the war so that ideas and experiences could be shared as quickly as possible throughout the Allied armed forces. As will be demonstrated later, his contributions to the Northfield Experiments were seminal. They include both the preparatory work he did on the nature of rehabilitation of soldiers and also his contributions to the later work done at the hospital.

Early in the war military psychiatrists and psychologists shared ideas and did not concern themselves with ownership. It was in this spirit that Rickman tended to efface himself, selflessly encouraging others to achieve advancement rather than pursuing his own. This was the cause of one of Bion's few critical comments about his mentor: 'Indeed, had he not been so careless of husbanding his resources I think it would have been not only better for him but for the causes he had so much at heart. But I never heard of

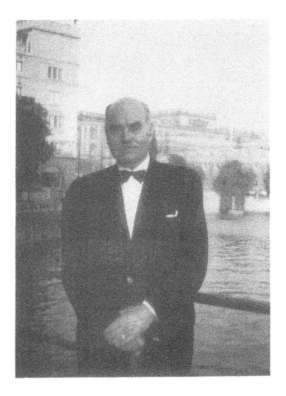

Dr Wilfred Bion c.1961. Reproduced by kind permission of Mrs F. Bion and family

anyone who was able to persuade him to consider his own welfare' (Payne 1957).

Rickman was evidently an inspiring figure who was greatly respected by those who knew him. This book will hopefully go some way towards re-establishing his reputation and his importance in the development of the therapeutic community movement.

A figure who crops up frequently throughout is Sigmund Foulkes. He arrived at Northfield a month after Bion and Rickman left and laid some of the foundations for the Second Northfield Experiment. His descriptions of his early days there elaborate on the atmosphere and environment, and so are important in shedding some light on the milieu of the unit that Bion and Rickman were familiar with. As mentioned above, Foulkes was also a pioneer of group therapy who made his own invaluable and distinctive contribution. However, his approach was in sharp contrast to theirs, and illustrates many of the attitudes to which they were opposed. As a result, when he figures in this book it is often as their counterfoil. Some readers may consider that this

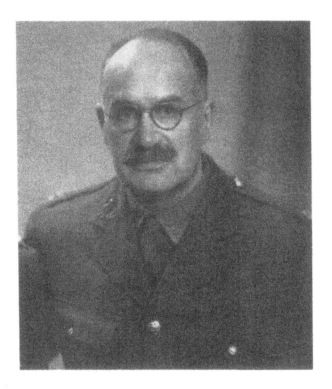

Major John Rickman, 1945. Reproduced by kind permission of Mrs Lucy Baruch

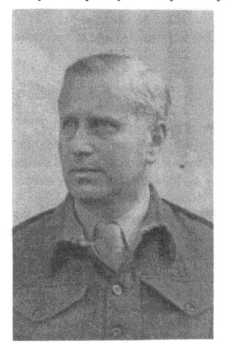

Dr Sigmund Heinrich Foulkes c.1944. Reproduced by kind permission of Mrs E Foulkes

undervalues his important contributions both to group psychotherapy and to the Second Experiment.

Tom Main and Harold Bridger also figure in the Second Northfield Experiment. Both acknowledged their debt to Rickman and Bion, following firmly in their footsteps and reinterpreting their work inventively. Both went on to establish major reputations for themselves after the war, the former as director of the Cassell Hospital and the latter in the Tavistock Institute of Human Relations.

Other individuals who were important in the subsequent development of psychiatry and psychotherapy also practiced at Northfield: in particular, Joshua Bierer, who later set up the Marlborough Day Hospital, and Laurence Bradbury, who was particularly significant in the development of art as therapy. Despite their importance in their fields, they are less directly relevant to this story, and are only referred to in passing rather than being accorded the attention they deserve.

CHAPTER 2

Social Fields
Social Psychological Theory before 1942

> I shall be fighting for the primacy of Man over the individual.
>
> (Antoine de Saint-Exupéry 1995, p.128)[1]

SUCH A COMPANY OF BROTHERS

The soldier's ability to fight depends on the small circle of men with whom he shares the sweat and drudgery of army life. Ellis argued that the soldier only fought for the 'tiny fraternity of comrades who shared his suffering'. They were his friends and the only tangible reality within which he could sustain a sense of his own self (1993, p.315). In his study of American troops in the Pacific theatre of war in 1944, Marshall found the same (1947, p.38). General Baynes analysed the nature of military morale in the 2nd Scottish Rifles in 1914 and concluded that 'Trust in the group is an essential part of the soldier's development' (Baynes 1987, p.102). This reliance extended throughout all areas of military life. After the First World War, Montague, who was much admired by Main and others (Rees 1945, p.18), wrote of his personal experience: 'whatever its size a man's world was his section – at most his platoon; all that mattered to him was the one little boatload of castaways with whom he was marooned on a desert island' (Montague 1929, pp.36–37).

During the Second World War, British military psychiatrists and psychologists assimilated observations of the importance of the group into their theoretical model of social integration. In essence, they comprehended that, emotionally, every individual was inextricably intertwined with those around them. Concurrently, Klein and Fairbairn were elaborating a psychodynamic theory that underpinned these conclusions. Their understanding of how the child's personal development is mediated through

---

1 This conclusion arose from his musings on why he continued to fly into almost certain death to no obvious military advantage.

relationships with others further confirmed the centrality of this interdependance. The conjunction of psychoanalysis, the exigencies of military life, and social theory led inevitably to the experimentation with group therapy on a wide scale within the British and other armies. The Northfield Experiments were a significant but relatively minor part of this.

In the previous four decades social psychology had developed from its tentative origins in the work of Le Bon and a few others into a discipline that supported two journals, *Sociometry* and the *Journal of Social Psychology*, and a flood of other publications. The understanding of human gatherings had evolved from a simplistic dichotomisation between the individual and the surrounding crowd into a dynamic theory which recognised the inter-relationships of groups and their constituent members throughout society. It was becoming increasingly clear that human beings exist through and are shaped by the social environments in which they live.

Three streams of theory exerted a strong influence on the protagonists of this story. The first two flowed from the British and American schools of social psychology and anthropology. Both traced their origins in European sociological thought.

The third confluence sprang from the work of Sigmund Freud and his followers. As Tom Main later stated: 'We were all keen on the psychoanalytic viewpoint.' (1984). Rickman was a fully-fledged practitioner, having been amongst the pioneering British group during the 1920s, and Bion was his analysand. Foulkes had trained in Frankfurt before arriving in the UK in 1933. Other participants in the Northfield Experiments were stimulated to become analysts later.

The history of ideas is a labyrinth, because the goal and success in reaching it are entirely relative. The debates raging over whether progress has occurred in psychiatry and which critera are valid measures are consequences of this (Scull 1991). The importance of a particular school of thought can only be demonstrated through explicit repetition of its conclusions by others. The effect of other influences can only be inferred from circumstantial evidence. There are no more objective measures. This is complicated by the fact that the influence of theory on the actual course of events is negligable compared with the effects of less rational economic and social forces. Individual actions are rarely, if ever, determined by pure thought alone.

Even when the goal of the enquiry is selected, the path is still seldom clear. No individual is conscious of all the influences determining the development of their conceptions. This is amply exemplified by Foulkes' varying views on the subject in his own case. In 1944, he described having read Schilder's book on psychotherapy (Foulkes and Lewis 1944). Later, in

1964, he claimed that he had only known of this work at that time through hearsay (Foulkes 1964, p.14). Another impediment was highlighted by Ernest Jones when he reported that 'nowadays far more Psychoanalysis is learnt from the spoken word than through the written word' (1936). Discussion went largely unrecorded. The contemporary written word only hints at this submerged history.

In this study it has been possible, through the published literature, interviews, reports and letters, to identify some of the most important contributions and some less expected ones. Where possible, reference is made to texts that are known to have been available to the participants. When there is no such evidence or certainty, such as in the case of Kurt Lewin's 1940s work on T groups, it has been assumed that the information was not known. A number of threads weave in and out, and it has not always been possible to follow through each one consistantly. Phenomenology, psychoanalysis, Gestalt ideas and Marxism interdigitated with the theories of Trotter, McDougal and Darwin. Each sought to provide holistic and dynamic explanations of the same social processes, leading to what de Maré described as a 'coherence of consistant thinking' (1972, p.43). The socio-political climate enabled different schools of thought, throughout Europe and North America, to arrive independantly at similar conclusions concerning the interdependence of human beings.

This historical exploration of group theory starts at the beginning of the century with Le Bon's classic work, *The Crowd*, published in 1896, which attempted to understand the popular uprisings of the late nineteenth and early twentieth centuries. The First World War led Wilfred Trotter, and less directly William MacDougall, to write their highly influential studies of the instinctual aspects of human behaviour. Sigmund Freud recast their findings, arguing that interactions in the social environment were determined by unconscious intrapsychic mechanisms. Developing this further, in some hitherto-neglected papers from 1938, Rickman was the first to apply the then novel ideas of Melanie Klein. Soon afterwards Fairbairn elaborated his position on object relations theory, rejecting instinct theory altogether.

American theorists, Moreno, Slavson, and in particular Kurt Lewin, were highly influential. Group therapy had been developing in the United States since the beginning of the century, starting with Joseph Pratt's work with patients suffering from tuberculosis. Foulkes was aware of the work of Schilder and Trigant Burrow, but stated that he was unaware of others until later on (1964, pp.14–17). Hargreaves introduced the ideas of Moreno to him in 1944.

There occurred, apparently independently, two significant realisations of social engineering that prefigured the Northfield Experiments. The first was the Peckham Experiment, an attempt to set up in London a 'real' health centre where people went in order to maintain their well-being rather than have their illnesses treated. The second was a series of communities embracing children and adolescents. Auguste Aichhorn's treatment of 'wayward youths' in Austria led to many imitations, including the Hawkspur Experiment. In the latter, 'delinquent' teenagers set up and ran their own community under the aegis of a remarkable man called David Wills. Both of these exercises were known to participants in the Northfield experiments.

MOBS, HERDS AND INSTINCTS

The turn of the century was marked by increasing concern about the threat of social upheaval. Le Bon encapsulated these fears when he predicted the 'Era of Crowds'. He emphasised the malignant behaviour of mobs, crudely characterising them as regressing to ancient and primitive modes of operation. The First World War exemplified this mayhem, and Trotter's examination of the behaviour of large groups in peace and war had to encompass this cataclysm. McDougall shared this preoccupation with the behaviour of people en masse, but also began to examine smaller groups. From his experiences of the same war he was able to demonstrate their potential for promoting great heroism, intelligent creativity and, indeed, the expression of some of the finest of human achievements. Le Bon, Trotter and McDougall provided the basic material for most British students of social psychology during the 1930s, including Bion and Rickman.

Underpinning all such theorisations, including those of Freud, was Darwin's instinct theory. Darwin argued that in addition to the primary urges of sex and survival there was one of socialisation. In his view, man was a social animal who inherited 'a tendency to be faithful to his comrades and obedient to the leader of his tribe' (Darwin 1871, p.112). Following his lead, Le Bon considered that the unconscious was created in the mind mainly by hereditary influences (1952). Adding to the drives Le Bon associated with self-preservation, nutrition and sex, Trotter introduced the 'Herd Instinct' (1919).

The psychoanalysts made great use of a related Darwinian theory: the notion of the 'primal horde'. This postulated that human social groups were originally dominated by individual men who kept all the other males in subjection. These primal fathers attempted to reserve all the females of their tribes for themselves. From this model Freud derived his perceptions of the incest taboo, exogamy, guilt and totemism (Freud 1940a; Rycroft 1972). In particular, he related this archetype to the sexual conflict between father and sons in the oedipal situation. In 1938, Rickman acknowledged his own debt to the theory when he elaborated on it in his analysis of Quakerism (1938b, p.384).

The crowd: Le Bon

As Freud pointed out, Le Bon stated nothing new, his importance lies in the fact that he provided a succinct account of thinking on group behaviours at the beginning of the twentieth century (Freud 1940b p.23). In particular, he identified the importance of the role of the unconscious, and although his characterisation of its development and manifestation now appears banal his insights were central to Freud's own theories of group dynamics.

Le Bon contended that the psyche, created in the mind from 'hereditary influences', played a key role in large-group behaviour. When an agglomeration of men and women forms a crowd it assumes attitudes very different from those of its constituents. In his view, a 'collective mind' emerges with very specific characteristics, albeit transitory in nature, which overwhelm individuality (1952). The crowd becomes a single organism, made up of cells working in unison, exhibiting a new set of behaviours. Intellectual judgement is suspended, and individual identity dissolves in the face of a 'racial' unconscious. Impulsiveness, irritability, inability to reason, suspension of intellectual judgement, and 'exaggeration of sentiment' replace rational consideration. These emotions, 'belonging to inferior forms of evolution – in women, savages and children, for instance', are expressed wherever crowds form (1952, pp.34–35). Their reasoning becomes magical, connecting ideas through apparent similarities and the immediate generalisation of particular cases, rather than logical induction. The association between ideas is not rational, and occurs through apparent similarities and the immediate generalisation of particular cases rather than logical induction.

This process is enabled by the sense of increased power and diminished responsibility that the person experiences when sharing a common cause with a large group. He advocated that a form of contagion, similar to hypnosis, in which the individual becomes an automaton who ceases to be guided by their own will, augments this. As a result, the activity of the brain is entirely paralysed, and each member of the crowd becomes the slave of all the unconscious activities of the spinal cord, which the hypnotiser directs at will. Conscious personality disappears entirely, a process which is accelerated by the sense of reciprocity amongst the group.

This frightening picture of mob activity reflected the bourgeois view of the upheavals occurring in France throughout the nineteenth century. Le Bon would have considered himself vindicated by the later cataclysms in

Russia and Germany. However, his simplistic notions were soon superceded by more complex theories.

The herd: Wilfred Trotter

Bion had contact with Wilfred Trotter whilst a medical student in Oxford in the 1920s. Seventy years later his wife recalled how he admired the author of *The Instincts of the Herd in Peace and War,* and how indebted he was to that particular book (F. Bion 1995). Trotter laid the foundations for British social psychology with the statement: 'All human psychology is the psychology of associated man, since man as a solitary animal is unknown to us' (1919, p.12). His pupil echoed this: 'no individual, however isolated in time and space, can be regarded as outside a group or lacking in active manifestations of group psychology...'. Later, in the same context, he was even more explicit, referring to humankind as 'a herd animal' (Bion 1961, pp.132–133).

Previously, in the works of Le Bon and others, the 'crowd' had been viewed as a special, transient phenomenon, in which people acted out of character under the influence of mass hypnosis. Trotter rejected this, insisting that the gregarious instinct permeates all psychological activity. He went as far to suggest that, as an example, the wolf pack could be considered as a single organism (1919, p.29). It was his view that people find that the company of others gives them 'an unanalysable primary sense of comfort' and warmth, whereas isolation leads to cold and terror. In order to avoid separation, the individual identifies with herd opinion; conformity to the group psyche underlies all human behaviour (p.33).

In Trotter's view, people avoid conflict by clinging on to non-rational beliefs that are in accord with the prevailing wisdom of their cultural group, even in the teeth of experiential evidence (p.32). Such beliefs are held to be self-evidently rational even when, objectively, they are entirely illogical. For instance, an English lady may smile at the barbarism of the African woman who wears rings in her nose when she herself has rings in her ears (p.38).

Such prejudices can be overcome by careful examination. One indicator of an a priori belief is the fervour with which it is defended. But despite the evident inconsistencies, this susceptibility to herd behaviour needs to be managed rather than eliminated. Human altruism is a natural outcome of this instinct, and the loss of gregariousness would diminish the human condition. Mental instability, he believed, stemmed from the conflict between real experience and herd suggestion (pp.56–58).

Above and beyond the ideas expressed in this thesis, possibly the most profound influence that Wilfred Trotter had on the Northfield Experiments was to introduce Ernest Jones to the ideas of Sigmund Freud, inaugurating the development of the British Psycho-Analytic movement (Jones 1959, p.159). This led in turn to Rickman's own contact with the leader of psychoanalysis, and to Melanie Klein's arrival in the United Kingdom, where she was able to freely elaborate her own particular model.

The group mind: William McDougall

A second influential British social theorist, William McDougall, sustained the instinctual approach when evolving his concept of the group mind (1920, pp.7–8). Despite his drawbacks as a scientist he is impossible to ignore. In the years between the two World Wars he was 'together with mental testing and psychoanalysis ... the working capital for a generation of psychologists' (Hearnshaw 1964, p.195).

In McDougall's view, the tasks of Group Psychology were fourfold. First, he determined to establish the validity and relevance of the group mind concept. After this, he aimed to identify the 'general principles of collective mental life' and distinguish them from those applying to individuals. The next tasks were to disaggregate different forms of group operation and then to describe and understand them (1920, pp.7–8). He summarised his purpose as being 'to establish the general principles of group life' and 'to apply these principles in the endeavour to understand particular examples' (p.8).

McDougall reiterated the dichotomy between the individual and the group, differentiating between a person's behaviour alone and that within a group. He followed Le Bon in believing that crowds behave in a less intelligent way than individuals because arguments and decisions have to be understood by the least able members. The crowd's intellectual ability is diminished still further by increased suggestibility, and each person's critical faculty becomes suspended in the face of powerful common emotions. It is under these conditions that successful orators can voice simplistic notions that sway their audience through the power of mass suggestion (p.41).

McDougall also agreed with Le Bon's perception that crowds are excessively emotional, impulsive, fickle, inconstant, irresolute, and extreme in action. However, he contrasted this with organised, smaller groups, which he believed could act less primitively. For instance, *esprit de corps* in the army gives rise to truly collective volition, leading to effective action and the enhancement of group intelligence, courage, endurance, trustworthiness and cheerful obedience (p.64). This environment encourages greater commitment and energy in the individual, as the consequences of action are direct and predictable, and recognition is more easily achieved (pp.83–84). This optimism about the functioning of small groups is very evident in Bion and Rickman's work and directly affected how they viewed issues of morale.

McDougall's anthropological studies led him to propose that the group spirit assists the evolution of responsibility within members of primitive tribes and increases the sense of individual, moral and physical support without which man finds it difficult to face the external world. Thus as well as providing the satisfactions and enjoyments of participation, the group spirit has a moral influence. An example of this is communal dancing, which he found reinforced group spirit, especially when each member carried out complex series of movements in unison.

Primitive societies that relied on such rituals were a lost Eden for McDougall. Life in the twentieth century compared unfavourably because natural conditions of social self-awareness had largely disintegrated. However, human beings still craved membership of groups 'in whose collective opinions and emotions and self-consciousness and activities they may share, with which they may identify themselves, thereby lessening the burden of individual responsibility, judgement, decision and effort' (p.77).

As a result, there is a vast skein of interwoven voluntary associations throughout a modern society. The successful ones contain a nucleus of people who identify themselves entirely with the group, making its interest their leading concern, making the desire for its welfare their dominant motive and finding in its service their principal satisfaction and happiness. In this situation the internal life of the group prevails over the achievement of any external purpose. Bion later elaborated on this in his theory of basic assumption (pp.77–78).

The reader is reminded again of Bion and Rickman's views when McDougall states that 'the definition of the group as such within the minds of the members is the prime condition of the growth of the group spirit, that spirit will be the more effective the fuller and truer is the knowledge of the group in the minds of its members' (p.86).

In McDougall's view, understanding alone was ineffectual unless accompanied by a sense of belonging; something that Tom Main whole-heartedly agreed with, arguing that it was a fundamental precursor of therapy at Northfield (see Chapter 8, in particular Main's contributions to the discussion groups). Both are promoted by internal openness and free intercourse between the group and other groups (McDougall 1920, pp.86–87). He classified groups along a spectrum ranging from organised to disorganised, with the implication that the latter was less valuable. Commenting on this later, Bion pointed out that order and chaos are characteristics of all groups.

Other influences

The work of the social psychologists described above were reviewed in Freud's analysis of group theory and were thus familiar to most psycho-dynamically orientated workers of the 1930s. The nature of the other influences on Bion and Rickman is either more or less clear-cut. Quaker worship is an ideal training for group therapy and Rickman's upbringing in that religion can only have helped him prepare for this kind of work. He was also in contact with W.H.R. Rivers in Cambridge, but it is not clear how familiar he was with the latter's ideas. However, the ways that each man is described by those who knew them bear an uncanny similarity, further emphasised by their preference for discussion seminars as a teaching method. Both had the ability to make the person they were listening to feel valued and interesting.

Quakers

Rickman's Quaker beliefs were part of his make-up. His experience of sitting in a congregation, often for considerable periods without anyone speaking, would have given him confidence in handling that most difficult problem for inexperienced group therapists: silence. Beyond this, Quakers believe that the experience of God is internal, and consequently worship is a very personal and intrapsychic exploration (Rickman 1938b). Listening for the expression of 'Inner Light' and awaiting its guidance is excellent preparation, both practically and theoretically, for psychotherapy. In both processes, calm reflection and trust enable the innermost thoughts to be expressed – in the former to the congregation and God, in the latter to the therapist. Both occur in the expectation of improvement in psychic well-being. This consideration of the 'here and now' experience and lack of explicit guidance from a leader are directly replicated in Rickman and Bion's approaches to group therapy at Northfield.

In 1938, Rickman reviewed the psychodynamics of the Quaker religion (which, incidently, is further evidence of his consistant attempts to integrate object-relations theory with wider social and ethnological thought). Religion, he argued, was an attempt to resolve symbolically tensions between the individual and internal representations of his or her parents. Quaker beliefs were important because of their concentration on intrapsychic events, and because they related better to the issues of early psychological development than did other religions. The early Quakers were driven by a sense of loneliness and wickedness that corresponded closely with the depressive position as outlined by Melanie Klein. Their belief that a relationship with God would save them from this overwhelming desolation was a symbolic search for an omnipotent parent who would save them.

Rickman's continued exploration of these beliefs right up until the start of the war confirm Main's observation that his religion was a significant factor in his involvement with group therapy (1977).

Rivers

The man who, in 1920, introduced Rickman to psychoanalysis was Dr. W.H.R. Rivers (Payne 1957). This polymath was then introducing the ideas of instinct and the unconscious to his students (Rivers 1920a). He had developed an understanding of Freud's theory whilst working as a psychiatrist treating War Neurosis during the First World War. His patients then famously included the poet Siegfried Sassoon. He stressed that military training was an essential element of a mental health promotion strategy. It had to 'fit each individual soldier to act in harmony with his fellows' and enable them to withstand the stresses of warfare (p.210). He argued that the chief aim was to 'enhance the responsiveness of each individual to the influence of his fellows', particularly his commanding officers (p.211). He recommended that the training should produce a state of mind close to that of hypnosis, in which the individual responds to the requests of the hypnotiser immediately and without question, preferrably before they are even articulated. This replicates the analysis of crowd mechanisms of his colleague McDougall, with whom he was in close contact at the time. It will become evident that Rickman, whatever he thought at the time, would later disagree profoundly with the concept that soldiers should be 'hypnotised' by their training into a state of mute obedience. He did, however, recognise the value of military training in inculcating effective *esprit de corps* and understanding of the soldier's role, made it an essential part of rehabilitation for those men recovering from neurotic disorders.

Rivers introduced the basic ideas of repression and sublimation, which he considered were mechanisms that could be manipulated to defend the individual against fear and other emotions induced by the battlefield. The promotion of *esprit de corps*, was an effective way of achieving this. The camaraderie of sharing common dangers meant that even a young officer fresh from school rapidly took on the role of father to his sons with the men in his unit.

Whether Rickman attended these lectures in uncertain. If he had, this probably would have been the first battlefield psychiatry he would have come into contact with, having spent the First World War as part of the Friends' War Victims Relief Unit in Russia (Payne 1957). He was aware of

Rivers' ideas and, in particular, took up the notion of 'manipulative activities'. These were psychological measures for protecting people experiencing threatening stimuli such as bombing. They both argued that ensuring that the potential victims were engaged in 'purposeful acts' which provided a sense of responsibility and engagement would provide a successful prophylactic measure against panic (Rickman 1937, p.55; 1939c, p.457; Rivers 1920b).

Rivers held the post of Praelector of Natural Science Studies, which he took as a mandate to set up numerous informal discussion groups at Cambridge University. These were attended by many visitors as well as staff and graduates (Slobodin 1978, pp.66–7). In the early years of the century he had been on an anthropological expedition with McDougall to the Torres Straits. A little later he participated in a famous experiment in the regrowth of nerves after injury with Henry Head (Hearnshaw 1964; Rivers and Head 1908). These experiences, along with his work during the war, led him to examine how these different disciplines could learn from each other. Rickman also followed this integrationist approach, investigating the implications of psychoanalysis for social and anthropological fields throughout his life.

As a result of Rivers' encouragement, Rickman went to Vienna to work with Freud, and thus embarked on his central role in the development of British psychoanalysis. He assisted Ernest Jones in founding the Institute of Psychoanalysis, edited the *British Journal of Medical Psychology* and the *International Journal of Psycho-analysis*, finally becoming president of the British Psycho-Analytic Society.

INSTINCTS AND OBJECTS: PSYCHOANALYTIC CONCEPTS OF GROUPS

Both in America and Europe, group theorists had to contend with psychoanalytic ideas. Many practitioners, such as Aichhorn, Homer Lane and Wills, came under their influence, and a number of Americans, Trigant Burrow, Slavson and Schilder, attempted to develop a group psychology based on them. Freud himself responded to the impetus from the other direction and wrote a number of papers and books on social psychology, of which the most relevant here is *Group Psychology and Analysis of the Ego* (1940b).

Melanie Klein and Ronald Fairbairn continued to develop their seminal theories of object relations and the paranoid-schizoid position during the period in which Rickman and Bion were engaged in army work. The Northfield Experiments and leaderless officer selection groups were the first applications of these concepts to practical social psychology. Though his work has been subsequently overshadowed, Rickman was also exploring the potential of this interaction during the 1930s. In this field, as in others, he had begun to formulate ideas that found their full expression elsewhere. In particular, his paper, 'Uniformity or diversity in groups' (1938a), contains many seeds of ideas later developed by Bion.

Group psychology and the ego

Freud's work on group psychology is pivotal to psychoanalytic discussion of the subject (Freud 1940b). Its influence is theoretical rather than practical; but his recognition of the unconscious forces at work opened the way for others to analyse them from a psychodynamic perspective. His main thesis was that the behaviour of the group is determined by the intrapsychic lives of its members.

Freud followed in the footsteps of Trotter when, in the introduction, he argued that 'only rarely and under exceptional conditions is Individual Psychology in a position to disregard the relations of this individual to others' (Freud 1940b, p.1). With this statement he began to overcome the dichotomisation inherent in the work of previous authors. However, as de Maré remarked, this seems to be only partially successful (de Maré 1972, p.52). Although Freud acknowledged this aspect of Trotter's work he was unable to accept the concept of the herd instinct – a conclusion later shared by Bion (Sutherland 1985, pp.66–7).

Group Psychology and the Analysis of the Ego is based on a detailed critique of the theories of Le Bon and William McDougall. Whilst admiring the former's account of the group mind, Freud argued that people do not manufacture new characteristics within such a situation, but instead express previously repressed manifestations of the unconscious. He stated in support of this that 'all that is evil in the human mind is contained as a predisposition', and that conscience, which he identified as 'dread of society' (soziale angst), attempts to conceal this (1940b, p.10). The barbarity of crowds, as perceived by Le Bon, results from repression of the intellect and heightening of affectivity (p.23). Le Bon's overwhelmingly unsympathetic view of groups stems, in Freud's view, from the fact that he was examining the manifestations of short-lived groups concentrated around a specific interest, for which the predominant model was the French Revolution (pp.25–26).

He then went on to reject McDougall's thesis that increased organisation raises the collective mental life to a higher level of functioning, arguing that unconscious mechanisms are far more potent. In developing this argument he reviewed some of the previous postulates. One of these was was the concept of suggestion used by the earlier authors to explain mass behaviour. After explaining his resistance to this explanation, he demonstrated how libidinal ties constrict and direct a person's actions within a group. These are the emotional bonds, the nature of which is dictated by the individual's previous experience, that maintain relationships between people. Usually these have a particular focus on a leader, who is similarly tied to the group. Freud contradicted completely McDougall's view that emotions are contagious, arguing instead that in a panic situation these connections evaporate, leaving the members subject to an overwhelming and senseless dread (angst). The terror comes, not from any perceived external danger, but from the threat of isolation. In order to prevent this, a considerable amount of energy is spent by group members in attempting to harmonise themselves with what they feel are the expectations and wishes of the whole group. It is this effort to remain part of the crowd that leads the person to behave in a more reactive and less rational manner, as Le Bon described. Bion later extended these propositions, arguing that Freud had not recognised the primitive nature of the individual's war against the group, contending that its origins stemmed from much earlier stages of psychological development (Sutherland 1985, pp.66–67).

Freud's main discussion concerned the large group, such as the crowd, army or church. However, in his introduction he did tentatively explore the differences that might occur in smaller groups, particularly families. Rickman later expanded on this when he examined the question of size in his article 'The factor of number in individual and group dynamics' (1950).

Relationships are always ambivalent. This is illustrated by Schopenhauer's famous analogy of the Freezing Porcupines, in which each animal's wish for the warmth and comfort of closeness is countered by the discomfort of the other's spines preventing this (Freud 1940b, p.54). Even in the closest familial relationships there remains a sediment of feelings of aversion and hostility, which have to be repressed. In looser relationships these sentiments may be less well disguised. This expression of self-love (narcissism) is a rejection of characteristics in the other that diverge from the individual's own ideals, which can be, temporarily, subjugated in favour of a libidinal tie. 'Love for oneself knows only one barrier – love for others, love for objects' (p.56).

The root force of libido, sexual love, carries with it another channel through which libidinal desires can be expressed: identification. In Freud's view, this was the earliest expression of an emotional tie with another person (pp.58–59). A little boy idealises his father, yearns to be like him and emulate him in every way; this contrasts with his wish for a straightforward sexual relationship with his mother. Later, in a regressive way, this can develop into a choice of dad as object, moving from wishing to emulate him to wanting to absorb him and introject him into the ego, with its direct sexual implication. Other emotional ties may arise later in life when a particular quality of the father is found in another person. This is a significant mechanism in the establishment of bonds between members of a group, and the intensity of the relationship is determined by the perceived importance of the identified common element. A doctor, whose father was medically qualified, may have a significant tendancy to select others in the profession to socialise with.

The development of the superego leads to the repression of the more overt sensual aspects of primary sexual love for parents (pp.68–70). What remains is tenderness, although earlier tendencies remain more or less strongly preserved in the unconscious. This separation may remain into adult life, resulting in a man's idealisation of the woman as an object of tenderness but not as an erotic object, and vice versa. The loved object enjoys freedom from criticism, and a sense of heightened worth beyond that of others (idealisation) (pp.73–74). This love may become so powerful that it consumes the ego and replaces the superego, thus enabling the individual to ignore their conscience in order to serve their paramour. Freud distinguished between identification and infatuation, arguing that in the former the ego has enriched itself with the properties of the object whereas in the latter it is impoverished and swamped by it. He then pointed to the parallels between being in love and hypnosis. The hypnotic relationship is the devotion of someone in love to an unlimited degree, but with sexual satisfaction excluded (p.77). In the case of groups, this explains the development of dependency on the leader and the group, substituting the group ideals for those of the individual. Bion would later incorporate these ideas into his concepts of basic assumptions, with the proviso that this may be only part of the process (Bion 1961, p.177). Introducing the concept of projective identification, he argues that a more profound and potentially more dangerous bonding can take place when the group and the leader identify with the communal phantasy (Sutherland 1985, p.67).

The importance of Freud's monograph is exemplified by Bion's explicit references to it in his own work (e.g. Bion 1961, pp.141–142). Foulkes also acknowledged it but was much more ambivalent about its practical value in group psychotherapy, initially dismissing it as irrelevant and then finding to his 'surprise, and satisfaction' that Freud was an ally with regards to his observations that the psychology of the group was more archaic than that of the individual (Foulkes 1964, pp.15, 59–60).

Melanie Klein and Fairbairn

Rickman was an important mediator of the ideas of Melanie Klein, although he did not always agree with her conclusions, for instance, he insisted on the importance of the father figure as well as the mother in early infancy (Bléandonu 1994, p.47; Rickman 1938a). He was in therapy with her from 1934 to 1941, and by 1938 was sufficiently conversant with her concepts to be delivering public lectures on their relevence to social psychology (Rickman 1938a; 1938b). During his time at Northfield he playfully referred to 'good' and 'bad' objects as 'lumps in the porridge' to help trainees to assimilate the ideas (de Maré 1985, p.111).

Fairbairn was working independently in Scotland, and though his ideas were known to both Rickman and Bion there is little evidence of his influence. This is surprising, as his rejection of instinctual theory was in close accordance with the theories of Kurt Lewin espoused by them both. The two papers describing the Northfield Experiment make no reference to any theoretical background and appear to deliberately eschew any psycho-dynamic analysis, and thus provide no extra clues (Bion and Rickman 1943; Bion 1946).

The work of Klein and Fairbairn is examined here as it stood between 1943 and 1945 and as it would have been known to the practitioners at Northfield. Any reference to theories that they developed later has been deliberately omitted.

Lectures and papers given between 1938 and 1941 demonstrate Rickman's grasp of object relations theory and his application of it to social situations, in particular groups. They often lack the precision of Bion's writing, but clearly prefigure the latter's later work. They also provide the most detailed account available of the psychoanalytic thinking that lay behind their work at Northfield. Because of this relevance, they are examined in some detail here, partly to cast new light on Bion's thinking, partly to elucidate the theoretical background of the experiments, and also to emphasise the significance of Rickman's role.

Throughout the following section, constant reference is made to 'objects' and 'object relations'. These terms refer to the fact that affect is always directed at another entity. They concern the fact that all feelings aspire towards another, whether it be human, animal, inanimate, or even phantasy. Such targets are known as 'objects'. In childhood, the most important of these are usually aspects of the parent, either in part or in total. For Klein and Fairbairn, the breast was particularly significant. The emotional bond established between the individual and their goal is designated the 'object relation', and is usually described from the perspective of the developing infant.

The destructive child: Melanie Klein

As stated earlier, the observations and ideas of Melanie Klein were central to the thinking of Bion and Rickman. During the 1940s, she was still forging her theories. She had been readily accepted by the British psychoanalysts on her arrival in 1926, rapidly becoming a member of the British Psycho-Analytic Society. Her ideas became largely accepted as the orthodoxy in the United Kingdom, and it was not until the later influx of refugees from the continent that this position was challenged by more traditional Freudians. This culminated in the acrimony and drama of the Controversial Discussions held at the Society in London during the years 1941–1945. The military psychiatrists were largely peripheral to these debates, but were acutely aware of them. Foulkes attended two of the business meetings and sent in written material for two other debates. He tended towards the Viennese point of view of Freud's daughter Anna; Rickman and Bion, by contrast, were clearly allies of Klein (King and Steiner 1991, p.xi). Rickman also attended a number of the business meetings, but more importantly took an active part in the reconciliation process after the war (King and Steiner 1991, p.xviii).

The work of Melanie Klein has been discussed elsewhere, and it is intended here only to outline the most relevant of her concepts that were current in the early 1940s (Grosskurth 1986; Hughes 1989; Segal 1973; 1989). These include the nature of anxiety and phantasy in early childhood, object relations theory, the death instinct and the depressive position.

Her first and most significant break with Freud came in the later 1920s with her observation that infants developed a phantasy of punishment and retribution, commonly described as the superego, in the first few months of life (Klein 1927, p.185; 1933, p.267). In his opinion, this was formed later on in childhood as a consequence of the dissolution of the Oedipus Complex; prior to that the child's behaviour was kept in check by fear of the authority of the real parents (Freud 1923, p.34). This initial schism then widened as Klein explored three different, intercalated threads: the early interaction of oral and anal stages, anxiety as the outcome of aggressive impulses, and the nature and importance of phantasy.

Klein became increasingly convinced of the psychodynamic importance of the early stages of life, in particular those described by Freud as oral and anal. In her paper 'Criminal tendencies in normal children' (1927), she emphasised the sadistic nature of these phases of libidinal development. She observed that the child's destructiveness was directed at his or her most loved objects, and the retribution threatened because of this became a primary cause of anxiety. She found evidence for this and for awareness of genital objects, even in the first few months of life (1932, pp.195–6). Oral sadism may be expressed not merely in the wish to bite the breast, but also to cannibalise the mother's body (1934, p.282). For her protégé Rickman, managing this aggression became an important theme, and was at the heart of his and Bion's co-edited paper on managing tensions in groups (Bion and Rickman 1943a). The different libidinal stages described by Freud were not, in Klein's opinion, as clearly sequential or as late in development as he described.

Unconscious phantasy was a central aspect of her theoretical position. As Susan Isaacs explained, this was the primary content of all mental processes in infancy (1943, p.276). All impulses and feelings, modes of psychological defence are expressed and experienced in specific phantasies. This is the mechanism through which they gain mental life and exhibit their specific direction and purpose. They are the psychic expression of instinctual drives and the reactions to them. Although Freud postulated that the infant satisfies his or her wishes in hallucinatory form, thereby intimating that such processes might occur, he himself did not complete this conceptual leap (Freud 1911, p.36; Isaacs 1943, p.278).

The phantasy is not an imagined scenario, like the word 'fantasy' in common parlance, but an experience that has the full impact of a real situation. The wish is immediately converted into a concrete fact. If the child in his anger desires to cut up his mother, it is a reality for him that he has done so. When he feels an emotion, for instance anxiety that the damage he has done has led him to lose his mother for ever, it is not expressed in words, but is an immediate 'here and now' event. The degree of differentiation between this all or nothing experience and a more accurate understanding of the reality is determined by the level of the child's psychic development and the intensity of the desire or emotion. Maturation leads gradually to a more realistic understanding of relationships, although intense feelings may distort this (Isaacs 1943, pp.274–280).

As part of her break with Freud, Klein increasingly recognised that infants experience the world in pieces rather than as a whole. They relate initially to parts of their parents, for instance breasts and penises, rather than to the mother or father as discrete entities. Their psychic development occurs through interactions with these objects, or part-objects. In phantasy they may be introjected, as punishing elements, into the superego, or as supports for the ego. Each object is either 'good' or 'bad', and is unable to contain elements of both. The breast, for instance, can be perceived as either a good, warm comfort that provides nourishment and security, or, in its absence, as a cold, destructive object that persecutes the child (Segal 1989, p.64; Klein 1934, pp.282–283).

Klein eventually described this early stage as the paranoid-schizoid position after the war, although Fairbairn had stolen a march on her by publishing his papers in the early 1940s. However, her fledgling idea that this initial period of development was associated with a psychotic process was expressed by her in 1934 when she accepted the validity of Glover's concept of the ego containing a number of ego-nuclei in infancy (Klein 1934, p.283).

Gradually, the successful development of the infant leads on to a stage where they are able to recognise the completeness of other people and their own distinct and separate reality. This leads to the development of a new form of relationship. Mother becomes a source of protection against persecutory attack, and her son wishes to incorporate her into himself to gain this security. However, as a result she is exposed to this danger and in turn needs to be protected. Simultaneously, by being a whole person the mother contains both loving and persecutory elements, and the child experiences ambivalence towards her. She thus becomes a victim of the boy's phantasised persecutors and also of his own sadistic, violent wishes for retribution. As she is constantly being introjected into his own psyche, this destruction becomes an internal one. Furthermore, the maturing child is establishing a fuller relationship to the external world and to real people. This brings with it a deeper understanding of the disaster created through his cannabilism and violence.

The loss and bereavement thus experienced brings on a new set of feelings: loss, sorrow, pining and guilt. This is the inauguration of the melancholic experience, and the child enters the depressive phase of emotional development (Klein 1934, pp.288–299). The mother's recurrent reappearance, and failure to be actually harmed by such phantasies, enables the child to recognise that his thoughts are not omnipotent and are containable. This process allows him to gain trust in his own abilities to love and care for himself and others (Klein 1940, p.313). This latter aspect is tested and retested in psychotherapy of all forms.

As far as is known, Bion had no contact of a significant nature, with Melanie Klein until after the war. During the war years and before, his knowledge of her work would have been gained primarily through his colleague John Rickman. This latter was in analysis with her until he joined the army, and was considered to be part of her circle at that time (King and Steiner 1991, p.xviii). His papers of the later part of the 1930s, as we shall see later in this section, are imbued with her ideas.

The concept of introjection – the incorporation of a representation of the object into the psyche – was examined in some depth by Foulkes in 1937. It is not relevant to examine this paper in depth here, except to state that he used the opportunity to review some of Klein's concepts and place them and British psychoanalysis in a European context. Tentatively, he tried to emphasise that Klein's use of the word was less of a break from traditional psychoanalysis than it seemed. Characteristic of the line he was trying to take is his discussion of the Oedipus complex. He agreed that, if the evidence showed it, the conflict could occur earlier than Freud had suggested; however, in his opinion its 'real importance' is during later childhood, when the genitalia take over as the primary source of pleasure (e.g. Freud 1922, pp.275–284). He was evidently trying not to offend, but still arguing the more classical Freudian case. His success in this was the evident high regard in which this paper was later held, as demonstrated by the frequent reference to it in the Controversial Discussions (King and Steiner 1991, pp.151, 319, 503, 554, 582).

Rejecting instincts: Ronald Fairbairn

Living in Edinburgh, Fairbairn remained largely on the periphery of the main circle of British psychoanalysts in London, particularly during the years of the Second World War. This 'comparative isolation', rather than having inhibited his productivity, may have even stimulated it (Hughes 1989, p.15). His first five papers on object relations theory are virtually contemporary with the Northfield Experiments, appearing as they did over the first half of the 1940s. These form the central corpus of his theoretical work (Rayner 1991, p.120).

He read his paper 'Schizoid factors in the personality' to the Scottish branch of the British Psychological Society in 1940, and published a summary of his position in the *International Journal of Psycho-Analysis* a year later (Fairbairn 1940; 1941). Reading a paper to this audience would normally have led to some bafflement, as few people in Scotland were knowledgable about psychoanalytic ideas then. However, the occasion was enlivened by the presence of a number of English psychotherapists who were working with the army, and there was a resulting 'lively, informed and friendly discussion' (Sutherland 1989, p.96). A second paper on the recasting of the libido theory was read in 1941, and met with a similar reception (Fairbairn 1941; Sutherland 1989, p.111). It is not certain who was present, but these first papers, which introduced his novel ideas, were written while Jock Sutherland, who was analysed by him during the 1930s, was working as the psychiatrist to the War Office Selection Board there. He was an active champion of his mentor's theories, and will thus have shared his enthusiasm with Bion, who was a close colleague in the same unit (Sutherland 1989, pp.64–65).

Both Bion and Rickman met Fairbairn in 1942, and the latter was aware of and impressed by the former's work on leaderless groups (Fairbairn 1943;

Sutherland 1985, p.47; 1989, p.122). Interestingly, Fairbairn's own awareness of the issues facing the two colleagues is explicitly referred to at the end of a paper he wrote in 1943, in which he contended that the 'war neuroses' were 'a problem of group morale' (p.81). He had had his own direct experience of assessing large numbers of soldiers with psycho-neurotic problems at Carstairs (Hughes 1989, pp.96–97).

Sutherland confirmed explicitly that, in his later writing, Bion was sensitive to Fairbairn's work (1985, p.47). The 1943 paper came specifically to the attention of Rickman, in his role as editor of the *British Journal of Medical Psychology*, where it was published. Thus, although no specific references are made to Fairbairn's work in Bion or Rickman's later writing, they were aware of his work and were indubitably influenced by it to some degree.

In writing on object relations Fairbairn stressed the break he was making with traditional instinct-centered psychoanalytic thinking. By replacing the Freudian concept of libidinal pleasure seeking with object seeking, he moved away from the Aristotlean explanation of cause by outcome and postulated a unitary underlying dynamic. Pleasure became a side effect of relating successfully to a particular object rather than an end in itself. Fairbairn himself explained that he was abandoning 'an argument based on the principle that *post hoc* necessarily means *propter hoc*' (1946, p.138). Freud and Klein followed Darwin in postulating that instinctual drives were the basis of human development. Whilst they did not go as far as McDougall in proposing twelve such impetuses, they both concluded that the pleasure seeking instinct (Eros) was counterbalanced by a death instinct (Thanatos). Fairbairn, by proposing the single motivation of exploration through relationships, followed Trotter's precept that all humans existed in groups, and demonstrated how this could be a primary explanation of psychic development. This obviated the need for further a priori causal factors. He considered that the so-called 'death instinct' could easily be explained as reactions to internalised objects that are perceived as 'bad'. Psychological development is the evolution from infantile dependancy on part objects to mature dependence on whole independent individuals (1946, p.34).

This dynamic world of interactions with internalised and external objects is an arena in which the infant tests out relationships. Through this, he or she gradually gains a sense of self, which in turn enables more realistic judgements to be made. Here is an evident paradigm for group therapy, particularly in the form of the 'here and now' explorations of interpersonal tensions that Bion and Rickman promoted. Fairbairn's other work is less directly relevant to Northfield, although it is significant in the later derivations, particularly Bion's exploration of object relations.

As noted above, Fairbairn anticipated Melanie Klein's later formulation of the paranoid-schizoid position and Rickman was aware of his theories, although there is no evidence on whether he accepted or rejected them. Fairbairn shared her idea that objects were perceived as partial in early infancy. Primarily, the breast was central to the first relationships established with the mouth (Fairbairn 1940, p.11). In its absence, thumbsucking was a vain attempt to replace it (1941, p.33). Two processes took place. First, the infant would incorporate a perception of the object, and second, she or he would identify with this. This primitive 'primary identification' led to the child being unable to differentiate the object from him- or herself (1941, p.42). These part-objects were experienced as either satisfying, comforting and supportive, or as rejecting. The former were loved and the latter hated (1941, p.35). This splitting of the part-objects into good or bad underlay the infantile schizoid position. Successful emotional development led to the increasing recognition of whole objects that could be perceived more distinctly as separate from the subject. Mature dependence involves a relationship between two independent individuals who are completely differentiated from one another as mutual entities (1941, p.42).

Melanie Klein was in the process of formulating her own views on these issues, and it is interesting to speculate on the part Bion, or even Rickman, played in transmitting Fairbairn's ideas to her.

'Unbearable impulses': Rickman and social psychology

Of the members of the British Psycho-Analytic Society in the 1930s, Rickman was the most concerned with the social consequences of Freudian thinking (Trist 1985, p.43). He explored their implications in a number of arenas, including group theory, the effect of air raids, religious experience and crime.

Despite his pacifist Quaker background Rickman clearly anticipated his military role. In 1934 he reviewed the origins of the aggressive impulse that led to wars (Rickman 1934). Later he investigated the psychological consequences of the Spanish Civil War, interviewing Langdon-Davies, who wrote a study of the effects of the German air raids there, and attending a lecture by Emilio Mira, a psychiatrist who had treated the war neuroses arising from that conflict (Rickman 1938a; 1938c; 1939a). In 1939 he wrote extensively on related subjects: in April on conscription, in May on evacuation and the child's mind, and in August on war wounds and air raid casualties (Rickman 1939a; 1939b; 1939c). During the same year he also edited selections from Freud on civilization, war and death (1939). The outcome of his prescience was that, within three days of the outbreak of war, he was able to write a memorandum for the army on the rehabilitation of soldiers suffering from psycho-neurosis (see Chapter 4) (Rickman 1939b). In this he demonstrated his awareness of the work done during the First World War.

Rickman's concern regarding the international situation was illustrated in a series of lectures given in 1938 on the operation of social systems. A significant subtext of these was interpreting the nature of authoritarian regimes in the Soviet Union and Germany. In a subsequent paper he proposed that developing a flexible, dynamic, democratic approach to group operation was a political issue that would influence the course of the impending war:

> Victory will go to the side which builds its group loyalties on the surest foundations – a Government which can identify itself with the people, and a community made up of individuals who have learnt to trust one another. (Rickman 1938d, p.372)

During this time he explored the application of object relations theory to social systems, in particular groups. This work, now largely overlooked, prepared the ground for the events at Northfield. Of particular interest are his lectures, unfortunately never published, on the psychodynamic theory of groups.

Managing aggression: Kleinian influences

The first paper in which Rickman appears to have confidently incorporated Klein's ideas was the Lister Memorial Lecture in 1935; typically, he applied them to a social system, namely that of the Quakers (Rickman 1935). However, a more significant paper, on 'unbearable ideas and impulses' appeared in 1937 which both harked back to W.H.R. Rivers, and also embraced the new ideas (Rickman 1937). Here he demonstrated his acceptance of Klein's theories of partial objects and their splitting into good and bad objects. In particular, he referred to the breast, which is 'loved with a consuming love or made the point of unbridled attack' (1937, p.56). The infant experiences these phantasies as reality, and regards them as dangerous because they will destroy the loved object. These morbid beliefs attenuate as the individual matures; but at some level all behaviour is determined by both objective understanding of the external reality and the internal subjective distortions engendered by these early experiences. He gave the example of the depressed person who suffers from an unbearable sense of sin, not from past deeds but from guilt over phantasied attacks on the person who in the past was 'most loved, most needed and most hated' (p.57). These discoveries, he believed, were momentous for psychology in that 'man's colossal appetite for destructiveness' and 'enormous capacity for guilt' could be seen in a new light. It explained the persistence and power of the impulse to create works that will last for ever as attempts at reparation (p.58). Those objects considered ugly can be interpreted as being reminders of these phantasms of infancy (Rickman 1940).

Uniformity and diversity in groups

In lectures given in 1938 and 1939, Rickman applied object relations theory to explain social systems. One of these, 'Uniformity or diversity in groups', was perhaps the first application of Kleinian ideas to groups (1938a). In this paper, a number of experiences and themes came together. He combined his observations of Russian village society made twenty years earlier with his concerns over the strengths and weaknesses of totalitarian states as opposed to those of democratic societies. Despite his claims of impartiality – 'its not my business to pass judgement' – his overall message is that democracy is a more mature, more integrated culture than the egalitarianism of the idealised agricultural village or the subservience of dictatorship (1938a, p.204). It enables creativity and supportive group ties, which in turn provide a healthier political, social and psychological climate.

In developing this implicit argument he applies his own amalgam of psychoanalytic ideas. These are evidently profoundly influenced by the work of Melanie Klein, with whom he was in psychoanalysis at the time. However, he did not slavishly adopt her theories, but used them as a casting-off point to explore how they might be applied in social settings, in particular to human groups. Unfortunately for the researcher he typically does not claim any ideas as his own, unlike Fairbairn or Klein herself. Thus identifying his particular contribution is rendered problematic, and any claims made here may subsequently be proved wrong. However, it may safely be stated that the unique constellation of thoughts he presented was a significant signpost for the future of group theory.

These lectures are explored in some detail because they provide a definitive account of Rickman's ideas at this time, many of which found fuller expression later, both in his own practical work and also in the theories of Wilfred Bion. The latter radically transformed these earlier propositions, but it is evident that they provided a significant starting point for his own intellectual advances. This account is supplemented by reference to some notes he made for another lecture, 'The individual and the group', in May 1939 (Rickman 1939d).

The following discussion elaborates first Rickman's psychoanalytic propositions, then his applications of them to group mechanisms, and finally some harbingers of the future.

'Lumps in the gravy': The psychoanalytic background

Psychoanalytic theory underpinned the lectures. Rickman aimed to demonstrate how psychodynamic mechanisms identified in individual psychological development operate in the wider social network. This directly iterates Freud's work on groups described earlier, updating it with reference to object relations theory. Rickman was aware of the relative novelty of this approach, noting that contemporary sociologists and psychologists were preoccupied with conscious levels of mind, such as organising group activity according to logic, rather than recognising underlying emotional conflicts. They tended to regard men as rational, acquisitive and reflexive. Rickman pointed out that man is actually disturbed by inner fantasy more than the real world (1939d, p.1).

Rickman's views were based on Melanie Klein's 'widened' concept of the superego, and echoed her belief that it began in early infancy as a means of managing infantile phantasies of destructiveness (Rickman 1938a, p.215). He rebutted those who believed that aggression was only aimed at people or things that are hated. The painful discovery of psychoanalysis was of the importance and prevalence of homicidal wishes towards loved ones (Rickman 1939d, p.2).

Objects perceived in the environment are split into good and bad representations, which are then incorporated into the psyche. The former, and he uses the father as an example, are idealised and taken into the superego, where they provide both a support for the ego, 'as does a loving parent', and a prohibition against evil action (Rickman 1938a, p.215). Normally this process progresses throughout life, with the addition of new objects such as schoolmasters and other exemplars. This enables the ego-ideal to become increasingly subtle and flexible, and to provide an 'inner treasury of experience on which the individual relies' (1938a, p.215).

The same objects can also be represented by malignant phantasies: 'The docile horse of our infancy readily turned into a brute that stamped and bit people to pieces' (1938a, p.216). These anti-social tendencies act as a foil for impulses of a constructive kind. Aggressive phantasies can also be projected outwards, for instance as 'bogies', or onto other objects. Thus the infantile world is populated with individuals who are either perfectly lovable or incredibly wicked, and this splitting protects people and things that are highly valued from being contaminated by what is feared and hated. If the anxiety generated by this interplay between good and evil becomes overwhelming it may result in paralysis. A safer and healthier process is sublimation, in which interest is diverted onto new objects. These, whilst less emotionally intense, provide more opportunity for satisfaction and resolution of conflict. Commonly, this occurs in play. These relationships are still subject to the original emotions overwhelming them, but provide more realistic opportunities for further psychic development.

In 'The individual and the group', Rickman pointed out that the child dreads the possibility that their blast of hate has destroyed good objects. Consequently, they search the outside world for good things that have survived their malice. Human curiosity becomes more than a simple impulse of enquiry, 'but is reinforced by the need for help against the forces of unconscious hate'. Thus guilt, derived both from the superego and from social sources, can drive the individual to acquire more knowledge of the outer world. These psychodynamic motives provided an explanation for 'that continuous, infiltrating and ever expanding drive to social action', which other psychologies at that time could not (Rickman 1939d, pp.2–3).

Rickman emphasised two aspects of this interplay. The first was that it was a multiple, dynamic process. The child is part of a psychic 'ballet' in which the relations between the main performers are reflected in the diverse nature of the 'minor characters who play in the background, each one catching some part of the main theme and colouring it with their own personality and characteristics, and reflecting back on the chief characters of the drama, features of the love and hate, the jealousies, doubts and cares...' (1938a, p.213). This variety is reflected in play, in which the child may take different roles from moment to moment, and toys are invested with new characteristics as rapidly. Second, the business of psychological development is never finished: the individual goes on through life exploring potentialities of pleasure to be found in the environment (1938a, pp.214, 224). As Rickman put it himself: 'Man may be described as an animal that is constantly seeking guilt free ways of being aggressive.' (1938a, p.203).

He elaborated on this complexity in 1939:

Ego plus its human and internalised acquisitions (Super ego, internal objects) is a composite creature containing images and impulses leading to constructive and destructive actions, and containing every variety of human type. Having incorporated many kinds we feel ourselves many-sided, and have many-sided interests and desires. This complexity of inner life is a reflection of the complexity of our outer environment, and if our relation to our primal love objects is good we shall enjoy and foster a many-sided development in ourselves and others. There is therefore a tendency for cultural complexity to perpetuate itself, but it produces its own crop of difficulties. (1939d, p.3)

Uniformity or democracy: Applications to social groups

Rickman's main thesis is that this continued exploration is essential to the health of group life. If it is systematically and prematurely terminated, societies become more rigid and less creative. The political squabbles of adulthood are not mere parallels of nursery behaviour, but the more or less satisfactory continuation of unresolved infantile conflicts. In order to illustrate this, he examined three types of cultures according to their uniformity or diversity of behaviour and beliefs.

The first, the Russian village, egalitarian and isolated, worked through consensus. In this apparently idyllic society, any individual who stood out was viewed with suspicion. The social group becomes the idealised parent, and the external world is seen as threatening and destructive (1938a, p.208). Hostile impulses, initially directed at progenitors, have to be projected outwards onto external authorities. As a result, a visiting government propagandist was beaten up and expelled. Whilst the group was found to be supportive and protective, it inhibited creativity. No new innovations were tolerable, with the consequence that the villagers were poverty-stricken and under the constant threat of famine because of antiquated farming techniques and poor equipment. No individual developed specialist skills, all work was the same for all the men. Even children's games were not allowed to be competitive. In this society, both behaviour and belief systems were uniform. Part of the aggression was turned inwards, taking the form of an increased vigilance over other members' behaviour and a readiness to accept authority unquestioningly. Rickman's description of life in a Russian village during and after the First World War makes fascinating reading, and it is unfortunate that a fuller account cannot be given here.

The second example results from the failure of the individual to adapt to new experiences and relate to other people. This fixation is a continuation of rigid infantile preconceptions; it leads to restrictions of choice and the incapacity to fuse love and hate impulses. Affection remains vulnerable to destructive urges. This dependence on idealised, inflexible parents leads to hero-worship and dependence on authoritarian leaders. The individual's own autonomy is sacrificed, and acts can be carried out that in other circumstances would be considered criminal. This is how Rickman characterised dictatorships. People are able to carry out individual trades, and thus there is diversity of activity but, they are overwhelmed by the uniformity of the belief system. Aggression is again diverted towards the external world, leading to expansionist wars; internally, it is directed towards other citizens with a culture of 'informing' and distrust.

Where the society allows for the continued mental development of its people, both culture and belief systems are diverse. Aggression is sublimated and expressed in relatively harmless ways. Political parties debate in state legislatures, and even rebels recognise that the needs of the state take precedence over their own grievances. Rickman gave the example of the Nore mutiny, in which the 'sailors suspended their business of hanging officers from the yard arm' to decorate their ship appropriately for a state visit of foreign dignitaries along with the other ships of the Fleet (1938a, pp.223–224). His sympathies are clearly expressed: 'The British, with their great capacity for maintaining internal quarrels for long periods of time, frequently disappoint their enemies in this respect' by drawing back from the potential incoherence of the diverse society and preparing for the organisation of war (1938a, p.223).

These three forms of organisation demonstrate Rickman's contention that the management of irrational emotions stemming from infancy is central to how society operates.

In 'The individual and the group', Rickman stated that another 'group-forming mechanism…is the diminution of guilt and anxiety if aggression is shared, and the access of feeling of power if constructive energies are shared' (1939d, p.3). This underpins the successful functioning of a military unit, and is also significant in group therapy. In the former, the ability of the leader to enable his men to direct their destructive impulses towards the enemy, and to share their sense of effectiveness, contributes to that most essential of military virtues, *esprit de corps*. In the latter, the sharing of emotions with others is an important aspect of treatment, especially when negative feelings can be managed in a constructive manner.

Signposts for the future

Through understanding the emotional dynamics of particular forms of organisation, Rickman contended that it was possible to face the task of shaping mankind's group life. However, at this time, apart from a few indicators, he largely left his audience to draw its own conclusions about how this might be achieved.

Perhaps of most importance was his recognition that group systems could be interpreted from the viewpoint of object relations theory. This was a sophisticated tool for analysing the apparently irrational conflicts and relationships that exist within a society. As Fairbairn pointed out later, object relations theory emphasises the interdependence of people. The inevitable consequence of the idea that individuals develop through their relationships is the exploration of ways of carrying out psychotherapy by exposing and analysing them within the group setting.

Particular aspects of the theory also have technical importance. The recognition that aspects of the superego can be projected onto the group and its leader enabled the observer to separate themselves from the maelstrom of emotions and take a more dispassionate view. Bion described this process, as it affected him, vividly in his later writing. Rickman also recognised that the greater the individual's dependency on the group, the more likely they are to endow it with phantasised characteristics of their idealised parents. In this lies the seed of the basic assumption of dependence (baD) so clearly delineated by his colleague (Bion 1961, p.105). Rickman also began to identify some of the symptoms of the basic assumption group when he described the projection of bad objects onto the external world outside the group and the phenomenon of scapegoating.

Rickman's anthropological observation of the leaderless group in the Russian village provided some of the groundwork for observing the leaderless groups in WOSBs and Northfield. This included dispassionate appraisal of the mechanisms, observing individuals' projections onto the group, and assessing their level of independence and objectivity. His dispassionate examinations of Quakerism reflected this same process.

Rickman recognised the value of work, as a purposeful activity, in resolving issues of aggression. Before creating something, preparation in the form of clearing the ground provides for the release for destructive impulses. This can occur even in philosophical tasks: 'the thinker must pull his own and other peoples' systems to pieces before he can find out how they are connected and construct one of his own.' (1938a, p.203). This concept of the 'constructive element in aggression' does not reveal his views of the libidinal impulses and the death instinct (p.221). However, it posits a potentially symbiotic relationship that is often not present in more classical accounts, and perhaps anticipates Fairbairn's melding of the two. Another of Rickman's observations was that communal work as experienced in the nursery contributes to the comradeship of war (p.203). These views are consistent with his emphasis on appropriate 'occupational therapy' in the rehabilitation of soldiers.

Significantly, these studies paved the way for the recognition that psychodynamic resolution of conflicts could be achieved through in social interaction, particularly reality testing. Curiosity and work are both mechanisms through which the individual develops less neurotic relationships. Thus, unlike many of his Freudian colleagues, Rickman began to visualise routes to therapy other than the psychoanalytic couch.

Air raids and religion: Other papers

In 1938, Rickman wrote two reviews of the psychological effects of air raids. After the publication of the first article in the *Lancet*, he interviewed John Langdon-Davies, the author of a book on the effects of air raids on the civilian population in Barcelona during the Spanish Civil War (Langdon-Davies 1938). The outcome of this was a further extended examination of the subject (Rickman 1938c; 1938d). In these two articles he examined group psychology under conditions of stress, emphasising the distinct and disruptive nature of panic. He wrote: 'Members of an organised group turn some of their affection towards other members of the group, but their hostility is in the main turned outwards, the cohesion of the group is thus maintained by the maintenance of bonds of affection and hate – safely distributed' (1938c, p.1291). A disorganised civilian population, on the other hand does not have this protective mechanism, and is vulnerable to chaotic responses. He suggested that whilst evacuation to special camps may have some benefits, it is more important to ensure that people have roles and duties to carry out when the attack starts (1938c, p.1294). This approach differed from the authorities' views at that time, who planned for mass panic and underestimated the courage of the average citizen (Harrisson 1976, p.30).

Confirmation of Rickman's views came from the unusual source of Slater and his colleagues observing the effectiveness of occupational therapy during air raids. In Mill Hill, the patients with mental disorders were found to be much better if they remained at work at such a time. If they were allowed to seek cover they became preoccupied with the fear of being caught out in the open, and this could lead to relapse (Debenham *et al.* 1941).

Rickman's papers examined the contribution of 'internal' factors deriving from infantile psychic conflicts, to the development of panic. Then he explored measures to reduce the risk of these disorders in populations exposed to air raids. Clearly derived from Rivers' ideas of 'manipulative activities', these measures included methods of supporting group formation and cohesion, and recognition of the protective effect of being engaged in purposeful activity. This progression from psychoanalytic understanding of a problem to recommendations in the sphere of social policy presaged the welter of changes that psychiatrists wrought in the structure and functioning of the army during the Second World War.

Rickman's pioneering role has rarely been recognised, and this oversight would have been reinforced by his own 'humility and diffidence' and 'readiness to urge a colleague to aspire to a position which he himself had an equal right to acquire' (Payne 1957, p.54). These articles support Main's contention that Rickman was a significant influence on Bion, on the work of psychiatrists in the army as a whole, and even in the Royal Navy (Main 1984). He further developed his concepts of relations between two or more people after the war (Rickman 1950; 1951). Rayner reports on this work that 'it was Rickman, of course, who first differentiated psychological theories on the basis of whether they were one-body, two-body, three-body or multi-bodied in nature. He was using a mode of thought that has become second nature to many Independent psychoanalysts' (1991).

A letter from Desmond Curran, Senior Psychiatrist in the Royal Navy, paid tribute to Rickman's influence on the recruiting measures in that service. He wrote in 1941: 'You may remember that at a recent meeting of the R.S.M [Royal Society of Medicine] I asked for guidance about a proposed scheme for Naval recruiting, and you will remember that you were the only person who really gave us any practical help' (Curran 1941).

SOCIAL CLUBS AND THE GROUP TRANSFERENCE: OTHER GROUP THERAPISTS
Waiting in the wings: Wilfred Bion

In contrast to his colleague's extensive list of lectures and publications, Bion's known output before Northfield consists of one paper, a little-known article on the 'war of nerves' published in Miller's summary of military psychiatry (Bion 1940). This book was intended to provide non-psychiatric medical practitioners with guidance on how to manage the neuroses arising in war (Miller 1940, p.105). It is evident that Bion overestimated the audience he was writing for: he launches into psychoanalytic theory in a manner that would have rapidly alienated many of his readers. This trait perhaps contributed to his sense of being misunderstood by many of those around him (e.g. Trist 1985, p.11).

Bion argued at the outset that psychological warfare is aimed at the infantile phantasy world of the opponent, aiming to separate individuals from one another in a miasma of fear. The two sides were engaged in a 'war of nerves'. Whilst he acknowledged that this somewhat precipitate explanation was crude, he seems quite unaware that his use of the word 'phantasy' without explanation appears quite inappropriate, especially given its very specific meaning, outlined above. He demonstrated none of Rickman's ability to move from the commonplace to the technical by means of a series of illustrations.

To succeed in this psychological field of combat, aggression had to be directed outwards towards the enemy, and supportive feelings maintained amongst one's own forces. He distinguished between the nature of soldiers' training and experiences in managing fear, and the lack of preparation for civilians. Recalling McDougall's ideas, he considered that the close ties of the small unit in which the soldier operates were of particular importance and were of greater benefit than the relative isolation of the civilian. This latter leads to the loss of social support that results in panic.

Bion's basic message reiterates that of Rickman two years earlier: that all civilians should have a role in an emergency, preferably as part of an existing organisation with well-recognised aims and purposes such as the Citizens Advice Bureau or the police.

The British pioneer: Joshua Bierer

Only one person is known to have been carrying out group therapy for people with psychiatric problems in the United Kingdom before the Second World War. This was Joshua Bierer. He thus has a justifiable claim to be the pioneer of British group psychotherapy. In 1938, he started running groups in mental hospital wards, expanding them later to the outpatient departments (Bierer 1948, pp.295–296). He organised both large groups of 50 or so individuals, which he called 'communities', and smaller ones of about ten people, called 'circles'. The latter were more intensive, dealing with personal and emotional problems. The psychiatrist, after studying the case notes in detail, would put forward a generalised history, which would then be discussed by all those present. The sessions were largely directed by the therapist and were based on Adlerian principles. In this he incorporated a technique that he described as 'situational treatment'. This consisted of creating artificial situations in which unconscious wishes could be acted upon – for instance, by letting a boy who had a strong desire to be like his father take a leadership role in the gardening gang (Bierer 1942).

'Communities' had open agendas, allowing the members to 'let off steam' both towards the authorities and about their own problems. The patients elected their own chairperson, 'but the psychiatrist directed the discussion'. This organisation in one instance elaborated into 'Social Club' meetings, which had a chair and club officers, all roles being taken by patients. Rules were formulated and activities decided upon. A magazine was published regularly (Bierer and Haldane 1941). This was a clear precursor of some of the activities of the Second Northfield Experiment, in which the soldiers took responsibility for a wide range of activities in the hospital. Incidentally, T.P. Rees, who showed a great deal of interest in the events at Northfield, reported that he had been involved in running a similar club for in-patients at Warlingham Hospital since 1938/9 (Rees 1943).

Discovering the group unconscious: Sigmund Foulkes

It is difficult to know quite where to place Foulkes in this summary of influences. Perhaps this characterised his experience at Northfield as well. He was an 'enemy alien' who came to the United Kingdom in 1933, having served with the German army in the telephone and telegraph services during the First World War (E. Foulkes 1990, p.6). Because of his strong German accent and habit of using 'entangled syntax' with truncated sentences, he was, at that time, not always easily understood by those he worked with (Lewson 1993; Anthony 1983, p.30). Although awarded the rank of Major, he was entirely outside the senior group of military psychiatrists, and was at times actively resented by some of them (Main 1945). This gap yawned wider because of his advocacy of traditional Freudian ideas in the Controversial Discussions referred to earlier, in contrast to Rickman and Bion, who tended to the Kleinian side. He also brought a rather different theoretical position to Northfield, stemming from his background in Frankfurt.

It is perhaps the measure of the man that he overcame such obstacles to become highly respected in British psychiatric circles; he was evidently much admired and warmly appreciated even by those who started off highly critical of him (Main 1989, p.197).

Two of his main influences, who are not easily included elsewhere, were Kurt Goldstein and Norbert Elias. He worked with the former for two years from 1934. This neurologist intercorporated concepts from Gestalt psychology and phenomenology into his thinking about the nervous system. The resulting theoretical position paralleled that which Kurt Lewin was developing concurrently. In Goldstein's opinion, neurological events could only be fully understood within the context of the whole organism and the environment in which it operated. Changes in one part of the system could affect it all. For a complete understanding one had to examine the whole and determine the underlying laws that were operating rather than concentrate on an individual aspect in isolation.

The biological system is always in a state of dynamic equilibrium, both internally and in relation to the external world. In the normal organism the whole body is in a state of moderate arousal, evenly distributed throughout. Whenever this is disturbed by internal or external stimuli it attempts to restore this average state. Fighting, fleeing, or satisfying hunger are all attempts to achieve this aim. Pathology disrupts this process, but does not prevent it. It is a 'shock to the existence of the individual caused by the disturbance of the well regulated functioning of the organism by disease' (Goldstein 1940, p.6). Treatment has to enable the patient to continue to exist despite the defects; in other words, to regain a satisfactory new equilibrium. Goldstein anticipated modern neurological thinking, recognising that function was not linked specifically to particular anatomical sites. If a man loses his right hand, he would not have to relearn how to write to be able to use his left, although there will be some initial difficulties with co-ordination (Foulkes 1936; reprinted in Foulkes 1990, p.49).

Goldstein, like the psychoanalysts, preferred qualitative, rather than quantitative, research, presenting individual cases in a holistic manner and attempting to understand their particular 'being-thus', or phenomenological moment of existence (Foulkes 1936; reprinted in E. Foulkes 1990, p.42). His disagreements with the Freudian way of thinking centred round the nature of the basic drive, which he considered to be an 'incessant process of coming to terms with the environment' rather than seeking pleasure (Goldstein 1939, p.333). This, of course, is entirely congruent with Fairbairn's understanding of development being mediated through relationships. Goldstein also considered that it was inadmissible to isolate the psyche from the whole human being; it was more acceptable to identify it as the conscious aspect of the totality (Foulkes 1936, p.53). The concept of sublimation, he felt, was unacceptable, being in his opinion a detour. Creative cultural achievement was already a potential in the primal state, as were all other abilities (Foulkes 1936, p.54).

Foulkes argued that the analyst had to step back from the total living reality of the therapeutic situation in order to to make observations, much in the same way that the distorted abstraction presented by an X-ray still provides new information to contribute towards the whole picture (Foulkes 1936, p.55). He believed that much of Goldstein's opposition to psycho-analysis stemmed from his limited understanding of it.

The importance of Goldstein's theories here lies in their similarity to the systems thinking that underlay all of the work at Northfield. His system tended to concentrate on the individual, but was readily adapted by Foulkes to the broader social fabric, in which the individual organism became part of the pattern in the wider weave (Foulkes 1946a). The single human being is analogous to the neural cell operating in conjunction with others within the overall communicating network of the nervous system. The latter cannot work on its own. Similarly, each person functions only in the context of the social system (Pines 1983b, p.268). Thus it provided Foulkes with an introduction to Gestalt psychology, in particular the concept of figure/ ground perception. This draws attention to shapes that can be perceived as one of two figures, depending on which part the viewer focuses on. Applied to groups, it emphasises how either the individual or the group can take centre stage whilst the other recedes into the background.

Norbert Elias was a sociologist with whom Foulkes had made friends in Frankfurt. Their ideas were in close enough harmony for them to consider co-authoring a book. In the end, this dwindled to an article by the former, 'Sociology and psychiatry', in a book edited by the latter (Elias 1969; Foulkes 1990, p.79). For Foulkes, Elias provided a sociological theory that was compatible with psychoanalysis, and indeed, extended its explanatory power. In principle he demonstrated, using a raft of examples, how, over the centuries, all normal functions have increasingly become subject to taboos and social constraints. Initially, the individual is relatively at liberty to express violence, being at the same time more vulnerable to the aggression of others. Laws and social restrictions have made society more stable; but have at the same time curtailed this freedom. These inhibitions have been inculcated into successive generations until they are internalised, with the result that aggression and fear are directed inwards into the individual. Internal life is constantly being modified by external social behaviour. Psychoanalysis actually demonstrates the mechanism by which they are passed on to the growing infant. It also analyses the process of how each person passes through stages of increasing repression of aggression similar to those which society has passed through over the years (Foulkes 1938). Elias, in a similar manner to Goldstein, was interested in exploring the underlying forces at play in the whole of society rather than examining parts in isolation. Over the centuries, societies change as a consequence of economic, geographical and demographic factors. This forces changes in behaviour on people, which then become internalised (Foulkes 1942).

Like Bierer, Foulkes had experimented with group therapy before arriving at Northfield. As he stated himself, he had long been exploring the possibilities of working with patients in groups. In the 1920s, he came across two papers by Trigant Burrow which made 'a deep impression' on him (Foulkes 1964, p.13). His interest was further stimulated by Gorki's play, *The Lower Depths*, which featured a group of people without a leader, pushed and pulled by overpowering forces (p.13). Pat de Maré added, from his knowledge of Foulkes, Wender, and a play by Pirandello, *Six Characters in Search of the Author*, to this list (de Maré 1983, p.221).

The opportunity for Foulkes to put these ponderings into practice came in 1939 when he took a position as a psychotherapist in Exeter (Foulkes and Lewis 1944). He was clear from the beginning that the actual reasons for taking up group therapy were practical. For successful traditional psychoanalysis, the patients would have needed more time than either they or he could afford in a time of war. He established, with Eve Lewis, groups of six to ten people meeting for ninety minutes on a weekly basis. They were single sex groups, following Schilder's prescription. These ran in a semi-open fashion in that people joined already established groups, so that a total of 50 people passed through in a period of two years. Selection was based on an assessment of whether the person's personality appeared to fit him or her to the group, whether they had reached a stage in their own personal treatment which meant that they were ready for the wider exposure, whether they might disturb the group, and their reaction to the proposal. He gave a detailed explanation of what to expect to each patient prior to them starting, and this was reiterated occasionally during subsequent sessions.

For Foulkes the key discovery was to allow the patients to talk in a free-flowing manner, using a form of 'free-association' (de Maré 1983, p.227). From this it became clear that the group was operating as a single organism, and that issues that arose were being treated by the group as a whole. This included group transfer reactions, which he distinguished from individual ones (Foulkes and Lewis 1944). This group unconscious became the key for therapeutic interpretations.

These initial experiments in Exeter formed the basis for Foulkes' first work at Northfield, and part of the interest of the Northfield Experiments lies in examining his painstaking development of group therapy from these beginnings.

ACROSS THE WATER: AMERICAN GROUP THERAPISTS

Many of the contributors to the Northfield Experiments had an idiosyncratic knowledge of group theory and practice in the United States. Foulkes and Bierer were variously interested in Slavson, Schilder, Burrow, Wender and Adler. Moreno was widely appreciated and respected, but it was the work of Kurt Lewin that had the most impact. It is not intended here to provide a comprehensive history of these sources, but to concentrate on those individuals whose influence on the participants at Northfield is well established.

Class methods: The pioneers

The first known psychotherapy specifically carried out in groups centred around the education of people suffering from physical illness. Joseph Pratt originated this 'class method' approach, which was emulated by many other physicians and laypeople alike (Pratt 1907). Bierer reported that the first use of this approach with psychiatric patients was by Lazell, who gave lectures on psychology as it applied to schizophrenia with reportedly beneficial results (Bierer 1948; Lazell 1921). An interesting figure is Marsh, who used similar methods to Pratt, but developed them to the extent that all the personnel of an institution were involved in a common effort to develop themselves to their fullest capability. He employed his military experience to explore methods of improving the morale of the whole hospital, in a manner which Corsini considered to be the first attempt at a 'therapeutic community' (Corsini 1947, p.14; Marsh 1933). Bierer was particularly influenced by Adler, who, although he never published anything on group psychotherapy, carried out individual therapy in front of groups. He started with children in 1921, and generalised this later. He believed that community was the most important and unavoidable factor in human life (Bierer 1948, p.289).

Tantalisingly, Strecker and Appel, in their treatise on army psychiatry, record that one of them used group therapy techniques during the First World War in the United States Army. However, they give no details of this, and from the other evidence of their approaches at this time, one can only assume that they tended to use a didactic method (Strecker and Appel 1945, p.42).

Fighting social isolation: Trigant Burrow and Louis Wender

It is difficult to estimate the influence of Trigant Burrow, who wrote prolifically. He was a pupil of Freud and an analysand of Jung who abandoned classical psychoanalysis because of its overemphasis on the individual. He echoed Trotter and others in reiterating the interdependence of people within groups. He considered that no analysis of the individual could be complete without real study of the group of which he or she is a part. Further than this, he believed that mental disorders were problems of social relatedness and consequently that research could only be carried out in a group setting (Burrow 1928b). Foulkes registered his own uncertainty about him. He had read some papers in the 1920s which, he wrote, 'must have made a deep impression on me'. They implanted in Foulkes the idea of group analysis as a form of treatment, but he later decided that he had overestimated the importance of Burrow's work (Foulkes 1964, pp.13–14). Burrow's theories were not popular because of the difficulty people had with his writing style. Corsini reports that he had no influence on subsequent group therapy and, indeed, that he gave up group work latterly (Corsini 1957, p.15).

Tom Main pointed out that Rickman was familiar with Burrow's psychoanalytic group work of the 1920s (1989, p.128). This is supported by the fact that as assistant editor of the *British Journal of Medical Psychology* he would have at the very least read Burrow's articles published there between 1925 and 1928 (e.g. Burrow 1927b; 1928a; 1928b). In these Burrow reiterated concepts that he had promoted previously. One was the idea of group psychotherapy being 'the analysis of the immediate group in the immediate moment' (Burrow 1928a, p.198). Elsewhere, he emphasised the importance of group therapy as a 'daily test of an actual living experience' (Burrow 1927a, p.223). This reality testing combined with a 'here and now' approach is identical to that carried out by Rickman and Bion in 1943.

Burrow, particularly with his attention to transference, revealed the unconscious elements at play in group therapy (1927c). In contrast with psychoanalysis, however, he argued that repression of sexual conflicts was not due to infantile experience, but the direct product of a society that 'blindly bullies the so-called neurotic into inviolable self-concealment and isolation' (p.273). He emphasised the relief that individuals felt when they found that their morbid conflict was recognisable in others. This was important in reducing the person's sense of isolation and allowing them to reflect more dispassionately on the issues raised. One of his theses, the dismissal of the 'ill' patient contrasted with the 'well' therapist dichotomy, was characteristic of Main's later contention. Burrow argued that the psychopathologist and the neurotic individual are in many respects neither more nor less sick than each other (p.271). Similarly, he believed that man's life is not static, but a continuous, dynamic and fluctuating process (p.274). Again, Tom Main's introduction to his essay on psychiatric rehabilitation almost repeats this word for word (1948, p.386).

Working in a hospital setting, Wender enlarged on this by reporting that it was a special property of the group to be able to help the individual to learn that his or her problems are not peculiar to him- or herself and that many co-members have similar underlying difficulties (1936). He identified specific dynamics working in the group: intellectualisation, transference between patients, 'catharsis-in-the-family' and group interaction. All of these had a role in the healing process. In contrast to psychoanalytic theory, he insisted that conscious processes could be marshalled to assist therapy. Intellectual awareness provided a reality testing apparatus whilst emotional storms were raging. A loud noise behind someone may cause panic, but not when it is possible to discover what caused it. He actively encouraged the identification of one patient with another, as this promoted transference towards the therapist and could also lead on to socialisation in settings outside of the group. His ungainly terminology 'catharsis-in-the-family' refers to the experience of the individual sharing previously unexpressed emotions with surrogate parents (the therapist) and siblings (the other patients). This setting allows for both free expression of feelings from earlier family experiences and re-enactment of these through emotional release towards other group members. In common with other theorists and practitioners, Wender emphasised the importance of social interaction in development, and believed that group therapy reinforces the conscious acknowledgement of this.

Bloch and Crouch contend that Wender was exceptional amongst pre-war therapists in that he was the first to identify such specific therapeutic factors within groups (1985, p.8).

Questionnaires and 'active groups': Schilder and Slavson

Others who applied psychoanalytic techniques to group therapy included Schilder and Slavson. The latter became very influential in group psychotherapy after the war, and many of the ideas that Foulkes took from him stem from that time. However, by 1943 he had only published two accounts of activity-orientated work with adolescents.

Schilder summarised his practice in 1938 (Schilder 1938, p.197–204). The patients were initially seen individually. He obtained their life histories both during these sessions and in written form. They then joined a group of patients at various stages of treatment. Here they were interviewed in turn, in a manner similar to that of individual psychoanalysis; the other patients were encouraged to give their own comments or associations in addition to those of the therapist. The transference was a particular focus for interpretations, particularly the negative ones towards the therapist. The sexes were not mixed, 'for obvious reasons' (p.202). As Wender and Burrow had found, discovering thoughts and feelings, which previously had isolated the individual to be similar to those of others was therapeutic for the patient (Schilder 1939, p.91). Schilder also devised a number of questionnaires to assist the therapist with collecting material about the patient. This was something Foulkes carried out in Northfield, although not to the same degree of detail. Schilder was explicit that this form of therapy was an economic way of carrying out individual therapy, and that this was the basic reason for taking this approach (1939, p.87).

Slavson initiated 'Activity Group Therapy' for adolescents in 1934; he reported on it in the early 1940s (1940; 1943). At the time he was unaware of psychoanalytic approaches, although he used these later. These earlier groups encouraged motor expression and projective activity with five to eight members. There was a careful selection procedure so as to ensure that the patients would 'have a desirable effect on one another' (Slavson 1946, pp.670–671). The setting was a simply furnished room with arts and crafts materials that the participants were free to use as they wished. They were able to express their destructiveness, aggression, and inhibitions as the whim took them. The therapist took a passive role, observing and only intervening if there was serious danger of significant injury or damage. At the end of the session the group was served with food, and again the therapist followed the lead of the participants in the discussion. His or her main role was to set limits and to prevent the group acting as a gang. Trips, picnics and excursions were all part of the programme. Members also had individual therapy to develop insight and promote ego-strength. The overall aim was for the individuals to have the opportunity to interact in a democratic manner, in the presence of a permissive and understanding adult, and form new and better relationships with their peers. Slavson later defined his differences with Foulkes' ideas, emphasising that his own focus of treatment was on the individual rather than the group (Slavson and Scheidlinger 1948, p.609). There were also parallels with other work being carried out with adolescents, which will be referred to later in this section.

Tele and spontaneity: Moreno and Sociometry

In October 1944, Hargreaves, following an earlier discussion, wrote to Foulkes enclosing papers by Moreno on Sociometry with the explicit request that he circulate them amongst his colleagues at Northfield (Hargreaves 1944). As a result, the latter gave a seminar which emphasised the author's 'structure of interpersonal relations and ... philosophy of group relations' (Foulkes 1944b). Illustrating the impact of this, Main later recalled the importance of the 'spontaneity' advocated by Moreno, in the activities of the hospital (Main 1989, p.133).

For Corsini in 1957, Moreno was most important individual in the history of group psychotherapy (Corsini 1957, p.14). He founded the original journal on the subject in 1937, and organised the first society of group therapists in 1942. Other major contributions were a theory to account for group structure and operation, and the institution of a new method of therapy in groups. He is attributed with coining the term 'group psychotherapy' in Vienna in 1932 (Whiteley and Gordon 1979, p.14).

Moreno rejected psychoanalysis for a number of reasons, amongst which were its concentration on the individual, its emphasis on talk rather than action, and his preference for a 'face-to-face' approach (Fox 1987, p.xiv). He believed in 'encounter' rather than transference as a basis for cure. His approach also removed the doctor as the final therapeutic agent, enabling each group member to become effective in the treatment of the others (Moreno 1945; reprinted in Fox 1987, p.34).

In the journal that Hargreaves lent to Foulkes, Moreno summarised the core elements of his system (Moreno 1937). First, he defined sociometry as the 'study of the actual psychological structure of human society' (p.19).

Central to this was the concept of the 'social atom', which is the skein of interconnected emotional relationships in which an individual exists (p.26). A connected idea was that of the 'tele', which he defined as the interpersonal experience of the web of feeling existing between two or more people. This provides the emotional basis for intuition and insight, and evolves out of personal relationships with others and objects from birth onwards. This non-verbal communion is the chief factor that determines the position of the individual within the group (p.10). The social atom stretches as far as one individual's 'tele' incorporates others, and its operation is fundamental to the formation of a society (p.26). Moreno and his colleagues elaborated on this by establishing methods of analysing the relationships between individuals in order to establish mutually satisfying groupings in schools and communities. Attempts to replicate this were carried out during 1945 in the Northfield Military Hospital, where some ward configurations were decided through sociometric questionnaires that identified which patients preferred to be together.

Psychodrama was a technique designed to bring the varying aspects of an individual's 'tele' alive in the therapeutic situation, through enactments of situations which he or she has experienced (pp.22–75). Spontaneity and catharsis were essential elements of the procedure. The first, defined as the propensity of the individual to develop new responses in old situations or adequate ones in new situations, was in Moreno's view older than libido, memory or intelligence (1953, p.42). It is a conditioning of the individual for free action, a release from restraints of social conformity. It is the moment when Beethoven conjured up the ideas of the Ninth Symphony, rather than the 'cultural conserve' of the final written form (Moreno 1940; reprinted in Greenberg 1974, p.167). This creative energy enables the individual to explore the complexities of his or her 'tele', with the outcome that Moreno described as 'catharsis of integration' (1953, p.85). He defined this term as 'a process which accompanies every type of learning, not only a finding of resolution from conflict, but also a realisation of self, not only release and relief but also equilibrium and relief' (p.546). By acting out a particular scenario in their life, the person could take on the parts of other members of their social and emotional network, or have others do this on their behalf. Through re-examining the interactions, and discussion with other participants, the individual could gain new insights into what had occurred and explore alternative ways of handling the situation in the future.

Foulkes' criticism was that this form of catharsis and acting out could not be the essence of psychotherapy, as Moreno advocated, because in his opinion it was necessary for 'verbal formulation and articulate comm-unication' to complete the therapeutic process (Foulkes 1948, p.153). He further refuted the 'social atom' concept in favour of a model in which the individual consciousness was a nodal point in a web of interconnections between the internal and external worlds (pp.14–15). In Foulkes' opinion, Moreno still overemphasised the individual modality as against the social context. In this he was heavily influenced by his mentors Norbert Elias and Kurt Goldstein.

Despite these reservations it is clear, on reading the discussions between the psychiatrists at Northfield, how profoundly Moreno's ideas infiltrated the system there. Psychodrama was the most obvious expression of this, but more deep-seated was the continuing attempt to enable individuals to make spontaneous readjustments to their environment.

After Galileo: Kurt Lewin and field theory

Despite Foulkes' assertions that Lewin was opposed to psychoanalysis, his psychiatric colleagues in the army found little difficulty in amalgamating the two theoretical positions (Foulkes 1946a, p.47; 1955, p.148). The leading activists of the Second Northfield Experiment leant heavily on his work. Bion and Rickman's paper 'Intra-group tensions in therapy' employs the language of social fields (1943). Later in the year of that paper's publication, Rickman was working on another article describing the work of the psychiatrist in the War Office Selection Boards. He added appendices which described field theory in some detail (1943b). Tom Main recalled that the neologism 'Lewinisation' was current in discussions at Northfield, and Bridger employed the terms 'Lewinfiltration' and 'phenotypical' in his 1946 paper for the *Bulletin of the Menninger Clinic* (Main 1984; Bridger 1946). Surprisingly considering his ambivalence expressed elsewhere, Foulkes specifically mentioned the value of field theory in his article in the same journal (1946c).

The key figure in introducing Lewin's ideas to his colleagues in the British Army was Eric Trist. He was a psychologist who had worked in America before the war and had made Lewin's acquaintance at that time. Through him, many psychiatrists and psychologists were kept up to date with Lewin's work (King 1994). With him, Rickman, Bion and Bridger were to cement the relationship with Lewin's team further after the war.

Ronald Hargreaves, at the Directorate of Psychiatry in the War Office, was again instrumental in bringing this work to the attention of those at Northfield. In his correspondence with Foulkes, he recommended a summary of Lewin's ideas presented in a book entitled *Psychology and the Social Order* by J.F. Brown (Hargreaves 1944; Brown 1936). The author described it as an introduction to the dynamic study of social fields, and considered that the methodological section was 'adequately presented in English' for the first time (Brown 1936, p.vi). He also specifically referred to the support of Karl Menninger, who in 1945 visited Northfield as part of an American delegation.

As with other theory examined earlier, the emphasis was on the dynamic interrelationship of the individual and the social group. Brown claimed that it was a 'scientific' approach to social psychology. The subject, including political science, was investigated using a methodology based on mathematical and physical concepts. At its philosophical heart was Lewin's distinction between Aristotlean and Gallilean modes of thought (Lewin 1935). He considered that contemporary psychology was riddled with superficial, valuative, anthropomorphic and entelechic conceptualisations. These stemmed from Aristotle, who believed that the highest forms of motion were circular and rectilinear, and only occurred in the movement of heavenly bodies such as the stars and the planets. Those in the earthly sublunar world, on the other hand, were less perfect. In psychology, parallel examples were the class concepts of instincts, the 'errors' of children and 'forgetting'. These classified actions according to valuation of their products rather than understanding of the underlying psychological processes involved. The dichotomisation reflected in the perception of actions as being either 'good' or 'bad' was present in other areas, such as the contrast between the individual and the crowd outlined by Le Bon (1917) and McDougall (1920). This consequently obscured the continuities and parallel processes present in both. Bion and Rickman strongly denounced this separation: 'Psychology and psycho-pathology have focussed attention on the individual often to the exclusion of the social field of which he is a part' (1943).

Lewin considered that modern psychology should identify underlying laws of behaviour that could be applied to all situations: 'The thesis of general validity permits of no exceptions in the entire realm of the psychic, whether of child or adult, whether in normal or pathological psychology' (1935, p.24). The forces that determine activity do not exist within the individual alone, but include responses to the social environment. In physics, the stone does not propel itself towards the earth but is subject to a gravitational pull that is exerted from without. 'Only by the concrete whole which comprises the object and the situation are the vectors which determine the dynamics of the event defined' (pp.29–30).

Galileo did not examine stones or the objects themselves, but the process of 'free falling or movement on an inclined plane' (quoted in Lewin 1935, p.29). Lewin and Brown employed this emphasis on dynamics by applying the physics of vectors to objects within the abstract space of the social field.

People are perceived as responding to forces that push them towards goals in psycho-social arenas that have boundaries and membership characteristics, and allow varying degrees of mobility and reality within them (1936, p.44–45). Main illustrated how central this perception was to his thinking in his paper 'Rehabilitation and the individual' in 1948. This began:

> Health and disease are not things, static or absolute in themselves; both are aspects of the dynamic process of biological adaptation between man and his environment ... [m]an's environment is, like himself, not a static but a dynamic system of relations. It is a socio-physical structure, itself reactive in one direction or another to the individual. Rehabilitation is not, therefore, a process which concerns only the individual, but an interreactive relationship between a dynamic environment and a dynamic individual. (Main 1948)

Because size was seen as significant in influencing the forces acting within them, Brown categorised social fields by their spread, as major, minor, primary and individual. The first included affiliations such as the Nation or organised religion, of which the second would include local sub-groups such as the local church. Smaller organisations might operate within the larger boundaries, such as the Bolsheviks within Russia before the Revolution. Only at times of social instability could these organisations become influential. Face-to-face groups such as families or gangs are seen as primary groups, and the person themselves is also a social field (1936, p.232). Main and Bridger recognised the importance of these levels operating within the hospital field. In their view, the failure of Bion and Rickman was to identify and counter the forces acting against their work in the wider order system of the 'hospital-as-a-whole' which resulted in their final dismissal (Bridger 1985; 1990a; 1990b; Main 1977; 1984).

Field theory as postulated by Lewin and Brown presented an optimistic view of the ability of changes in the social field to influence the people in it. Their work offered another view of the neurotic personality, regarding it as capable of responding beneficially to an appropriate social environment. This contrasted with the traditional psychiatric view, as implied by Eliott Slater in a letter to John Rickman, referring to his pioneering work at Wharncliffe:

> the greatest weakness of your scheme is that it has to be applied pretty universally, and therefore to unsuitable cases. My report criticises the results as being over-optimistic ... The whole subject is exceedingly difficult as fundamentally I maintain the view that the great majority of neurotics do not make good soldiers, whatever is done further, and that

they constitute (or more than 50 per cent of them constitute) a source of weakness rather than strength to the army. (Slater 1941)

Brown found that in any situation, the aims of the participants with regards to original goals are constantly shifting. Thus barriers in the social and psychological field of the individual should be placed so that that person raises their expectations of themselves and achieves tasks in 'such a way that the personality is enriched' (Brown 1936, p.294). At the Northfield Experiments, Bridger learnt that in all groups, of whatever size, 'the individual contribution has a value only in so far as it has a significance for the community'. He endorsed wholeheartedly Brown's optimism regarding the possibility of manipulating the environment so that it becomes enabling: 'the individual can only experience full freedom and satisfaction in a society that recognises his worth, and gives him the opportunity to develop in a spirit of warm human relationships' (Bridger 1946, p.76).

Lewin, with a colleague Ronald Lippitt, investigated this interaction between individuals and the social field experimentally by placing a number of schoolchildren into two groups. The first was run in an authoritarian manner, with all decisions being made by an appointed leader. This individual remained impersonal and largely uncommunicative about the future direction being taken. The second was described as democratic, and all policies were a matter of group determination. The methods of carrying out the tasks in this latter group were as far as possible decided upon by the members of the group, with advice and a number of alternatives being offered by the leader. Over a number of areas the findings demonstrated that the democratic group scored more highly in the areas of cooperativeness and creativity, the members became more objective in their outlook, and there was an increased sense of 'belongingness' (Lewin and Lippitt 1937). This paper was amongst those that Foulkes received from Hargreaves in 1944, noted above.

Lewin and Lippitt's work was extended by French, who published a paper on groups without leaders in 1941 (French 1941). Trist, Bion and Sutherland were aware of this study when they were designing officer selection procedures later that same year (Harris 1949, p.26). French studied the behaviour of two types of groups, organised and unorganised, faced with the task of solving insoluble problems. The organised groups were either college sports teams or neighbourhood groups, and consisted of six members each. The first finding was that they varied widely in their responses: one almost split into two, whilst another contained a great deal of aggression, but remained effective and friendly. Previously organised groups tended to promote more social freedom, interdependence, interpersonal hostility, disorganisation, equality of participation and determination to win through. Increased social freedom was positively associated with increased aggression. Every group had 'within it the seeds of its own destruction' in that it had the capacity to dissolve itself. Increased interdependence between group members increased the levels of frustration expressed. French then proceeded to examine the groups topologically, using Lewin's social field model to demonstrate the tensions within them. The disruptive forces fell into three classes. First was the failure of group members to agree on the preferred method to achieve the goal. Less commonly, members were unable to agree on the goal, and occasionally personal ambition overwhelmed the task. This examination of the dynamics of a group and their relationship to morale was seized upon by Bion as a significant tool for understanding his and Rickman's own task. Its impact is amply illustrated by its incorporation into the title of their first paper on the Northfield Experiments: 'Intra-group tensions in therapy' (1943).

HAWKSPUR AND PECKHAM:
EXPERIMENTS IN COMMUNITY

Two sources of inspiration deserve more attention than can be paid to them here. The first was the work of some psychoanalysts with adolescents, in particular their association with David Wills in the Hawkspur Experiment. The second was the birth of the 'Health Clinic' in Peckham.

Wayward youth: Communities for juveniles

Throughout the nineteenth century there were varied attempts to provide democratic learning experiences for young people who had earned themselves the soubriquet 'juvenile delinquents'. Starting with the work of August Aichhorn in Austria after the First World War and Homer Lane in America and then England, there was a steady trickle of communities established to enable distressed young people to acquire the art of forming mature relationships with their fellows (Aichhorn 1936; Wills 1964).

Aichhorn serves as an example of this approach. He was a psycho-analytically-orientated director of an institution for boys with behavioural disorders in Vienna immediately after the First World War. It proved difficult to manage twelve of the most disturbed and disturbing juveniles in the home. He was aware from discussions with them that they had not had the opportunity of a normal emotional development, and had been left with feelings of intense bitterness and hatred towards one or both of their parents. His response was to place them in a separate hut, where they were allowed to do whatever they liked. The attitude of the adult staff was to remain impartially friendly and kind. The first few weeks proved predictably destructive and chaotic, with the property being vandalised and fights breaking out regularly. Increasingly, the aggression became 'staged' for the benefit of the staff, and when even apparently life-threatening gestures were ignored the behaviours began to change. A period of intense instability with intermittent violence and good behaviour ensued. Eventually, the behaviour improved enough for the young men to be transferred to a newly-decorated house with good furniture. The relationship that Aichhorn had established with the leader of the group allowed him to begin a period of re-education for them all. He claimed that all became useful citizens and remained so after leaving. His book describing this was published in English in 1936 and was known to many psychoanalysts (Aichhorn 1936).

Most of these initiatives had at their centre someone of more than usual patience and reflectiveness who allowed the children to express their aggression and work through the consequences of it. Their ideas were not dissimilar to those behind Slavson's in 'Activity Group Therapy' described earlier. This work was supplemented by the increasing interest of psychoanalysts in working with children. During the 1930s, Melanie Klein, Anna Freud and others developed child guidance clinics. From the clinical experience thus gained they were able to elaborate a theoretical background for the understanding of the psychology of young persons.

Members of the Tavistock Clinic and the British Psycho-Analytic Society, through the agency of the Institute for the Study and Treatment of Delinquency (ISTD), supported another of these experiments. This latter organisation was founded in 1932 to provide a base for co-ordinating the assessments of the psychiatrist, psychologist and social worker in cases of adolescent disturbance, and was influenced by the ideas of William Healy. Healy had demonstrated the importance of working with the whole family in juvenile cases rather than concentrating on the individual alone, as had been the case previously. He also recommended the use of a multi-disciplinary team, including psychiatrists, psychologists and social workers, working from specialised clinics (Friedlander 1947, p.195). In his opinion, criminality was not an inherited trait, although a more generalised tendancy to instability might be (p.103). J.R. Rees acknowledged the importance of Healy's approach in tackling delinquency in the British Army (1945, p.31).

The institute was closely interwoven with the psychoanalytic movement, and had many psychoanalysts working closely with it. One of these, Marjorie Franklin, had become aware of the positive effects of a cheerful and encouraging atmosphere on mental illness. It was her contention that, with skillful support and psychoanalytical intervention, such an environment could be established and achieve improvements for socially disfunctional young people. She became aware of the plans of a psychiatric social worker called David Wills, who wished to set up a community for young offenders (Bridgeland 1971, p.181). They then co-operated to establish the Hawkspur Camp in 1936.

Drawing from his knowledge of Homer Lane and August Aichhorn, and also his own experience at a farm training colony, Wills became 'Camp Chief'. He had to set up the organisation on a site which, although large (26 acres), with good soil and natural springs, had nothing else. As Marjorie Franklin put it, they were 'in clover', there being little else! (1943b, p.11). The camp opened in May, and all the members and staff lived in tents until the wooden buildings that were to serve as proper living quarters had been built by the youths themselves (p.12). Responsibility for running the camp and day-to-day decisions about management were shared between all involved. The members, those young men who had been selected because of their previously disturbed behaviour, formed a Camp Council along with the staff. This body, initially presided over by Wills, served as a focus for discussion and democratic decision making over how the camp should function. Later, it was chaired by the members themselves. Any punishments for misdemeanours were instituted by this council, there being no other established penal code (Franklin 1943c). Consequently, there was a tendancy for anarchy to prevail. At one point anarchy was formally declared, with the Camp Chief declaring his support if it cooked the dinner. This eventually culminated in the expected disorder, and the members themselves, in the absence of Wills, decided to reinstate a 'constitutional government' (Wills 1943a, pp.26–27). Over a period of time, the young men began to take on a sense of personal responsibility and diverted their aggression into more creative roles, including gaining education. Wills was consciously aware of his role in the community as the centre of an 'emotional vortex'. He expressed this in psychoanalytical terms, describing the feelings that members had towards him as 'transference' (1941, pp.125–127). However, he did not carry out psychotherapy himself; this was left to members of the ISTD where it was thought necessary.

No formal, controlled trial of such an experiment could have been carried out, and examining outcomes was further complicated by its closure at the outbreak of war. However, Wills did follow up many members, and found that clear improvements in behaviour had occurred in men who otherwise would most likely have spent the rest of their lives in and out of prison (1941, pp.13–15; 1943b, pp.39–41).

During the 1930s, Bion both worked for the ISTD and was a board member for a short while, and Rickman was both a medical officer and on the Scientific Committee in 1944 (Bléandonu 1944, p.44; Glover 1944, p.2). His colleague Dennis Carroll, commanding officer at Northfield a year later, was closely involved and supportive (Wills 1941, p.9). Whilst at the hospital, Carroll had the amusing experience of his commanding officer approaching him with a booklet on the Hawkspur Camp and suggesting that he try out the ideas, evidently ignorant of the fact that he had already been part of it (Franklin 1966, p.6). The consulting psychiatrist to the army, J.R. Rees, would have been referring to this work when he emphasised the importance of previous work with adolescents in his review of military psychiatry after the war (1945, pp.31–32).

The ideas of Madame Montessori were better known in the United Kingdom. She worked with children in the slums of Rome, and the ideas derived from her experience there had a profound effect on the development of infant schools elsewhere (Lawrence 1970, p.327). She believed fundamentally that 'the school must permit the *free natural manifestation of the child*' and should promote 'such liberty as shall permit a development of individual spontaneous manifestations of the child's nature' (Montessori 1912, p.115). Unlike Wills, Aichhorn and Homer Lane, she was not an advocate of limitless liberty, and considered that there can be no freedom without limits. In her view, the purpose of education was to enable the child to gain independence. She fought against the adult wish to do things for children, recognising their need to master activities for themselves. Children only learnt by means of their own activity, guided and encouraged by the teacher. Discipline of a genuine nature can only be achieved when the child works willingly because it appeals to their innate needs and interests (Lawrence 1970, p.331). The following statement anticipates Bion's approach to this issue at Northfield:

> Discipline is reached always by indirect means. The end is obtained, not by attacking the mistake and fighting it, but by developing activity in spontaneous work ... The child disciplined in this way is no longer the child he was at first, who knows how to be good passively; but he is an individual who has made himself better. (Montessori 1912, p.352)

Montessori was known to workers at the Tavistock Clinic, where she taught on a course on child psychology (Dicks 1970, p.76). Her influence also extended to the authors of the Peckham Experiment. They were particularly impressed by her understanding of the development of fine co-ordination in the infant (Pearse and Crocker 1943, p.317). It was their intention in 1939 to develop an educational programme with her there, but of course the intervention of the war prevented this.

A real health clinic: The Peckham Experiment

Harold Bridger read the report of the Peckham Experiment as part of his preparation for Northfield, and evolved his concept of the hospital social club from the earlier venture (Pearse and Crocker 1943; Bridger 1990a). Following a discussion in 1944 with one of the authors, Innes Pearse, Rickman was impressed enough to passionately advocate her project after the war was over (Pearse 1944; Rickman 1944). Like many others before her, Innes enjoyed their 'stimulating' talk, and wrote in further explanation of her work:

> The practical and important meaning of Peckham for this moment lies I believe, in the fact that through the experiment we have found a means of canalising and tapping the growth energy of the family, and in such a way that through the 'Centre' we have now the means of enabling the people to educate themselves through their own drive.
>
> I must say again that one of the poignant disclosures of the Centre was the quite extraordinary fund of good sense and good will which exists pent up in the ordinary man. If at this critical moment in time we could realise that, we could ensure the future for our own country – and perhaps for the world – by giving it outlet. (Pearse 1944)

This enthusiasm for the abilities of the ordinary person would have been wholeheartedly reciprocated by Rickman and Bridger.

The Health Centre was a biological experiment set up to examine the responses of individuals and their families to changes in their environment. Certain precepts were formulated that were echoed by the Northfield Experiments and their participants. First, it was considered that the 'organism' is any 'entity capable of performing the full cycle of its specific existence'. Thus an ant is part of the 'organism' of the whole anthill. Similarly, to understand the human 'organism', one must study the family. Second, there is a dynamic mutuality between the organism and the environment it exists within. It has already been emphasised that in the army the individual soldier cannot act without the support of his comrades. Foulkes also acknowledged this: 'The healthy organism functions as a whole and can be described as a system in a dynamic equilibrium' (1948, p.1). Finally, the individual can only be understood within the context of its organism. Thus the group became the central focus for many workers in the hospital.

Members of the Health Centre agreed to undergo regular health checks in order to participate in its activities. At the heart of the building was a swimming pool, which symbolised the whole, emphasising the role of individuals in keeping themselves well. This was paralleled by an 'information pool', which was a repository for the information gained from the health checks and also a resource for learning how to maintain the 'organism' in a healthy way, which members could 'dip into' when they needed to. Many activities were created and maintained by the members themselves. Members planned the purchase of requisites, or even brought them in themselves. The cafeteria was 'self-service', a terminology that adumbrated the purpose of the building itself. It was intended to be a 'self-service' health centre, not a sickness centre where others provided all the care. The scientists who collected the data were there to be questioned, and were responsible for sharing the knowledge they were acquiring.

The similarities between this work and that at Northfield cannot be entirely explained by direct influence. Bion and Rickman's work was carried out before the book on the Peckham Experiment was published (Pearse and Crocker 1943). It is evident that there were other less overt influences at work, which had their effect on both groups as well as on the intellectual climate in other areas.

IN THE SOUP: THE SOCIAL
AND POLITICAL BACKGROUND

Throughout the first half of the twentieth century an intellectual primeval soup was fermenting. Reminiscent of Rickman's 'lumps in the gravy', more or less successful group-life forms precipitated out. Some were able to multiply, of which one was Northfield.

The accumulation of evidence and theory outlined here was evidently an expression of underlying currents in the social and political fields. The fact that apparently unconnected theoreticians and practitioners were convinced of the intimate connections between the individual and his or her social milieu indicates that such ideological vectors were operating throughout the Western world. The increased preoccupation with Marxism in the universities of Europe was another illustration of this. It is not coincidental that a number of the protagonists of this story were themselves left-wing by inclination. The turning of their talents, in the form of the Tavistock Institute, towards commerce after the war was a classic expression of socialism, which saw industry as the anvil on which capitalism was forged.

Northfield was yet another expression of this ferment, enabled by the collaboration of a particularly energetic, enthusiastic and articulate set of individuals, all of whom shared the idea that the individual human being existed only as part of the social network in which he or she lived. This predicated the necessity for forms of therapy which acknowledged this. It was the exigencies of army life that provided the final link in the chain, and whether group therapy would have ever gained such recognition without this fillip is uncertain. Clearly, there were individuals promoting this form of activity before the war; but they were largely operating in isolation and in a more or less charismatic manner. The war led to ordinary psychiatrists experimenting with these new ideas, and in some cases performing a complete volte-face, such as that of Maxwell Jones.

CHAPTER 3

Battle Fields
Military Psychiatry

The soldier is not chiefly a military figure; he is primarily a social figure.

(Viscount Montgomery 1946)

THE 'INVISIBLE COLLEGE': PSYCHIATRY
AND PSYCHOLOGY GO TO WAR

At this distance in time it appears inexplicable that group therapy and therapeutic communities could have flourished in the British Army. Commonly, the military is characterised as subject to unthinking and slavish adherence to machismo, 'Bull' and 'the old school tie'. Independence of thought in the ordinary 'Tommy Atkins' seems entirely incompatible. Part of the fascination of exploring the history of the Northfield Experiments is the dawning realisation that they were an integral part of a complete re-examination of the whole structure of the military machine, which culminated in the rejection of such stereotypes. The conjunction of a number of influential figures, in particular General Sir Ronald Adam (Adjutant General of the British Army) and Ronald Hargreaves, with the recruitment of more mature soldiers, as well as psychologists and psychiatrists influenced by the Tavistock Clinic, led to social psychiatry transforming the whole organisation (Ahrenfeldt 1958; Harrison and Clarke 1992; Harrison 1997; King 1989; Privy Council Office 1947).

Colonel Baynes has already been quoted in the previous chapter with regards to the necessity for trust between soldiers and the importance of the social environment to morale. Whilst acknowledging the importance of the platoon, company, battalion and division, he asserted the particular importance of small groups such as the section (Baynes 1987, p.102). Although people live with others, such as in the family, at work and in clubs, throughout their lives, he argued that the collective loyalty of the soldier is stronger than in any social groups in civilian life. This is partly because the training and milieu demand it, but more importantly because on active service each depends on the other for their very existence. Robinson emphasised the same points when asserting the validity of group therapy in the army:

> Military service enforces close relationships. It thus provides a setting which encourages and invites the trial of group psychotherapy. In the first place, military patients have a great deal in common as members of the military services. They have lived, trained, played, travelled and in many cases fought together... (1948)

The last chapter demonstrated the growing recognition of the fact that people are enmeshed in relationships with each other. It became increasingly obvious, as the war progressed, that group therapy was a logical extension of army life. This, allied with the large numbers of men requiring help and the relatively few staff available, led inevitably to widespread experimentation with the new technology. As a result, it was employed both in hospitals and in exhaustion centres next to the battlefield (Jones 1942; Robinson 1948; Sutherland and Fitzpatrick 1945; Wilson, Doyle and Kelnar 1947).

However, the sway of the psychiatrists and psychologists spread far beyond the field of therapy. Concern about morale catalysed reform of selection procedures, training, discipline, and the involvement of psychiatrists in combatant units. This increasing range of operation led the sceptical Sir Winston Churchill to launch an enquiry into their military involvement, with the aim of curtailing their activities. He was deeply suspicious and hostile, stating to Parliament that their work should be restricted because of the harm he believed that they would do (Ahrenfeldt 1958, p.26). Probably to his intense chagrin, the investigation inaugurated by his remarks concluded that 'the contribution of the psychiatrists has been important and indispensable' (Privy Council Office 1947). His response is not known.

The foundations of Second World War military psychiatry were laid down during the First, although many of these early lessons were neglected in the interim. After a slow start, military psychiatrists and psychologists drew on this reservoir of information to initiate advances on all fronts. Not all were immediately relevant to events at Northfield, except in that they demonstrated further the wide applicability of social psychology.

Bion and Bridger's work in the War Office Selection Boards and Rickman's implementation of a system of rapid rehabilitation in the treatment of neurosis were, however, directly germane. The latter's work was complemented by the introduction of early treatment centres in theatres of battle, known as 'forward psychiatry'. He was also involved in the training of psychiatrists and the institution of intelligence testing for recruits. Tom Main, on the other hand, became involved in the issues of morale, in training and the planning of the invasion of Northern France. These four, along with other recruits from the Tavistock Clinic, formed the social psychology powerhouse of the army, which came to be known as the 'invisible college' (Dicks 1970, p.107).

This section concentrates on those activities which led to the development of group therapy at Northfield Military Hospital; consequently, the story may appear somewhat skewed to those readers who are aware of the full impact of psychiatrists within the military setting.

HIDDEN CASUALTIES: PRECURSORS OF SECOND WORLD WAR MILITARY PSYCHIATRY

Hardly noticeable: Neurosis and the soldier before 1914

An anonymous contributor to the *Journal of the Royal Army Medical Corps* in 1951 lamented the high wastage of men as a result of psychiatric causes during the Second World War. His view was that, in the previous 2000 years of conflict, psychological problems had been 'hardly noticeable' (*Journal of the Royal Army Medical Corps*. 1951). His historical knowledge was superficial: a more rigorous examination exposes the speciousness of this view.

From antiquity, through the Crimean War, and up to the Falklands War, it has been the officially maintained view that British soldiers are made of 'stern stuff' and do not succumb to nervous problems as a result of battle. On each occasion this has been exposed as inaccurate, but only after many men have suffered. This studious ignorance was most explicit during the First World War, with the consequence that many men were shot for cowardice. However, during that conflict some lessons began to be learnt, only to be entirely forgotten by 1939.

Desertion, suicide and drunkenness: The hidden costs of military stress

Homer, in his account of the siege of Troy, gave a vivid description of a panic state: 'A coward changes colour all the time; he cannot sit still for nervousness, but squats down, first on one heel and then on the other; his heart thumps in his breast as he thinks of death in all its forms, and one can hear the chattering of his teeth' (1964, p.241). The effects of panic on Hellenic warfare could be dramatic: 'Sometimes an army, weaponed and drawn up for battle, has fled before a spear was raised' (Euripides 1976, p.201). Clearly, psychological problems have been part of warfare since battles were first fought, but it was not until the American Civil War that anyone attempted to tackle systematically the issues they raised.

The costs for the British Army were enormous. Morselli recorded that between 1862 and 1871 the suicide rate among British soldiers, 0.379 per thousand, was three times the rate of civilian men of the same age. In the army in India this rose to 0.468 per thousand. With regards to the latter he stated: 'We may suppose that here nostalgia and the fatal influence of the climate play a large part' (Morselli 1883).

These figures, however, are dwarfed by the rates of desertion. Between 1816 and 1836, 5.8 per cent of the entire force (3994 men) deserted from the Canada command. In the late 1850s, stimulated by the fear of being sent to the Crimean War, this rate rose to 18 per cent. Whilst proportionally less, even in Britain during the period of the Crimean war the figures reached 4.2 per cent (Burroughs 1985). Of course, not all of these were suffering neurotic conditions; however, it is reasonable to speculate that many were severely emotionally unsettled. This contention is supported by the testimony of Fortescue, the military historian, to the Southborough Committee in 1923. He reported of the British Army in the nineteenth century: 'No doubt there were men who, from one cause or another, broke down in every campaign; and I have little doubt that this was one of the causes that led to desertion' (HMSO 1923, p.9). Further confirmation of this was forthcoming in the Second World War, during which men under sentence for military crime, including desertion, showed a high incidence of psychiatric disorder (Crew 1955, p.486).

Excessive alcohol consumption was endemic. The recruiting sergeants usually entrapped their prey with the King's shilling at inns and taverns. 'The doors of the beerhouse and the brothel were the common gates of admission into the military service of the State' (Onslow 1869). Between 1847 and 1854, 1.1 per cent of the army in Britain had been held in prison on drink charges. During the years 1865–1867 4626 men were court-martialled for being drunk on duty and 25,710 for habitual drunkenness. This made up 39 per cent of all offences (Burroughs 1985, pp.555–556). What made the situation worse, as a Royal Commission reported in 1868, was that many other offences were associated. Drunkenness was 'connected with the vast majority of crimes tried by court martial' (Parliamentary Papers 1868; quoted in Burroughs 1985, p.556).

Although, as the anonymous commentator in the *Journal of the Royal Army Medical Corps* stated, psychological problems remained unrecognised, and punishments were meted out liberally, it is clear that such problems resulted in enormous wastage of men, loss of morale, defeat in battle and absorption of resources throughout the centuries.

Heroism or cowardice: Shell-shock and the First World War

During the First World War, 'nervous disorders' began to be recognised as a military problem. Although the French had begun investigating neurosis at the battle front in 1915, the British authorities only took significant action later, in July 1916, after the battle of the Somme. Whilst the leadership prevaricated, the pharmaceutical industry was less equivocal, advertising popular remedies for 'Nerve Strain' on 'active service' in popular newspapers such as the *Daily Mirror.*[1] Over and above the slaughter, several thousands of soldiers were withdrawn from the front line with mental health problems, many of whom were evacuated to Britain (HMSO 1923, pp.1–7). Despite the dire nature of the situation, there was little agreement about appropriate responses. The term 'shell-shock', coined at this time, reflected many of the controversies that raged about the nature of war neurosis. For a generation of young men brought up on ideals of masculinity that eschewed such 'feminine' attributes as fear, the terrors that affected them and their comrades were perplexing and shocking (Showalter 1987, p.171). The evolving understanding of these issues profoundly influenced the subsequent clinical, organisational and theoretical development of psychiatry.

The first line of debate was whether the affected individuals were cowards. Amongst the records of those men shot for cowardice there is clear evidence to suggest that a number were suffering from mental health problems (Richardson 1986, pp.282–286). Brigadier Rees reported in 1945: 'Those of us who had to have first-hand experience of the men who were shot at dawn in the last war feel that ... these men were in many cases quite obviously suffering from an acute neurosis' (1945, p.113).

Doctors and psychologists struggled to find a less condemnatory formulation of the problem. Where the concept of nervous disorder was accepted the discussion shifted to the cause. Following his earlier work on the psychological effects of head injuries, Mott, later to work at Hollymoor in the 1920s, found microscopic damage to the central nervous system in two soldiers who had been killed in an explosion. This was in the absence of any other obvious major physical damage. From this he concluded that 'Shellshock' had an organic origin (Mott 1917). This stance had both the advantage of providing the ordinary medical officers with a tool for distinguishing between illness and non-illness, and a rationale for describing those men afflicted as being 'sick' or suffering 'debility', thus avoiding the

1 Phosphorine: 'This keen and efficient Lance-Corporal says he can get more and more out of his day since Phosphorine saved him from the menacing nerve collapse provoked by his 15 months of continuous duties'. The advert goes on to state that a special form has been made for sailors or soldiers on active service (*Daily Mirror* 1915, p.15).

stigma of mental disorder (Merskey 1991, pp.246–260). At a propaganda level it supported the view that 'England's finest blood' were not tainted with madness. (Ahrenfeldt 1958; Stone 1985)

As the war progressed, it became increasingly evident that most cases were psychological in origin. The Southborough Committee, reporting in 1922, concluded that about 5 per cent of cases were organic, or 'commotional', in origin, 15 per cent had features of mixed organic and emotional factors, and the remainder were entirely emotional (War Office 1922, p.112). However, even amongst those doctors who accepted this, there remained a divide between those of a perjorative inclination and those who were less condemnatory. Some regarded hysterical phenomena 'as something closely akin to malingering'(Elliot-Smith and Pear 1917, p.30). Colonel Burnett made this statement in his evidence to the Southborough Committee: 'Although a man's nerves may break down we must look upon it as a disgrace, otherwise you would have everybody breaking down as soon as they wanted to go home' (War Office 1922, p.45). The practice of Adrian and Yealland was a direct consequence of this viewpoint. They made their mute patients stand in line in the treatment room watching the first one receive painful electric shocks to his larynx. This continued until he made a noise, at which point he was informed that he had recovered his voice and the next man took his place (Adrian and Yealland 1917).

Those who espoused the psycho-neurotic formulation became very influential. Whilst they recognised that individuals vary in their ability to cope with the strain of the battle front, they also emphasised that appropriate recruitment, training, morale and improved working conditions could improve this (War Office 1922). Many found, as did Lt. Col. Rogers, that 'as a rule you will find that bright volatile people – people who are willing and anxious to do dangerous work, battalion runners, men who are anxious to go out on raids and patrol – are even more liable to this anxiety condition than others' (War Office 1922, p.62). The widely used term 'psychotherapy' usually reflected treatments which were orientated towards a more discursive and didactic approach. Although the psychiatric profession was becoming more familiar with the theories of Freud, full-blown psychoanalysis was frowned upon as being unnecessary and impracticable. (War Office 1922, p.129)

Simple short-term psychotherapy was recommended by Elliot-Smith and Pear, amongst others (Elliot-Smith and Pear 1917, pp.56–75; War Office 1922, p.129). This largely consisted of discussion in private with the doctor, accompanied by suggestion, re-education and persuasion. Most advised against being too sympathetic and recommended the early introduction of military discipline and training in the convalescent period. Myers recommended hypnosis for exploration of the traumatic event and subsequent recall of repressed material (Myers 1916, 1940). Many of these techniques were recommended again at the beginning of the Second World War. For example, Hadfield outlined techniques of suggestion and hypno-analysis in his paper of 1940, referring specifically to his experience in the previous conflict. (Hadfield 1940)

The increasing body of evidence supporting psychodynamic techniques led to 56 doctors being trained in these skills under the guidance of R.G. Rows, at Maghull (Shepherd 1996, p.447). The *British Psycho-Analytic Society* emerged from its relative obscurity before the war to become a rapidly expanding organisation of increasing influence, and by 1925 it had 54 members (Pines 1991, pp.215–216; Rayner 1991, p.11). The Tavistock Clinic, after its foundation in 1920, also promoted psychoanalytic ideas and succeeded in securing as honorary vice-presidents Field Marshall Haig and Admiral Beatty (Stone 1985). Members of both these organisations had been drawn to the ideas of Freud through their wartime medical experiences. Although these two institutions did not find it easy to work together, they formed between them a focus for the promotion of, and research into, psychodynamic theory and its application until the Second World War.

Difficulties with identifying the cause of war neurosis and finding suitable treatment strategies were mirrored by the problems organising appropriate services. As a response to the mounting psychiatric casualties of 1916, Lt. Col. Gordon Holmes, a neurologist, and Lt. Col. C.S. Myers, a psychologist, recommended that special units be established in each army area. These were for diagnosis and treatment of nervous disorders, and were placed within the battle area but out of danger zone. Brought into service in late 1916, they were organised in such a way as to separate the different forms of disorder for immediate therapy, until the patients improved enough to move to a common convalescent area where normal military activity was reinstituted. Patients were admitted within 48 hours of their breakdown in the front line. Myers shared the common view that early treatment and 'maintenance of strict discipline' would lead to early return of the recovered soldier to active duty (1940, pp.61–62). This echoed another of Myers' recommendations to the War Office Committee of Enquiry into 'Shell Shock' of 1922:

> The centre to which these slighter shell-shock cases are first sent should be as remote from the sounds of warfare as is compatible with the preservation of the 'atmosphere' of the front. (Myers, in War Office 1922, p.124)

Those soldiers who did not respond to this were evacuated to the base hospital. Many of them ended up in psychiatric hospitals in England. However, much to Myers' disgust, the scheme was never fully implemented.

Learning from history? Reports on shell-shock

The lessons of the First World War were encapsulated in the 1922 War Office Committee of Enquiry into 'Shell Shock' (War Office 1922). In all, 59 witnesses gave testimony, including such names as W.H.R. Rivers, Bernard Hart, A.F. Hurst and Professor G. Roussy from the Faculté de Médicin de Paris. The Committee presented five pages of recommendations in the areas of classification, prevention (including training), recruitment, treatment and rehabilitation (pp.190–194).

Some of these recommendations were central to the developments of the Second World War. For example:

- Under the aegis of training: 'Every possible means should be taken to promote morale, esprit de corps and a high standard of discipline'. The report stressed the need for co-operation between medical and regimental officers in observing for signs of 'mental or nervous instability' amongst trainees, and the requirement for medical officers to study psychiatry.

- Early intervention and treatment for those showing signs of nervous breakdown or exhaustion, and early return to the front line for those whose disorders are easily treated.

- The use of limited forms of psychotherapy, and, in convalescence, the use of 're-education and suitable occupation of an interesting nature'.

- Assessment as to whether it is possible to retain those soldiers who are unfit for front-line duty in some form of auxiliary duty.

- The value of proper assessment of new recruits was emphasised, as was the need for medical personnel to be able to make appropriate examinations to ascertain their nervous and mental conditions.

These recommendations were then studiously ignored in the British Army, so that by 1939 there were only six medical officers who had some understanding of psychiatry, and a new leadership in the field had to be recruited from civilian organisations. However, the existence of the report provided material for the next generation of practitioners to learn from. Indeed, its importance was such that Emanuel Miller reiterated the conclusions wholesale in *The Neuroses of War* (1940, pp.211–224).

A second highly regarded source of information concerning military psychiatry during the First World War was the report of Dr. Thomas Salmon for the United States Army (Salmon 1929). He distilled his recommendations chiefly from the British experience, and came to the same conclusion as Myers and his colleagues over the necessity for early treatment, with treatment centres near the front line to support this. His systematic account of the services established during this time provided a wealth of information for his colleagues in the later conflict (Rees 1945, p.20).

Finally, C.S. Myers himself wrote of his experiences in the hope of preventing the senior administrative officers of the Army Medical Service and the Adjutant General's Department from 'repeating the same mistakes – errors of commission, omission, and especially of wasteful procrastination – as arose in the last war' (1940, p.viii).

ESPRIT DE CORPS: ORGANISING PSYCHIATRY AND PSYCHOLOGY IN THE SECOND WORLD WAR

Since the days of Socrates, generals have accepted that the crucial element in battle is morale. Xenophon, leading his Greek troops through Persia, anticipating fighting an enemy whose forces hugely outnumbered his own, came to the conclusion:

> it is not numbers or strength that brings the victories in war. No, it is when one side goes against the enemy with the gods' gift of a stronger morale that their adversaries, as a rule, cannot withstand them. (Xenophon 1951, p.104)

General Montgomery echoed this message at the end of the Second World War, when he stated that the 'morale of the soldier is the greatest single factor in war' (1946, p.706).

The failure of morale inevitably results in psychiatric casualties (Richardson 1978, p.172). This observation goes to the heart of the military psychiatrist's and psychologist's role. The primary issue was prevention, and this involved a wide range of initiatives. Tom Main's lectures to officer students and commanders of infantry battalions attending Battle Schools during the first half of 1942 exemplified the breadth of this concept-ualisation. His subjects included measures for excluding unsuitable men before battle, the principles of group feeling, the place of discipline in mental health, *esprit de corps*, the effects on morale of enemy weapons, 'battle inoculation', and the function of leadership (Ahrenfeldt 1958, p.197; Privy Council Office 1947, p.58). Similarly, the handbook issued to army psychiatrists covered selection procedures, leadership, battle school training, morale, the soldier as patient, and disciplinary cases (War Office 1946a).

Shaping military psychiatry: The leadership

As has already been stated, at the outbreak of war in 1939 there was extremely limited mental health expertise in the British Army. As a first step towards remedying this, two senior psychiatrists were appointed as 'Consulting Psychiatrists'. The first was Henry Yellowlees, who worked with the British Expeditionary Force during its retreat to Dunkirk, but took little active role thereafter.

The invitation to J.R. Rees, commonly known as 'J.R.', to act as the second Consulting Psychiatrist to the army in the UK was at first sight an inauspicious move. He had been director of the Tavistock Clinic and was imbued with the psychodynamic viewpoint. In Tom Main's acerbic view, the Senior Service (the Royal Navy) and the Royal Air Force had been able to take their pick of the neurogically-orientated psychiatrists, and it appeared that the army had to make do with second best (1984). This view is supported by the statement, in the Report on the Work of Psychologists and Psychiatrists, that in the other two services 'psychiatry and neurology are regarded as two aspects of one subject closely linked to medicine' (Privy Council Office 1947).

In the event, the appointment was inspired. From the outset Rees used his previous management experience as director of the Tavistock Clinic to take an overview of the needs of the army. He was also able to recruit colleagues who shared a similar viewpoint. Indeed, many of those psychiatrists and psychologists who were at the heart of the reforms came from this source, including Ronald Hargreaves, 'Tommy' Wilson, Eric Trist and Wilfred Bion (Dicks 1970, pp.104–105). It is not evident how carefully he chose the original command psychiatrists, but the linking of Hargreaves and Adam in Northern Command gave rise to a crucial partnership that continued throughout the war.

In some people's view, Rees never quite understood the full implications of some of the events he had set in motion. In particular, Bion and Trist felt that he had not resolved the difficulties that occurred at the end of the First Northfield Experiment to their satisfaction. He appeared to them to be building medical dependencies, bottling up psychiatric resources by using them to maintain organisations rather than initiate self-sustaining systems (Trist 1985, p.17). However, if there was truth in this view, it was well offset by the high morale evident throughout the psychiatric services in the army, which can only be attributed to Rees' leadership. He became Consulting Psychiatrist to the army as a whole later in the war.

The lack of medical manpower limited achievements during the early years. However, by July 1943 there were 197 serving psychiatrists, and by 1945 there were over 300 (HMSO 1947; Rees 1958). This dramatic expansion led to the formation of a Directorate of Army Psychiatry within the new Army Medical Department (AMD 11) at the War Office to oversee their various activities. This department consisted of three branches:

1. AMD 11 (A) was concerned with the psychiatric aspects of morale, discipline, training and equipment.

2. AMD 11 (B) related to the selection, training and allocation of army psychiatrists, the psychiatric aspects of recruiting, selection, grading, allocation and transfer of officers and other ranks, and psychiatric liaison with the Ministry of Labour and National Service.

3. AMD 11 (C) had responsibility for clinical policy and research, psychiatric clinics and hospitals, psychiatric liaison with the Ministry of Pensions, Ministry of Health (EMS), and boards of control, and psychiatric aspects of discharges and medical boards.

AMD 11 was responsible for these activities in the British Army both at home and abroad. At this time, the other disciplines of medicine and surgery were subsumed within the Directorate of Hygiene.

The first Director of Army Psychiatry was a regular Royal Army Medical Corps officer, Col. H.A. Sandiford. He was supported by three majors, who were specialists, as Deputy Assistant Directors. Despite his evident seniority he features very little in accounts of the development of army psychiatry. He appears to have been largely sidelined by the other participants.

Particularly important in the expansion and influence of psychiatry and psychology in the army was the backing of Lieutenant General Sir Ronald F. Adam, who became Adjutant General to the Forces in 1941. At this very senior level in the army he was able to implement a wide range of policies, both in psychiatric and other fields. Rees said of him: 'His vision and courage led to the development, not only of selection procedures of various kinds in the Army, but also of a great number of other sociological experiments ... and his deliberate contribution to social medicine and social psychiatry as well as to winning the war is difficult to overvalue' (1945, p.11). In his history of officer selection boards, Harris acknowledged Adam's 'constructive and prophetic foresight' in initiating and 'fostering the War Office Selection Board as a psychological and scientific procedure for selecting leaders in the military field' (1949, p.3).

Whilst Rees was Commander-in-chief of Northern Command in April of 1940, a colleague from the Tavistock Clinic was appointed as his command psychiatrist. This was Ronald Hargreaves. In Bridger's words, he was 'the anchor man throughout the war at the Directorate of Army Psychiatry' (1990a).

During this initial phase, Rees and Hargreaves led the experimentation with and development of selection procedures. When appointed to the War Office, they continued by supporting and inspiring the whole psychiatric effort in the army. Trist and Murray considered that this relationship was 'of critical importance' in inaugurating and sustaining innovations in army psychiatry (1990a, p.3).

Hargreaves contributed directly to Northfield. He was keenly aware of what was happening at the hospital, keeping in both postal and direct contact with its staff. He briefed both Harold Bridger and Tom Main before they took up their posts there (Bridger 1990a; 1990b; Main 1984). A letter he wrote to Foulkes in August of 1945 is illustrative. After referring to the recent visit by the American delegation, he discussed the papers that both Foulkes and Bion were to write for the *Bulletin of the Menninger Clinic*; this section demonstrates his acute grasp of what was occurring, and, incidently, his diplomacy in handling the conflict between them:

> The Northfield Experiment to my mind is not limited to group psychotherapy; it is the fundamental integration of group psychotherapy with an attempt to structure the hospital field in a purposeful and therapeutic manner. Your own work in the field of group psychotherapy is, of course, in no way derived from Bion's concepts... But the total pattern of the Northfield Experiment as I have summarised above, is part of a long chain of developments in the army which originated from Bion's work with the leaderless group tests. (Hargreaves 1945)

A second highly-placed supporter was Lieutenant General Sir Alexander Hood. When he became Director General of the Army Medical Services in 1942, the *Lancet* reported:

> His innovative quality is revealed most clearly, perhaps, in the support he gave, often against advice, to the development of psychiatry at a time when this had to contend with opposition not only from powerful military authorities but also from powerful members of our profession. (*Lancet* 1948)

As referred to above, this animosity included that of the Prime Minister himself. One of the apparent anomalies of the Northfield Experiments is explained by the backing of Adam, Hargreaves and Hood. Their endorsement explains how such anti-autocratic ventures were sustained, despite the inauspicious failure of the first one.

Main, when describing the events at Northfield, was at pains to emphasise that they were only a small part of what was happening in the army as a whole. He considered that the real creativity and intelligence lay with the group of people referred to subsequently to as the 'Tavistock Group' or the 'invisible college'. Without their commitment, support and vision he considered that the army psychiatric services would have been left to the likes of Aubrey Lewis, who he saw as wanting to treat casualties only (Main 1984). Hargreaves was central to this group. Other members included

A.T.M. (Tommy) Wilson, John Bowlby, Eric Trist, Ronald Hargreaves, Harold Bridger, Jock Sutherland, Bion, Rickman and Tom Main himself. They were all psychoanalytically-orientated, shared many theoretical viewpoints and were in regular communication with each other. Members of this group, whilst never exclusive, tended to cultivate each other. Without rancour, MacKeith recalled that he was asked to return from Italy, where he had successfully overseen the establishment of psychiatric services, in order to carry out a similar task in preparation for the opening of the second front in northern Europe. Once he returned he was politely informed that Tom Main was to do this job instead (MacKeith 1994). An ex-Northfield officer-patient, who worked with Trist and Wilson in the first Civilian Resettlement Unit, related that they were very friendly to him, but that he was aware of their mutual understanding and co-operation (Interview: Mr K.1994).

After the war, the group was involved in the formation of the Tavistock Institute of Human Relations. As one explores the expansion of psychiatric activities during the war, it becomes clear that more often than not members of this group inaugurated and promoted the transformations. MacKeith gave an instance of how subtle and influential these could be when he described how the important term 'non-combatant guilt' was widely accepted amongst psychiatrists as influencing their feelings about their work. He related how Hargreaves had, during informal discussion, relayed this explanatory and helpful term to him (MacKeith 1994).

The developments in military psychiatry throughout the war relied on the creativity of all the psychiatrists employed in the army. As an example, forward psychiatry required acumen, the skill to relate to combatant officers, the ability to survive under difficult conditions and sheer hard work from those doctors involved. However, the inspiration and support of the group of officers described in this section was crucial. They created the expectations and either actively participated in or nurtured the changes. Their example and involvement promoted the *esprit de corps* that they aimed to engender in other sections of the army.

Cannon fodder and old school ties: Selection procedures

Not everyone carries a field marshal's baton: Sorting of conscripts

At the outbreak of the war little attention was paid to the abilities of the men recruited as soldiers. Discipline was considered to be all that was necessary to sort out any behavioural problems. As a result, psychiatrists, when called upon to assess soldiers referred from the training schools where they were placed, continually complained that many were quite incapable of carrying out any form of military duty as a result of low intelligence, personality difficulties or mental ill-health. Most of these had to be discharged from the army as unfit (Gilman 1947; James 1944; Tredgold 1942).

The implications of these reports were resented in some quarters, because they undermined the myth that 'every soldier carries a field marshal's baton in his knapsack'. This romantic fantasy, widely current in the British Army, kept alive the notion that it was possible for every man to achieve the highest rank if they just worked at it (Rees 1945, p.25). The resilience of this idea, in the teeth of the evidence, is quite remarkable in retrospect. The conclusion of both the Southborough Committee and the United States Army was that selection would prevent the entry of many men who would be harmful to the service. Cautions about the effect of recruiting men with mental disorders were sounded by Ross in the *British Medical Journal* in 1939 (Ross 1939). J.R. Rees and Alec Rodger, a psychologist, drew up a scheme for selection procedures for the army in April of the same year. All this was ignored, and it was not until 1941 that the mounting problems of disposal of men who were evidently either not clever enough or too disordered to manage army life led to the introduction of a more appropriate system of filtering people entering the army.

This was not a case of psychiatrists arguing for some idealistic notion of efficiency. Their concerns were shared by combatant officers, who were well aware of the damage that a soldier could cause if he were unable to understand the complexities of manouevering, weapon training and mutual support in the frontline unit (War Office 1942; Rees 1945, pp.26–27). The First World War had taken soldiering from a blind obedience to authority to an increasingly sophisticated exercise of personal skill. Responsiveness to orders had to be supplemented with the readiness to react to new and unpredictable situations, the technical expertise to work with complex equipment and the ability to anticipate the actions of one's fellows.

After some research carried out on new recruits in Scotland by Bion, Trist and Sutherland, and in Yorkshire by Raven and Hargreaves, the latter wrote a memorandum in January 1941 (Ahrenfeldt 1958, pp.33–36; Vinden 1977). This recommended the setting up of appropriate selection procedures that not only identified whether or not individuals could function satisfactorily in the army, but also where they might be placed to best utilise their skills (Ahrenfeldt 1958, pp.37–38).

As a result of Brigadier Adam's support, in July 1942 the General Service Corps intake scheme was established. This ensured that all recruits were subjected to a series of intelligence and aptitude tests and that individuals were posted to the duties most appropriate to their abilities. Most of the work was carried out by by a large force of technicians given a small amount of relevant training. By October of 1943 they had assessed 47,000 men (Privy Council Office 1947, p.67). Part of the procedure was psychological testing of recruits using Ravens' Matrices (Raven 1942). When actually put into practice this, in combination with psychiatric examination of about 14 per cent of problem cases, began to abate the influx of people with mental health disorders and learning difficulties (Anon 1942c; Rees 1945, p.48). Furthermore, there was evidence that selection into specialist roles was more successful. Using the example of drivers, before selection procedures up to 20 per cent of men were failing the training, whereas afterwards this fell to less than 3 per cent (War Office 1947, p.458).

Although Rickman's involvement lay elsewhere, his knowledge and interest in these developments is reflected in a letter that Desmond Curran, senior psychiatrist in the Royal Navy, wrote to him in 1941:

> You may remember that at a recent meeting of the R.S.M. I asked for guidance about a proposed scheme for Naval recruiting, and you will remember that you were the only person who really gave us any practical help.
>
> Their Lordships have now passed our scheme *in toto* and we are just about to have a trial run at six combined recruiting centres. If this is a success it will be applied to all the centres where men are accepted for the Navy. Wrens are to be employed to do group intelligence tests, simple colour vision testing and some supplementary interviewing on the basis of a questionnaire. (Curran 1941)

This seems to be characteristic of Rickman's role throughout the war. He was aware of everything that was happening and was able to give advice behind the scenes on fields as far apart as personnel selection and rehabilitation.

Dreams or science? Officer selection

From 1939, increasing alarm was being expressed about the apparent lack of potential candidates for officer training (Ahrenfeldt 1958, p.53). Traditional methods of appointment had relied on a 10–20 minute interview that tended to concentrate on the background of the individual candidate, and in particular the public school that they went to. There was no specialised testing, and the board made up its mind on the basis of the subjective impression that the applicant made, a lack of objectivity described damningly by Ahrenfeldt as 'oneiromancy' (or divination by dreams) (1958, p.52). This resulted in a very high drop-out rate during training of up to 50 per cent of candidates (Adam 1949; Gilman 1947; Murray 1990; Rees 1945; Vinden 1977; Vernon and Parry 1949, pp.52–53).

In order to overcome this perceived shortage Bion, with his psychology colleague Eric Trist, made the proposal that in addition to the traditional recommendation from the senior officer in a unit, the rank and file should also take part in nominating individuals. This, the Regimental Nomination Scheme, was carried out in a Scottish unit where the number of candidates increased by 1500 per cent, effectively scotching the myth that there was only a limited supply (Trist 1985, pp.12–13). The Army Council rejected this approach, although many other units, including a full army division, wished to take it up. Despite this, the result was that from 2000 candidates being put forward in the first quarter of 1942, there were 6000 in October of that year alone (Murray 1990, p.61).

The War Office Selection Boards were the next to come under review, and were strengthened by the introduction of psychological assessments, more comprehensive interviews and discussion groups. The most significant breakthrough was the establishment of the leaderless group procedure, which became the pre-eminent focus of interest subsequently. It has been commonly accepted that this was Wilfred Bion's initiative; however, Vinden painted a more complex picture. He credited the invention to Colonel Delahaye, the president of the pioneering Edinburgh Selection Board. As this artillery officer was accompanying a test group past a stack of granite blocks, he spontaneously ordered the group to take the top block off the stack, without nominating a leader as had previously been the practice. He then recounted his experiences to the psychologist and psychiatrists in the team, including Bion and Trist (Vinden 1977). They were aware of previous work on leaderless groups. Harris stated that the technique was developed by Bion, Sutherland and Trist, who knew of the studies on such groups by J.R.P. French and Paul Schilder referred to in chapter 2 (Harris 1949, p.26). This difference of opinion as to the true originator of the concept reflects tensions that were present within the group at the time. The relationship between Col. Delahaye and Bion became more and more strained. The latter was concerned that the Board president was increasingly behaving like an 'amateur psychiatrist' by trying out various time-wasting experiments (Sutherland 1985, p.51; Trist 1985, p.7).

In the established form of the group tests, the candidates carried out a series of unstructured group interactions that included a discussion, outdoor practical task-solving and an inter-group game. These evolved into four phases of assessment: exploration, competition, co-operation and discipline. Initially, the members of the group sized each other up and gave a short account of themselves. This led on to a free group discussion. The next phase was entered through the short practical tests, in which each man had the opportunity to exercise his leadership skills. The progressive group task, characteristically that of carrying a heavy and awkward load over a series of obstacles, tested the ability of the candidates to co-operate when under physical stress. The final test aimed to assess the individual's ability to identify himself with the group decision and accept a role assigned to him during a group game in competition with another group (Murray 1990, pp.55–56; Research and Training Centre 1944).

The Board personnel acted as observers, without interfering in any manner once the task had been set. The candidates' actions provided a basis for the assessors to discuss each individual's capacities. Bion's account, even if he was not the progenitor, is important as it established both the rationale for the process and his own mode of thinking. He held that the procedure provided a scheme in which the selection staff could assess how well the candidate could maintain personal relationships in a stressful situation which encouraged him to consider only his own needs:

> It is not the artificial test, but the real life situation that has to be watched – that is, the way in which a man's capacity for personal relationships stands up under the strain of his own and other men's fear of failure and desires for personal success. (Bion 1946)

> If a man cannot be a friend of his friends, he cannot be the enemy of his enemies. (Bion 1948, p.88)

Rickman echoed this view. The psychiatrist's role was to assess the individual's capacity for compassion, because military officers needed to be able to maintain good relations with their own men, whilst promoting aggression towards the enemy:

> What we need to know about these men is their capacity to endure and manipulate intra-group tensions so that hostile impulses will be turned out towards the enemy and their friendly impulses will strengthen morale in their own unit. (Rickman 1943c)

The Military Research and Training Centre produced a technical memorandum entitled 'The method of leaderless groups', which would have been directly influenced by Bion, if not actually written by him (Research and Training Centre 1944). This asserted that the social role and 'adaptability to persons' was central to the officer's job. The nature of this social contact is expounded upon in detail; the memorandum emphasises that good leadership engenders confidence in ordinary soldiers under stressful situations. To achieve this the officer had to pay attention to such apparently trivial matters as the men's pay problems, showing concern for their welfare and that of their families, and reinforcing the belief that if they were wounded or killed they would be properly cared for. The distinction was made between technical proficiency, i.e. whether an officer could do his job, and his behaviour, i.e. whether he always would. Poor social contact with others means that the officer would not be sensitive to his men's needs. One statement directly reflected the views of Rickman and Bion quoted above: 'if an officer's ability to preserve a friendly relationship with his own side is a matter of doubt, his ability to preserve a hostile relationship with the enemy must be equally suspect' (Research and Training Centre 1944, p.3). These attitudes were considered to be the natural result of mature behaviour, and the document went in to some depth explaining how previous group experiences, such as the family and school, contributed to this.

At Northfield, Rickman and Bion replicated the passivity and receptiveness of the observer/psychiatrist in these selection procedures. There, their understanding of the group process took account of the individual's role in promoting group cohesiveness or disruption. They took this a stage further by experimenting with ways of intervening to enhance individuals' understanding of how groups operate and skills in improving them. The selection boards were thus a particularly important stage in the advancement of group therapy during the war and significantly influenced the work at the hospital through the interactions of participants and the shared psycho-social theoretical basis.

As a sidelight on Bion's career before going to Northfield it is worth recording his transfer to the headquarters of the WOSB organisation. This was the Research and Training Centre that was set up to co-ordinate and evaluate the procedures. It did not act as a selection board itself and was eventually unable to make progress in its original intentions. Later, it concentrated on evaluation and other aspects of selection. Bion found this bitterly frustrating, as, incidentally, did Sutherland and Trist, who felt that they had been moved away from the centre of developments. Consequently, Bion requested a transfer which led to him joining Rickman at Northfield (Murray 1990; Trist 1985).

Table 3.1 Comparison of officer selection methods		
Grading of candidates	Old methods	WOSBs
Above average	22.1%	34.5%
Average	41.3%	40.3%
Below average	36.6%	25.2%

(*Source*: Adapted from Ahrenfeldt 1958, p.73)

The success of the War Office Selection Boards over previous methods of officer selection was demonstrated in research quoted by Lord Piercy during a parliamentary debate on the procedures after the war. A study comparing large numbers of men selected for officer training by traditional methods and through the WOSBs demonstrated a 12 per cent rise in the number of successful candidates, with this increase occurring as a result of the promotion of those who were of above average grade.

Later research, carried out in 1949, was less conclusive that WOSBs had been successful. Reeve followed up some 2500 candidates who had gone on to further officer training, and found that there was only a low correlation between grades achieved at the selection board, and those being achieved six months later. He stated that there was as yet no better selection method, however, and also that his study was biased because of the impossibility of assessing those individuals who had failed (Reeve 1971).

Wishart gave an unsolicited testimonial when he wrote in 1944: 'I have still to meet a case of neurotic breakdown in an officer who passed through the modern WOSB procedure' (p.6). The special commission covering psychiatric policy and practice in the United States Medical Corps specially commended the system after their examination of it in 1945 (Bartemeier *et al.* 1946, p.523). Further evidence of the selection board's success was the adoption of their techniques after the war by the Civil Service, the police, the Church in Scotland, the Royal Navy, the Royal Marines, the Royal Air Force, the National Fire Service, the governments and armies of several other countries, and many industrial firms (Murray 1990; Murray, undated).

Battle inoculation, mutiny and fifth column work for amateurs: Aspects of morale

> In battle a man has to think and act for himself – to think without other guidance than his own, to act on instantaneous appreciation of a situation. (War Office 1922, p.206)

So wrote the authors of the Committee on Shell Shock in 1922. In order to achieve this the individual soldier had to be able to manage that most deadly enemy: fear. The new technologies of battle involved weapons with a powerful psychological component. For instance, the German 'Stuka' dive bomber was rated by 20 per cent of the American soldiers in North Africa in 1943 to be the most frightening weapon they had faced. However, its effectiveness in terms of actual physical casualties was rated by the same soldiers as much less (Stouffer *et al.* 1965, pp.232–233). The discrepancy was due to its effectiveness in instilling panic through its shrieking sound and sinister silhouette (Craigie 1944; Holmes 1987, pp.209–211). As

'Tommy' Wilson reported, victory depends less on the number of soldiers killed than the number demoralised (Wilson 1942, p.2). There were repeated instances of this in the Second World War; for instance, Rommel's victories at Tobruk were carried out by fewer men and less weaponry than the British had, but with more determination and confidence (Dixon 1979, pp.126–129; Fraser 1983, pp.222–227; Liddell Hart 1973, pp.284–289).

In order to help the individual to maintain his equanimity under fire, attempts were made to inoculate troops against the expected noise, physical conditions, exhaustion and bewilderment of the battlefield. The first Army Battle School was formed in 1942. Its purpose was 'to provide a new, realistic battle drill and to condition soldiers to the noise and fog of war' (Privy Council Office 1947, p.55).

Whilst never neglecting the primary task of confronting soldiers with their onerous and dangerous responsibilities, the psychiatrists involved in training sought methods that encouraged and supported rather than humiliated or frightened. This was not out of misplaced sympathy, but because the methods they introduced were demonstrably more successful. The aim was to enhance the soldier's own enthusiasm. J.R. Rees described how the morale of new recruits deteriorated after four to five weeks in certain primary training units. Old-fashioned instructors spent many hours training them how to strip, clean and reassemble guns, long before they were allowed to fire them. Men were not inspired by this copy-book approach. What Rees believed was necessary was to involve them in appreciating the purpose of the task through first using the weapons and then ensuring their efficacy (Rees 1945, p.79–80). A further example of this pragmatic approach was provided by Eric Trist, who recalled Bion's intervention in one training school. Bion was asked to give psychiatric advice on simulated battle conditions in which soldiers had to go over an obstacle course amidst the sound of gunfire, with the ground covered in animal entrails and gore. His intervention consisted of taking a rifle from one man and pointing out that the muzzle was choked with mud. Bion commented that in his view 'A soldier's first job is to look after his weapons so that he can use them against the enemy. This form of training had failed to teach him that' (Bion, quoted in Trist 1985, pp.10–11).

The technical memorandum on Battle School Training and Battle Inoculation circulated to all psychiatric personnel underlined this. It stated:

> Many of the questions asked about the Battle School movement reveal serious misconceptions of its nature and purpose. A Battle School is not merely a school for toughness, where muddy soldiers spend their days leaping through sheets of flames, wading rivers or advancing through a hail of bullets over mountains of barbed wire ... An infantry platoon is no

longer a flock of sheep moving in an unintelligent mass. Each man has his own job to do and can take pride in doing it, knowing the part he plays in the work of the group as a whole… Battle Schools are not merely increasing the soldier's technical competence, but by giving individual soldiers a new sense of responsibility and purpose, and a new spirit of attack, they are making great contributions to high morale. (War Office 1946a, pp.1,7)

It was recognised that this could prepare men for battle and prevent mental breakdown. Tom Main became the psychiatric adviser and exerted 'considerable influence' (Ahrenfeldt 1958, p.198; Privy Council Office 1947, p.55). He vehemently opposed the sadistic approach to training that exposed men to large quantities of blood thrown about, displays of atrocity photographs and other methods intended to arouse hate, which the battle school instructors had instituted initially. Indeed, it was found that some of the best and keenest students ended up depressed and ineffective as a result of these methods (Rees 1945, p.80). He demonstrated that a gradual build-up of real battle conditions was more effective. In March of 1942, the Director of Military Training invited him to a demonstration of 'noise training' (Privy Council Office 1947, p.53). Explosions were set off at varying distances from the men, and Main was able to report that those who had a milder initial experience were calmer throughout the rest of the test. He suggested a further experiment, which was carried out in May of the same year. In this, the effects were gradually increased by bringing the blasts closer and increasing their power to the maximum of the previous trial. The new recruits who were the subjects of this test were less restless, showed no fear and were ready to re-experience the most severe charges. They had become habituated to the experience. The clinical observations provided graduated scales of the distance and force of the explosions for further training. The training developed the principle of graduated exposure to enable men to cope with low-flying aircraft, tanks, and rifle and mortar fire, and was described as 'battle inoculation' (Rees 1945, p.81; War Office 1946a, pp.5–6).

Despite some opposition, this approach was adopted in all Battle Schools subsequently. This was encouraged by Main visiting some 20 of them in June and July of 1942 (Privy Council Office 1947, p.56). Later, when he was working in North Africa, he was able to interview some of the officers who had passed through the new training. He found that 'they were emphatic that their first experience of a set battle at Alamein had been well prepared for in Britain, and that they had been the steadier for it' (Ahrenfeld 1958, pp.203–204; Privy Council Office 1947, p.56).

This empathic method of determining how to approach problems characterised Main's investigations of the Salerno Mutiny in 1943. During the early stages of the Allied invasion of Italy, 172 troops, Eighth Army veterans with excellent combat records, refused to join the divisions they were allocated to. They were eventually court-martialled for mutiny (Ellis 1990, p.262). Main interviewed these men and reported impartially on their attitudes and points of view. He found that the draft involved were expecting to join their own formations, and were willing to face whatever the future held for them as long as they were with the units to which they had strong group loyalties. During the transit from Tripoli in North Africa to Salerno, they received no information about their destination or what the plans were. They became increasingly suspicious of outside authority. When they arrived and found out that they were to be drafted to entirely different divisions they rebelled. After they had been convicted and given suspended sentences, they were subjected to a succession of humiliations and injustices, which further stoked their rebellion, resulting in imprisonment. Main's observation was that the rehabilitation of this group of men had been poorly implemented, their morale had been damaged, and this had culminated in their loss of discipline. Eventually, because of increasing uneasiness about their fate, their sentences were reviewed in the light of the psychiatric evidence and revoked. Most of the men eventually rejoined their units (Ahrenfeldt 1958, pp.215–219).

This investigation into the failure of morale reflected the wider attempt to understand soldiering from the men's point of view. It assumed that successful discipline was internally imposed, not externally exacted. As the Southborough Committee had identified in 1922, the modern conscript soldier had to be able to 'think and act for himself'. This meant that soldiers required information, and needed to understand what was expected of them. Keeping them ignorant, even unintentionally, was a failure of leadership.

'Tommy' Wilson elucidated this in his brief guide to unit morale (Wilson 1942). Entitled 'Suppose you were a Nazi agent: Fifth column work for amateurs', he demonstrated how poor leadership effectively assisted the enemy. He gave other examples of how to damage morale:

By display or abuse of officer privilege at a time when conditions for the men are bad.

By failure to give praise where its due.

By breaking up groups of friends in platoon barracks rooms, detachment, or by blind posting e.g. on an alphabetical system.

By refusing to listen to men's grievances, or better still, by paying little attention to them when they do come with them. (Wilson 1942, pp.12–13)

This pamphlet laid the foundations for the 'Tavistock Group' approach to morale. He outlined a balance between the group, the individual and the leader in a manner that anticipated the framework of task, team and individual later advanced by the Industrial Society (Adair 1994, p.12). Routine drill was an essential element of group performance. 'In the recruit, it is a cane to hold up a growing plant', and in the trained soldier it assists the effective movement of the team from place to place and reinforces the sense of combined action (Wilson 1942, p.5). Regimental tradition also had its place in fostering a sense of belonging and expectation.

However, these were inadequate on their own. Team spirit required the individual to have the capacity to adapt and modify their work to fit in with the methods of others. To be able to submerge one's individualism in this manner, one has to feel valued and to take ownership of the process. The Fascist method of exerting control through fear 'leads to apathy ... or to rebellion' (Wilson 1942, p.2). Thus leadership consisted of demonstrating concern for and interest in the group members, keeping them informed of plans and reasons, and sharing the hardships of day-to-day military life, whilst ensuring effective and efficient execution of tasks.

Overzealous sympathy: Critics of military psychiatry

Not everybody was happy with these reforms. As well as the Colonel Blimps, many of whom were doctors, there were also some more informed criticisms (*British Medical Journal* 1947).

The 'At Random' commentary in the *Journal of the Royal Army Medical Corps* in 1951 perhaps characterised the tendancy to dismiss wartime psychiatry with a few statements of 'common sense' that had little or no grounding in evidence (*Journal of the Royal Army Medical Corps*. 1951). The author criticised the system of psychiatry on the grounds that too much emphasis was placed on 'possible' disorders and the consequent wastage that resulted from the exclusion of these individuals from the forces. Apart from neglecting completely the effects of unstable individuals on their colleagues in battle, no reference was made to the immense waste of resources, decline in social and work performance, and sheer misery of those individuals who were accepted and then were invalided out of the service on psychiatric grounds (Lewis 1943; Guttman and Thomas 1946). Finally, the writer referred to men being excluded from service through 'overzealous sympathy' with the individual (*Journal of the Royal Army Medical Corps* 1951).

It is easy to see how the work of Wilson and Tom Main can be simplistically interpreted in this light. The complexity of leadership, which has to combine stern discipline with fairness and concern, can easily be skewed. However this article completely misrepresented the views of the Directorate of Psychiatry, which clearly recognised the primacy of military requirements.

More effectively, L'Etang concatenated a limited experience of poor psychiatric practice, unsupported assumptions about military psychiatric policy and evidence stemming from before selection policies were instituted to support his criticisms. His view is best summarised by his assertion that:

> If a man's discharge from the Army is related to his nuisance value, it seems that recalcitrancy might become epidemic. (1951)

Apart from neglecting to consider the time and effort wasted in trying to manage such men and the effect that they have on their colleagues, the time-honoured supposition lying behind this was that externally imposed discipline and punishment would prevent mass defections from the army. L'Etang failed to examine critically the available historical literature, commenting that no reports of psychiatric disorder are given in accounts of the campaigns of Wellington or the Crimean War. First-hand accounts of these give limited but clear accounts of suicide, desertion, drunkenness, depression and even psychosis.[2] More impressive, however, are the statistics on these subjects quoted earlier in this section.

He then uses 11 cases to demonstrate, from his experiences as a Regimental Officer in the invasion of northern Europe, that the Corps Psychiatrist did not keep in contact with the combatant officers and himself. This clearly was a failure not of the policy but of individual practice and training. Whilst the technical memoranda circulated to psychiatrists do not make specific reference to liaison work with the combatant officers, it was well recognised that a key role of the psychiatrist in forward areas was to maintain and develop these links (MacKeith 1946a; Wishart 1944). However, L'Etang saw this as an indictment of the organisational strategy. He later recounted his experience as a general practitioner. Of the 30 cases

---

2   L'Etang was wrong. In the personal accounts of many soldiers there are brief reports of mental disorder, e.g. Henry 1970, pp.118–119, 139; Ward 1971, p.268; Warner 1977, pp.36, 181; Wheeler 1951, pp.18, 39, 108, 133, and 136. However, they are often telegraphic, and would appear to be relatively uncommon. There are many possible interpretations of this. The first, of course, is that nervous problems were rare; in view of the statistics of suicide and other problems, this is not supported by the evidence. The second is that reports indicating that the British soldier was anything other than the foremost in the world would have been suppressed, either officially or by the soldiers themselves.

he used as examples, one might suffice to give an indication of his arguments.

> A specialist stated that how as mentally self-centred, hypochondriacal, and of low intelligence (50 per cent of normal), that he was a feeble unstable personality who did not succeed in adapting to ordinary army life, but had long sick periods, and broke up completely at the first slight strain. (L'Etang 1951, p.238)

He argued that this man had presumably given good military service in peacetime, as he had been in the army since 1931. This was with a record of recurrent headaches and anxiety attacks, and then, finally, of cracking up on coming under fire in 1940. Again, little or no attention is paid to the effort involved in maintaining this man in the army, or the fact that he was discharged before appropriate treatment and reallocation services were put in place. L'Etang also criticised the service for failing to 'make any provision for rehabilitation or treatment of these cases' (1951, p.325). The Northfield Military Hospital and the Mill Hill rehabilitation unit were established to do precisely this; however, he either chose to ignore or did not know about this. He also echoed Menninger's view that when armies were expanding rapidly, psychiatrists were often inadequately trained, failed to appreciate the importance of the person's social environment and concentrated on the individual (Menninger 1948). Again, these were precisely the views of the Tavistock Group and the Directorate of Psychiatry. If L'Etang had read the technical memoranda circulated by this directorate he would have recognised that this is exactly what they were proposing; however, he makes no allusion to this explicit statement of army psychiatric policy, preferring instead to attack a shibboleth of his own making (War Office 1946a).

One of those who L'Etang quoted as inspiring his enquiries was Herbert Moran. Moran worked as the president of a medical invaliding board in Colchester up until his retirement through ill-health in 1945. In a book called *In My Fashion*, openly described as being written from 'odd notes' and without reference to military documents, he fired off a number of broadsides against psychiatrists (Moran 1946). His criticisms often stemmed from hearsay and rumour, and can best be illustrated by such nuggets as:

> The psychiatrist will spin with ease a dozen different theories, all as unsubstantial as the rings from a smoker's pipe (p.162).

> The Freudians ... postulate as a cause for hysteria ... the fixation of the sexual emotions at an infantile level. Nevertheless it has been observed that a little hysteria adds some spice to an otherwise dull life, although an overplus may convert the daughter of a vicar into an Emily Brontë (pp.118–119).

Moran complained that the first weakness of psychiatrists was to 'wish for every soldier with the slightest abnormality to be invalided out of the army' (p.139). This line of argument is remarkable only in that it triggered off a correspondence in the *Daily Telegraph* and evidently represented a viewpoint that had little public expression until the end of the war.

Despite how poorly addressed these arguments were, they had some worth. L'Etang himself quotes a number of critics, including psychiatrists such as J.R. Rees and G.W.B. James, who recognised the crudeness of the selection methods and the fact that it was not possible to determine precisely which neurotic traits led to success or failure in battle. Some reflected on the fact that many successful commanders in the past had gross psycho-neurotic problems. However, even this argument was posed somewhat dis-ingenuously by Pozner (1950). He referred to the WOSBs trying to establish a 'universal standardisation', which is not at all what they attempted to achieve. Indeed, a greater range of experience and character was made available as potential officer material than ever before.

The real impact of these criticisms was that they led to a reduction of the role of army psychiatry after the war. Though the arguments of the critics were poorly substantiated, they held sway as they reflected traditional military values. After the war, instead of the issues of selection being more stringently evaluated, the psychiatrist was relegated to the role of 'invaliding officer' confined to examining the misfits and alcoholics, and his service ended up as the 'Department of Odds and Ends' (Pozner 1961).

Uniformity and diversity: From 'Bull' to self-discipline

The 'invisible college' argued for nothing more or less than a cultural revolution throughout that most hidebound of organisations: the British Army. The extent of their achievement was reported by the very instrument that Churchill established in order to uproot them: the Expert Committee on the Work of Psychologists and Psychiatrists in the Services (Privy Council Office 1947). The conclusions of this report 'emphatically' vindicated the value of the work done by these two professions (*British Medical Journal* 1947). It went on to argue for an extension of their role throughout the three services. In the event, however, these recommendations suffered the same fate as the Committee of Enquiry into Shell Shock after the First World War: studious neglect.

The tentative arguments put forward by Rickman before the war had now been tried and tested. A diverse society, in which individuals were encouraged to continue facing the unconscious conflicts stemming from childhood and explore reality-based experiences, was able to survive more successfully than one in which the population avoided these anxieties and remained dependant on an idealised leader. Of course, this wasn't anything like a sufficient explanation: the huge impact of the world's leading industrial country joining on the Allied side was crucial, although it could be argued that the success of this economy was precisely the outcome of such diversity. Moreover, the nature of psycho-social theory itself had changed dramatically, with the result that Rickman's earlier paper now sounded archaic, both in language and content. Instead of relying entirely on psychoanalytic theory, Rickman needed to incorporate a whole range of socio-psychological concepts and experiences.

However, 'morale' remained a significant factor, and the United States, despite its resources, has since been humiliated by a less technically advanced society than Hitler's Germany because of just that issue.

The word 'discipline' conjures up many, usually unpleasant, connotations. Yet for any team of people to achieve an objective there has to be a subjugation of personal wishes to outside regulations. Where this cohesion is consistently essential to life, many of these actions need to become habitual, almost unconscious in their execution. The parade ground inculcates a sense of group co-ordination, and further military training has to emphasise this almost mindless ritual activity. It is quicker to move a large body of men from one area to another if they fall automatically into organised ranks and march in unison rather than all attempt to make the same moves at once or run chaotically in all directions. Yet it is all too easy to see this as the only purpose of training and ignore the necessity for the soldier to be able to think on his feet, or flat on his face as the case might be. Rees' example of the sergeant trainer mechanically ordering his men to strip and rebuild their guns without giving them the opportunity to understand their purpose by firing them illustrates this. Leadership can also be expressed in a similar manner when men are treated like numbered robots and their personal welfare is neglected.

It was this next level of discipline that the psychiatrists and psychologists concentrated on: the ability of the ordinary soldier to develop self-discipline. That he would do so given the opportunity they rarely doubted, and all their enquiries, experimentation and observations confirmed them in their confidence. Main, examining the mutineers at Salerno, was quite clearly impressed by their integrity and intention to do what was right. They expected to be treated appropriately and their loyalty to be respected. They believed themselves to be doing what was correct and expected this to be corroborated once the evidence was examined properly. It was only after they felt that no one had made any attempt to see their point of view, and after they had been exposed to ridicule and humiliation, that they became delinquent. It was to avert these situations that the question of officer selection became so important. The key leadership ability that Bion identified, the capacity to consider other's needs when under stress oneself, would have enabled these men's grievances to have been dealt with immediately, thus preventing the situation from developing into the shambles that it eventually did.

The task, as has been reiterated, was to maximise the human resources available for the war effort. The approach, as exemplified by the selection and training, was to enable the individual to understand what was expected of him, to encourage the development of self-discipline and enhance team-membership skills, either as a leader or a follower.

'Tommy' Wilson argued that morale was a 'state of mind which grows in strength and can be maintained, no matter how difficult conditions are' (1942, p.1). Achieving this is based on activity in three areas: leadership, group spirit and individual confidence. Each level interacts with the other, and the socio-psychological concepts of the 'field' and 'tele' both contribute to the conceptualisation of this process. Thus the theories of Lewin and Moreno provided the intellectual basis for the Tavistock Group's particular brand of systems theory, and provided the techniques of experimentation and enquiry.

What is impressive about these workers was their mobility. Bion, Rickman, Bridger and Main all worked in different units, whilst Hargreaves and Rees visited different countries and services. This nomadic penchant was also intellectual, manifesting itself in the exploration of different techniques and issues. Thus Rickman worked in rehabilitation, organised psychiatric conferences, carried out officer selection and edited the *British Journal of Medical Psychology*. Main gave lectures on morale, researched the Salerno Mutiny, worked in hospital and advised on battle school training. Others have commented on the very strong sense of co-operation that there was throughout the war amongst the medical and psychological professions, further exemplified by the widespread interest in psychosomatic medicine that developed as a result of physicians and psychiatrists being thrown together in field hospitals and similar environments (Lewsen 1993; MacKeith 1994; Markillie 1993).

This was the key to the whole reorganisation, its internal theoretical and ideological consistancy. What one group of psychiatrists and psychologists were carrying out in one arena was co-ordinated with work being done in other fields. Officer selection provided men who had both the intelligence and the capacity to understand the needs of their men. Personnel selection excluded those who did not have the capacity to understand either the technical requirements of modern warfare or the responsibilities they would have to their fellow soldiers. Training emphasised personal motivation in the context of the social requirements of a society at war. It was organised so that the overall task became central – for instance keeping weapons clean was for the purpose of keeping them effective rather than being part of an overall attempt at humiliation.

Northfield was another field of enquiry, in the same values, ideas, theories and practices were re-evaluated – in this case with those people who had become casualties. They were seen not as failures, but as individuals who still wished to contribute to the war effort but who had lost faith in themselves and others. Morale and discipline remained central, and Bion's first deliberations, after arriving there, addressed precisely these issues (Bion and Rickman 1943).

CHAPTER 4

The Mind Field

Clinical Military Psychiatry

'Bill, you're in a hell of a funk.'

'Yes,' said Bill, 'I am. If you were in as big a funk you'd run away.' (Anon, quoted in Culpin 1940b, p.40)

TREATING THE HIDDEN WOUNDS: THE DEVELOPMENT OF A TREATMENT SERVICE

Psychiatric disorder in a conscript army arises from different sources. Not every man is able to accommodate himself to the responsibilities and self-effacement of communal living. As a result, soldiers may exhibit anxiety, depression, alcoholism or disciplinary problems. Exhaustion, bewilderment, and fear are companions of the battlefield, whereas boredom shares the periods of idleness. Physical disability from trauma or infection is commonplace, and carries with it psychological concomitants. Those who have been incarcerated in prisoner- of-war camps experience their own unique difficulties. Finally, readjusting to civil life afterwards is traumatic for many.

Strecker and Appel emphasised the variety of situations that men could experience in the Second World War compared with the First (1945, pp.3–5). They argued that increased mobility, variety of geographical locations and technological sophistication had increased the sense of instability and lack of security for soldiers. Even their loved ones at home were no longer safe. The war was fought mainly by non-professionals, men torn away from their civilian occupations, given three months training, and expected to manage complex mechanical and tactical technology (Ellis 1990, p.10).

Despite these differences, few would have disagreed with Bion when he recalled his own experience of the 1914–1918 war: 'I didn't know what was happening, or what had happened. The war had become a terrifying game of chess in which we had to participate' (1986, p.207).

The consequences of these problems overwhelmed the flimsy service that was set up initially. Strategies had to be developed that made the best use of the psychiatric manpower available. Despite the screening methods set up to try to reduce the number of men incapable of service or inappropriately placed, the sheer scale of the problem was enormous.

The system had to be rebuilt from top to bottom, on the lines recommended during the First World War by Myers and his colleagues. The initial groundwork was carried out in England, but gradually spread to forward psychiatry developing in theatres of war overseas. Northfield Military Hospital came at the end of the line, both in time and function. It opened after most of the other developments had occurred, in order to field those men who had the capability of giving further useful service but had not benefited from the other facilities.

The clinical approaches also underwent a radical transformation, in nosology, treatment and aftercare. Some approaches were derived from earlier work, whilst others were entirely new. War gave a boost not only to the development of psychotherapy but to radical physical therapies as well.

Emptying the ocean with a spoon: The first years of military psychiatry in the Second World War

The importance of psychiatric disorder during the Second World War cannot be underestimated. The scale of the problem in the British Army is illustrated by the facts that between April 1941 and October 1943 a total of 342,729 psychiatric outpatients were seen (Rosie 1952) and that, during the whole war, about 118,000 men and women were invalided out of the services on mental health grounds (Cope 1952, p.340). This latter figure represented between one-third and one-half of all medical discharges from the services. Half of those who left on mental health grounds were suffering from anxiety neurosis (War Office 1948). Psychiatric disorder made up 50 per cent of all medical discharges in men under 28 years old (Hogben and Johnstone 1947, p.161).

The lack of appropriate professional manpower in the earlier years meant that it was only after the appointment of the first Command Psychiatrists in April 1940 that significant numbers of soldiers with nervous disorders began to be seen by military psychiatrists as outpatients. Previously they could only be managed as in-patients in the Emergency Medical Service (EMS) hospitals. This new development allowed patients to be filtered more effectively. Military psychiatrists referred to hospital care only those who would benefit by it, discharged from military service those who were not fit and advised on the management of those who could remain with their units.

Later, with the introduction of the Annexure scheme, the possibility of reallocation to more appropriate employment within the army was added.

Editorials in the *Journal of the Royal Army Medical Corps* give evidence of the nature of care at that time. Men from the Battle of Flanders with acute neurosis were 'left to languish for long periods in general hospital beds under an organic label with no other treatment but a placebo', and psychiatrists 'were at times over-pessimistic in their assessment of a man's military fitness' (1942a). Criticisms were made in the early days of the war that 'many Army Psychiatrists were young and inexperienced in both life and their special subject' (1945).

The workload was excessive and there was no specialist training for the conditions appertaining in the army. Those who had worked previously in mental hospitals usually had little or no experience of neurotic disorders (Ahrenfeldt 1958, p.17). Initially, the main task was to provide outpatient services for all establishments where there were troops and visit different units to advise on mental health issues (Ahrenfeldt 1958, pp.17–18). Gilman described how, working as an area psychiatrist in June 1940, he was told that there were not many cases and it was in the face of some opposition that he set up clinics. Soon he was overwhelmed by the numbers of men sent, seeing between 30 and 100 men a day. His work was made more difficult by the lack of appropriate places for disposal of individuals who were not fit for full duties. It was also evident that selection procedures had not kept out those who quite clearly could not manage army life because of intellectual difficulties or lifelong nervous problems (Gilman 1947).

The increase in psychiatric personnel throughout the war went some way towards alleviating such difficulties, as did more appropriate selection of men and systems for the disposal of individual cases. Outpatient work, however, continued to expand and remained a key element of psychiatric practice throughout. With the introduction of divisional psychiatrists from 1943 this was taken virtually to the front line.

The EMS hospitals were established early on in order to treat the expected casualties from air raids. They were never actually required for this purpose in the numbers that were predicted. Indeed, Hollymoor, the site of the Northfield Military Hospital, in its first year as an EMS hospital, treated both civilians and soldiers mainly for such minor physical complaints as colds, coughs and measles (Hollymoor Hospital Records 1942). A few EMS hospitals were allocated to the treatment of mental ill-health, including that of service personnel, the most famous being Mill Hill Hospital, where Eliot Slater, William Sargant and Aubrey Lewis worked. These were civilian units, often treating soldiers in a manner that bore little relationship to any military environment.

From the beginning of the war until 1942, hospital-based military psychiatry relied almost entirely on this hotch-potch of services run mainly by civilians. Some initiatives occurred to encourage development along more appropriate lines, but this was largely the product of individual inspiration.

The only exception was the first unit set up to go with the British Expeditionary Force to northern Europe in 1940. However it did not have the opportunity to even cross the channel before the evacuation from Dunkirk. It remained in Sussex for a while before moving to Bishop's Lydeard in Somerset in October 1940. The personnel associated with this moved to the Middle East in 1941, but the hospital continued as a military psychiatric hospital concerned with the treatment of psychoneurosis. Subsequently, other units were requisitioned for a similar purpose, adding 150 beds in Shenley, 300 in Scotland at Bellsdyke and a further 40 for officers in Dumfries. However, this smattering of units was insufficient, and finally Hollymoor Hospital was taken over in April 1942 with potentially 800 beds. The 300 beds in Bishop's Lydeard were closed as a result (Crew 1955, pp.471–474).

Haymeads and Wharncliffe: Rickman and rehabilitation

One person who had a strategic view of how this system could be better organised was working as a civilian doctor in an EMS hospital in Bishop's Stortford. From the start, Rickman concerned himself particularly with the recovery of psychologically-traumatised soldiers. Within three days of the commencement of war he had written a short piece subsequently referred to as the Haymead's Memorandum. This referred to his work in the Haymeads psychotherapy department (Rickman 1939c).

Principally, Rickman aimed for rapid intervention and effective, appropriate occupational therapy:

> The aim of treatment is to short circuit the chronic stage and get the patient as quickly as possible to the stage of resolution which is characterised by resumption of social contact, response to command, realisation of responsibility, return of self-confidence and therefore return to work... Since the aim is to restore the patient to normal life, the period of full-time residence in the hospital should be reduced. The patient's energy must be turned outwards to work and normal life (not to inturned neurotic brooding). (Rickman 1939c)

This emphasis on meaningful activity echoed points he had made in an earlier article on air raids, in which he recalled the advice of his early mentor, Dr. W.H. Rivers, that 'a mind occupied in *doing* something was more resistant to fear than one that is idle' (Rickman 1939b). Thus the Occupational Therapy Centre should be close to the treatment unit. This would

> afford a two-stage return to normality: first stage – sleeping at the Hospital and working at the Occupational Therapy Centre, i.e. on half-time parole; second stage (if the billeting can be managed) – full time parole with visits to the hospital for final treatment and part-time work at the Occupational Therapy Centre. (Rickman 1939c)

It is difficult to see from this distance in time how radical this approach was. Psychiatrists before the war fell into two groups: those who worked solely in the large asylums, where their main concern was with severe and long-standing mental illnesses such as schizophrenia, and, on the other hand, those psychotherapists who were preoccupied with treating paying patients over long periods of time with psychoanalysis. Few, if any, were interested in dealing with neurosis on an in-patient basis, and the Mental Health Act of 1899, which was in force at the time, largely precluded it. The report on shell-shock, which outlined the necessity for rapid treatment and rehabilitation, had been largely ignored. The lectures by Emilio Mira, mentioned earlier, concentrated on acute treatment and paid little attention to recuperation (Rickman 1939a).

As noted earlier, Rickman had for a long time been concerned with the social and practical application of psychoanalytic ideas, often ahead of his other colleagues at the Institute of Psychoanalysis. Before the outbreak of hostilities he had been concerned for some years about the psychological preparation of people for war. This practical bent went back as far as his work in Russia in 1918, where he trained peasant girls to work as nurses treating the typhus epidemic that was raging (Payne 1957).

Some brief notes on a lecture he gave to nurses, probably at Haymeads, illustrate Rickman's continuing concern with the training of other staff. In these, entitled 'Mental rest and mental pain', he tried to assist them in understanding the unconscious projections that patients place on them.

> The patient transfers onto the nurse a role which has no relation to present needs; but is dictated by his past or infantile needs… the nurse must not play the role the patient wants her to play. (1940b, pp.4–5)

To achieve this they had to attempt to create a realistic relationship based on 'mutual respect or love' (p.6). He deprecates attempts to treat the patient using the 'psycho-therapeutic methods now so much in vogue', as they encourage him to regress to more infantile modes of thinking and acting.

> The nurse's privilege is to stand near to the patient in his suffering and not behave unreasonably (as the relations do) nor to fall into the offensive-defensive partnership with infantile attitudes (as the relations

do) but to keep a steady path of conduct becoming to the relationship of one adult to another. This of course does not win an hysterical outburst of grattitude; but if the nurse is sympathetic it evokes from the neurotic that rare but prognostically favourable sign – his respect. (p.7)

This approach emphasised the constraints on resources in wartime, and the necessity of resisting the temptation to carry out inappropriate and time-wasting psychotherapy. Rickman's own approach at this time is discussed later; but essentially it was a psychoanalytically-informed pragmatic one that built on the patient's abilities whilst taking immediate steps to overcome recent traumas.

From Haymeads, Rickman moved to the EMS hospital at Wharncliffe in Sheffield at the beginning of 1940. There he was able to put his ideas into more practical effect, largely with the help of Sergeant Major Bryant, who ran the Rehabilitation and Training Centre.

Rickman described how this worked:

In the hospital there was a system of 'para-military training' in which military exercises, the equivalent, for soldier patients, of occupational therapy, were blended with psychiatric testing of the patient's responsiveness to situations calling for various degrees of quickness, assertiveness, exertion and discipline. Under these conditions his improvement as a soldier could be watched with the same care as his progress as a patient. (1941)

One particular soldier demonstrated how he was recovering:

For a week or two he remained depressed and then took up his military interests again. His pleasure in small arms drill, its briskness, those resounding right-hand slaps on the butt of his good rifle, proved a stimulus to recovery. (1941)

By 1941 the fame of the unit had reached Eliot Slater at Mill Hill Hospital, he visited in January, and described, somewhat sceptically, what was happening:

At this hospital a new system has been worked out for the occupational therapy of soldiers suffering from neurosis. It consists in the widest possible application of the principle that, as the occupation of the soldier is soldiering, the best occupational treatment should be soldierly activities. For this purpose, extensive use is made of graded classes in physical training, grenade practice, route-marching, classes in map-reading, strategy, signalling, etc. (1941a)

This differed from Slater's own hospital, in which the occupational therapy department had various workshops including one in which a woman officer held 'classes in rug-making, basket and leather work, weaving, painting, embroidery etc.' (Minski 1941). Trist recalled meeting in the corridors there in 1940 a 'large punch-drunk ex-boxer, now in the Guards, forlornly carrying an absurd peacock painted on glass' (1985, p.5).

It is not clear whether Rickman was treating his patients in groups at this time. However, it is certain that he and Bion were contemplating how all the relationships and activities of the hospital could be used in a therapeutic manner. As a result of this collaboration, Bion wrote the Wharncliffe Memorandum, a document that is now lost (Trist 1985, pp.5–6; Bridger 1990b). Rickman's attempt to implement these ideas was resisted by the medical and administrative staff of the hospital, and as a result he had to defer further developments until he arrived at Northfield.

J.R. Rees recognised the importance of Rickman's work at Wharncliffe, in particular the use of military instructors in occupational therapy. This use of real-task-orientated activity in helping recuperating soldiers to prepare for their future roles was in his view seminal (Rees 1966, p.64).

Forward psychiatry: At the battle front

This pragmatic approach to the treatment of neurosis was reflected in developments in areas of active service. Taking military psychiatry up to the battle front was indicative of how the whole of the system was taking on board the lessons of the First World War. Northfield was part of this policy, although its relative isolation meant that it was never closely associated and the sense of urgency was not as evident.

Against much resistance, the lessons of the First World War were eventually being taken note of. In 1943, in North Africa, a new form of service was developed by James in Egypt and Wishart in Tunisia (James 1952; MacKeith 1946b; Wishart 1944). The Southborough Committee and C.S. Myers had recommended that treatment be administered quickly and as near the battle front as possible. The cognomen 'forward psychiatry' epitomised these new services (Ahrenfeldt 1958, p.8).

A description by MacKeith gives an idea of what the treatment of psychiatric casualties was like in Tunisia and Algiers before these services were developed. They 'travelled, without sedation, by slow stages along the winding valley routes from the front. In turn they were bullied, ignored, and mollycoddled' (1946b). By the time they reached the psychiatrist many cases had deteriorated, gaining new symptoms, showing signs of their original ones becoming more entrenched, and accumulating more reasons to stay ill. In some cases they developed a 'hysterical stupor very difficult to distinguish from psychosis' (1946b).

The scheme was organised into four tiers. The first line of treatment was provided by the Unit Medical Officer, usually someone without psychiatric experience trained by the Corps Psychiatrist in simple forms of assessment and treatment. For Brigadier James this teaching was summarised in the phrase 'Fluid, food, sleep and stool', which listed the basic needs that had to be attended to (1944). Very mild cases would be returned to their units after firm, sympathetic guidance. Those that the Unit Medical Officers was unable to treat were referred on to the Exhaustion Centre.

The location of this unit was best '"just behind the noise" – distant gunfire did not worry the patients unduly' (Wishart 1944, p.4). It was considered by some that a 'little bombing' helped the patient and the medical officer decide on the results of therapy (James 1944).

Exhaustion Centres were set up with some difficulty and relied on the improvisatory skills of the psychiatrist and his staff (Hunter 1945). The numbers at these centres fluctuated from under ten to 65, the maximum that one psychiatrist could cope with. Ideally, these were divided into three 'wards' for admission, treatment and convalescence.

Assessment identified those who would recover quickly with rest, sedation, general hygiene measures and simple psychotherapeutic measures. These included cases of physical exhaustion, the less severe anxiety states and mild hysterical conditions. The remainder were evacuated to the Advanced Base Psychiatric Units (MacKeith 1945; Wishart 1944).

Treatment at Exhaustion Centres was simple and usually included 'a hot meal, a clean up of his usually dirty state and attention to his bowels' (Kenton 1946). This was supplemented by a psychiatric interview, which included discussion of the individual problem, reassurance, encouragement and sometimes re-education (Wishart 1944). Wishart warned against carrying out more complex treatments. Except in the admission ward, military discipline was maintained strictly, but the rehabilitative measures included arrangements for entertainment, exercise and the chance to write letters (Wishart 1944). About a third were returned immediately to active service (Kenton 1946).

The more intractable cases were evacuated to Advanced Base Psychiatric Units where a third level of triage was carried out. In Italy, these were two small 100–bedded 'expansions' of general hospital units in forward areas (Ahrenfeldt 1958, p.186; MacKeith 1994). Those casualties that were expected to recover within a fortnight remained for further treatment whilst those with psychosis, severe neuroses or personality disorders were evacuated further on down the line to Rear Base Units, which were placed well to the rear in the army base area (Kenton 1946; MacKeith 1946a).

Northfield acted in this capacity for the early part of the campaign in northern Europe.

The Advanced Base Units provided therapies which were more individually-orientated and specific than those of the Exhaustion Centres. Here treatments included further rest, sometimes reinforced by sedation, modified insulin therapy, abreaction, continuous narcosis, and psychiatric interviews. There was a programme of occupational and diversional activities, physical training and 'group activities of the leaderless group type' (Kenton 1946). This lasted between 8 and 16 days, after which there was a period of about 4–6 weeks of rehabilitation. Again, the aim was to treat milder syndromes rapidly before secondary symptoms developed. A few patients were returned to their original units, and most were downgraded in their medical category. These latter patients were then referred to the personnel selection service, from where they were reallocated to other duties (Ahrenfeldt 1958, p.186; Kenton 1946; MacKeith 1945; 1946b).

At all levels there was some form of rehabilitation. This was widely considered to be a key element of the whole system. The model was similar to that of John Rickman at Wharncliffe and later at Northfield. Those recovering from their disorder were placed in a separate unit, run by non-medical staff, to avoid retaining patients in psychiatric beds after the strictly medical part of their treatment was completed and to prevent further deterioration in morale (MacKeith 1944, p.2). In the Advanced Base Unit this included a rehabilitation centre which provided three weeks of essential military training and 'toughening'. This was not a medical unit, and was run along military lines. As a way of making this more interesting, examples of new and enemy weapons were demonstrated. In the Eighth Army, Brigadier James emphasised its importance, and Palmer described how a paramilitary atmosphere promoted physical health and reinstituted the men's sense of duty and pride in their profession (James 1944; Palmer 1945b).

Those cases that were unlikely to improve were evacuated further away from the field of combat to the Rear Base Psychiatric Unit. These were a minority of the overall group of cases. Here, long-term treatment of up to six weeks was carried out, or the patients were held prior to their evacuation to the United Kingdom by ship.

Altogether, in the North African and Italian campaigns, the results showed that by these methods 83.6 per cent of the men treated were retained for duty in the theatre of war and 16.4 per cent were invalided home (Kenton 1946).

Forward psychiatry was a demonstration of how hospital-based psychiatry was jettisoned in favour of a form of social medicine, and as such formed a template for military clinical practice as a whole (Palmer 1946). It

was at the sharp end of clinical practice. Northfield never faced the acute
pressures of the Exhaustion Centres. It was larger and employed numerous
psychiatrists, some of whom never went near a battlefield. This led to
significant inertia, and Northfield was slow to develop a more active
approach. However, the widespread existence of social psychiatry in other
parts of the army meant that there was continued pressure for it to respond in
a parallel manner. Its role was further emphasised by the formation of the
32nd General (Psychiatric) Hospital there, prior to transfer to northern
France after D Day (Lewsen 1993). Northfield's responsibilities increased
during the Normandy landings, when it needed to react as if it was close to
the front line, serving as a base hospital for the British invasion force.
Notably, this was the period when Harold Bridger, having been appointed
as a non-medical officer to the rehabilitation centre, established the Second
Experiment, emphasising the role of the 'hospital-as-a-whole'. Foulkes
commented on the clear sense of purpose that the hospital had then, in
comparison with the later uncertainties during demobilisation (1946a).

Trick-cycling with a rifle: Military psychiatry as a system

This section has concentrated on the in-patient services, because that is what
Northfield was part of. It must not be forgotten, however, that most
psychiatric care was carried out on an outpatient basis. For the practitioner,
this was often in combination with an advisory role to other medical staff
and the commanding officer of the unit they were attached to. Initially their
activities were viewed with some suspicion, but more often than not they
performed their duties effectively enough for them to become seen as
valuable allies. J.R. Rees phoned one general to ask him to relinquish the
services of one who was working with him. He was gratified to find that this
officer was reluctant to give him up, because when wrestling with
administrative and executive affairs 'this chap, who is always thinking about
what he calls the human factor, throws a most astonishing light on many of
these problems. No, for heaven's sake don't take him away' (quoted in Rees
1945, p.27). After telling Wishart, the psychiatrist attached to his division,
that he was the most unwanted man in the corps, General Cantlie revised his
opinion when he found that he soon proved his worth (Cantlie 1948).

This practical, 'reality-based', orientation of psychiatrists was enhanced
later in the war when their training incorporated a month's experience in a
combatant unit. There they acted as observers and participants in the unit's
activities (Cope 1952, p.341; Privy Council Office 1947, p.18). This
involved going on marches and assault courses, 'humping shells, firing
weapons, servicing guns, or indeed any other of the multifold occupations of

the soldier in which they can share' (Rees 1945, p.24). Fidler gave an account of his experiences as a trainee. He explained that he learnt how to assemble a Bren gun 'to understand the degree of intelligence required for the task'. He recounted how he had spent a week of intensive mulepack training in co-operation with Indian troops and worked with the stretcher bearers in getting patients across a river by rope. He found this experience 'very useful indeed' (Fidler 1946).

As in the other activities of the psychiatrists, a number of core values underpinned the clinical approaches. Again, the 'human' approach lay at the heart of their work. This aimed to enable potential casualties to regain their pride and dignity by returning to their original roles or by finding others that continued to serve the war aims. A systematic approach was adopted in order to provide a coherent strategy for managing the loss of manpower as efficiently as possible, with the central aim of ensuring that as many men were retained for effective active service as was possible.

EXHAUSTION AND ANXIETY: THE SOLDIER AND MENTAL DISORDER
'What slow panic':[1] The nature of war neurosis

The range of mental disorders that a soldier can suffer is identical to that of any civilian. The difference is that soldiers can undergo experiences that rarely occur away from the battlefield. Most soldiers in therapy at Northfield were classified as suffering from neurotic disorders. Unfortunately, no official patient records are available, even concerning the numbers of diagnoses. What information that does exist is scanty: a few participants published research papers, Foulkes recorded some clinical information, and recent interviews have yielded a little more. The nature of the patients' problems have to be largely inferred from other sources outlined here.

Classification was a major hurdle. Among many doctors, the lack of adequate nosology led to a free-for-all in coining new terms or reintroducing old ones, leading to what Laudenheimer called a 'babel of psychiatric nomenclature' (1940). Foulkes himself was not free of this, utilising the outmoded term 'effort syndrome' in his clinical notes (1943). Despite their rejection by the Southborough Committee in 1922, other relics of the First World War were resuscitated. Shell-shock gained a brief vogue in some areas, such as Hollymoor whilst it was an Emergency Medical Service hospital in May 1940. Of the 1010 soldiers returning from Dunkirk who were treated

---

1   From 'Mental Cases', Wilfred Owen 1973, p.98.

there, 25 received this diagnosis and a further three were designated 'effort syndrome' (Hollymoor Hospital Records 1939–1942). Idiosyncratic terms such as 'wind up' and 'loss of grip' came into vogue (Palmer 1945b). Symonds considered that the word 'fear' was 'excluded from the vocabulary of the soldier' and thus 'wind up' was aceptable as an alternative as it did not have the same sense of severity (1943).

The drawing up of an official nomenclature didn't bring these problems to an end; indeed, it brought some discrepancies of its own (War Office 1943a). Hadfield pointed out correctly that it failed to contain a satisfactory category for depression (1942, p.282). However the offical nomenclature was widely circulated from 1942 and served as the main tool for classification (*see* Appendix 1).

Later writers have found it easy to criticise the quality of the research during the war, ignoring the conditions under which the authors were operating. Trimble expressed his regret that personal views were expressed and data were not easily verifiable (1981), and Healy was even more dismissive, finding them very naïve (1993, p.100). This derogatory stance ignores the fact that the work was carried out under difficult conditions by individuals who were rarely trained researchers (Bartemeier *et al.* 1946, p.359). They themselves often recognised the lack of scientific rigour in their work. Information needed to be disseminated as quickly as possible, at a time of national emergency. As a result, information about the psychiatric casualties from Dunkirk, the Middle East and the Far East was widely available within a few months. Censorship prevented the publication of many details. For instance, J.R. Rees stated, in his summary of war psychiatry, that 'it was inadvisable to give exact figures or percentages of the psychiatric disabilities' (1943). Most papers do not reveal the location of the hospital or unit from which they were derived. The problems of diagnosis have already been referred to. Follow-up studies were virtually impossible, because the individuals from any treatment centre were sent far and wide into new placements, or left the service. As a consequence, the results are not strictly comparable: individual perceptions coloured different contributions and the science is distinctly sketchy. Despite this, there is a wealth of information, dependent largely on the clinical expertise of the individual collecting the data.

That diagnoses were not always recorded with an eye for the scientific truth is well illustrated by Culpin's story of one soldier treated for deafness after a motorcycle accident. The usual conversational gambits met with a stare, and finally, after some consideration, he said, 'Well, Sonny, you've got yourself into a bit of a hole.' The patient agreed, and then launched into a story about his sick mother. 'I couldn't bear to think of her crying, ' he said, 'and when I had this bit of an accident I thought if I let on to be deaf I might get a drop o' leaf, but I didn't get no leaf, and once I'd let on to be deaf I couldn't go back on it.' After reassurances, he returned to his unit, as nobody wanted to get him into trouble, with a diagnosis of 'Deafness found to be functional; cured by visiting psychotherapist'. He was also instructed to say that he had been hypnotised and was unable to recall anything about it (Culpin 1940a).

This story also demonstrates how an appropriate pragmatic response to the individual was more effective than relying on strict psychiatric criteria, a course that would have been taken often throughout the war. Braceland, in reviewing US naval psychiatry, emphasised that diagnostic labels 'were to count for little'. What was important was the functional capacity of the man (1947).

Some of the more common diagnoses that would have been treated at Hollymoor are described here. This is both to illustrate what the patients themselves would have been through and to demonstrate what the treatments were for. First, however, some studies on the frequencies of various conditions are outlined.

Some measure of misery: The statistics of psychiatric disorder

Three categories are discernable amongst the studies of neurosis in soldiers carried out throughout the war in disparate theatres of operation. There were those who had not seen combat, largely recruits in the United Kingdom before the opening of the Second Front. Then there were the men who had had battle experience, and as a result were experiencing both acute and chronic stress reactions. The papers on these usually stemmed from overseas: North Africa, Italy, the Far East and then Western Europe. The final group were the returning prisoners of war. A particular subset that stimulated a great deal of interest were the psychosomatic disorders. Psychotic illness occurred in every situation, but its frequency was low. Main embellished this arid schema with his own characteristically lucid view of the casualties he saw:

> The lonely homesick man, overwhelmed by insecurity, showing anxiety and hysterical illness, is sometimes met before he has even been in battle, together with the men who have carried out their social obligations in the face of fantastic dangers until their sense of security too has gone. There are others who have contained their anxiety, supported by comradeship and affection until the death of their friends has left them bereaved, to face further dangers alone. The man who has killed too much, the officer who has lost his men through an error of judgement, the tank commander who escaped alone from a burning tank – present pictures of

guilt and depression that may be psychotic in depth. Fleeting schizophrenic screens may be drawn for a few days over anguish too gross to be borne. (1946b)

It will become clear that, although there was discussion about details, psychiatrists and many of their medical colleagues found that they broadly agreed on most issues, for example selection, the frequency of the disorders, and the need for early and rapid treatment. The disagreements were over the form of treatment, causation and the likelihood of improvement. All the varying forms of disorder were represented, and the debates reiterated, at one time or another at Northfield.

The overall impact of psychiatric disorder in the army has been referred to earlier. Crew, in 1952, gave a perspective on the incidence of specific diagnostic categories, giving detail to the bare-bones statistics of crude discharge figures. He compared the distribution of different diagnoses occurring in men discharged from the army with mental health problems. The figures are given as percentages of the total for each group of men and compare ex-prisoners of war (POWs) from different theatres with all other discharges from the army.

Table 4.1 Percentage of specific disorders in men discharged from the army with mental disorders			
Disorder	Non-POW	POW from Europe	POW from Far East
Manic depressive psychosis	3.9	1.7	3.1
Schizophrenia	6.3	5.6	6.3
Anxiety neurosis	45.5	76.2	62.3
Hysteria	19.3	10.2	6.8
Psychopathic personality	16.3	2.8	1
Mental deficiency	6.5	0.5	0.5
Other psychiatric disorders	2.2	3	19.5
TOTAL	100	100	100

Source: Crew 1953, p.450

For reasons mentioned earlier, it would of course be foolhardy to claim that these figures were entirely accurate; however, they agree largely with the rest of the published literature. They demonstrate the preponderance of neurotic disorders over all other diagnoses and the significant problems posed by personality disorders in the army in general. It is noteworthy that personality disorders and learning difficulties either were not captured or failed to survive concentration-camp conditions. The latter explanation is the most likely.

Before a gun was fired in anger: Non-combatant disorders

In the early years of war, until the opening of the Second Front in northern Europe, the psychiatric services in the United Kingdom mainly saw men who had had little or no combat experience. The early studies tended to reveal the consequences of inadequate selection procedures at the time of recruitment, which resulted in a high incidence of severe and incapacitating neurosis, personality disorders and psychosis (Leigh 1941; Slater 1943; Stalker 1941; Sutherland 1941). These authors added their voices to the ever-growing demands for adequate assessment of recruits.

A couple of papers illustrated the role and experience of the ordinary military medical officer in the United Kingdom. Leigh found 58 cases of psychiatric disorder amongst 2814 men during four months in a large driver-training centre (1941). A year later, Jones found 40 cases of neurotic disorders presenting on sick parade in six months. After treatment, 15 remained on full duties, whilst five were invalided out of the service. Only nine were referred on for specialist help, suggesting that the psyciatrists were not seeing all the cases that presented (Jones 1942).

As already reported, the specialists began to see large numbers of cases. In 1940, Sargant and Slater reported on men who had broken down before they experienced combat. These had obvious problems with 'personality deviations, constitutional instability and lack of stamina' and constrasted sharply with those who they saw immediately following the retreat from Dunkirk (Sargant and Slater 1940). Two large studies of 2000 and of 700 patients reached similar conclusions about the frequency of diagnoses (Slater 1943; Hadfield 1942). Neurosis was overwhelmingly the most common. In the former study this made up 62 per cent of cases (anxiety 31.8 per cent; hysteria 18.9 per cent), and in the latter 82 per cent (anxiety 53 per cent; hysteria 24 per cent). Slater also found that a fifth had lifelong disorders of either intellect or personality and should not have entered the army. Hadfield further identified that 60 per cent of the cases had been exposed to very minor trauma or none at all. In his opinion these men had trouble with managing army life itself.

The problems were not confined to the ranks alone. One study of officers revealed that the prevalence of neuroses was the same as in other ranks, but hysterical disorders were less common. Doctors were over-represented, and had a high incidence of psychosis and psychopathic disorders, probably due to the less stringent selection criteria that they were subject to (Roberts and Moore 1947). In India, officers at base units became psychiatrically unfit more often than those in the forward units. Some who had been demoted to work in the former areas 'had never been anything but a menace to an efficient office' (Tredgold *et al.* 1946).

From the language used in many of the reports, it is clear that sympathy for this group of men was stretched, if not entirely lacking. A 'mother's darling', or unresolved Oedipus Complex, was how Culpin viewed one case who never saw any action (1940a). Similarly, Slater described some of the survivors from Dunkirk as showing 'weakness in fibre' (1941c). In a letter to Brigadier Rees suggesting the 'Annexure' scheme, Lewis identified two groups of soldiers suffering from neurosis: '(i) Men who are too timid, immature, or otherwise psychopathic to endure any danger and discomfort, camp or campaign life, discipline, and separation from their home, (ii) Men who have been put on jobs for which they are unsuited and which therefore they dislike' (1941).

Tayleur Stockings described the clinical picture. According to him, those men 'with mild degrees of mental defect, psychopaths of the emotionally inadequate and anti-social types, the hysterical, and the anxious, worrying over-conscientious type' were subject to neurotic depression. This would take one of two forms. The first would be found in the man whose 'expression is dejected, mask-like and miserable, and the conjunctivae often injected as if red with weeping'. He would appear sullen, hostile and uncooperative in attitude, giving monosyllabic answers to questions. Symptoms were exaggerated and dramatic. Often he would take to his bed in a semi-stupor, ignoring his surroundings. The second type of depression was marked by acute anxiety and agitation. The sufferer would complain of being 'browned off', 'fed up' or 'miserable', and being unwanted or thought odd by his comrades, He would be unable to concentrate properly and subject to transient periods of confusion, often described as 'black outs' or 'turns'. Worry and irritability would predominate, often associated with fears of crowds, handling live ammunition, bombing, guns or air raids. Complaints of lack of sleep, often exaggerated, would be the rule.

These soldiers would recover rapidly in hospital, within two or three days. However, in the long term they rarely returned to full duty; at best they were able to cope with more sheltered conditions of service. Tayleur Stockings distinguished members of this group from those with psychotic depression who had been keen and efficient soldiers before their illness (1944).

Men with difficult personalities figured highly (see Crew 1953, p. 450). There were few descriptions given of these, as they were of little or no interest academically. Individuals with severe obsessional traits could have a particularly difficult time. Anderson gave an account of a 27–year-old corporal who had headaches, dizziness, blackouts, an inability to concentrate, and poor sleep following a head injury. This man, who had 'always been conscientious, punctilious and a worrier', worked hard at his duties, mulling them over when off duty. Keen to be promoted, he was constantly fearful of making mistakes and losing rank. He fretted about his work, his wife's attitude and his officers' opinions, and was in a 'permanent state of indecision about his activities, beliefs and ideals (Anderson 1942).

Logan identified a number of men suffering from a 'pernicious behaviour disorder, an instinctive emotional instability, a continuous or episodically recurring pattern of conduct showing social inadequacy or social deviation, treatment-resistive'. One, who took an overdose because he was fed up with Malaya, enjoyed being in detention as it relieved him from any duties. Another deserted, without any planning, and had to pawn his boots to raise money. He borrowed from some Malays the fare to travel some 500 miles around the country by train before giving himself up. A third, with a lifelong tendency to impulsive behaviour, was re-referred because he had yet again stolen a car, gone to a restaurant, ordered an expensive meal and when requested to pay said calmly, 'Call the police'. Others deliberately injured themselves, were delinquent or had problems with poor anger control (Logan 1941). A similar group figured prominently amongst those cases of amnesia that developed, following little or no trauma, during the retreat to Dunkirk. In 9 cases out of 32, deliberate lying was observed, or there was a strong suspicion of malingering (Sargant and Slater 1941).

The effects of inappropriate placement of men with long-standing psychological difficulties on their colleagues are easily inferred from a paper by Haldane and Rowley. When ordered to advance they were unable to 'refrain from flight'. They became disordered in behaviour, leaping from the trenches and running 'about wildly while mortar bombs are bursting around, sometimes rushing towards instead of away from the enemy's guns'. By the time they arrived at the treatment centre, however, they would often be showing little or no evidence of difficulties (Haldane and Rowley 1946).

Malingering, though hotly debated, appeared to be rare, with a few sporadic cases being reported. More commonly found was the tendency for individuals, once they had developed a disorder, to exaggerate the symptoms in order to remain sick. Thorner explained that soldiers were ready to accept that they were ill because it conferred certain advantages on them, such as removal from the battle front. Once in hospital they would exaggerate their symptoms, and this escape into illness relieved them of internal tensions. He was clear that this did not constitute malingering, but was an effect of hospitalisation itself which could be countered by manipulating the environment (Thorner 1946).

At the sharp end: Combatant disorders

In describing the appalling conditions facing soldiers in battle, it is easy to lose sight of the fact that the majority survived their ordeal with great valour. It was only the minority who reported sick. Soldiers had to cope with torrid physical conditions, often as bad as or worse than those of the First World War, and the psychological stresses of imminent death or incapacity. Exhaustion was the most common cause of breakdown. In the Middle East this made up four-fifths of the casualties evacuated from the fighting (Craigie 1944).

The experience of extreme exhaustion is rare in peacetime activities, and it is difficult to comprehend its pervasiveness in war. Personal accounts only hint at its all-encompassing severity, with images of soldiers nodding off standing, resting their heads against a wall, or a regimental Sergeant Major placing a bayonet point upwards under his chin, whilst marching, to prevent himself dozing off (Ellis 1990, pp. 234–239). In the United States army the associated unblinking look was described as the '2000 year stare'. The fatigue, compounded by emotional enervation, led to a feeling of deadness and visual hallucinations. As Bellamy, a medical officer, described it:

> the desperate craving for sleep may stultify all sense of duty, all aggression, all comradeship, all leadership, and cases of battle exhaustion, however temporarily will multiply by leaps and bounds. (1945)

This led to a fatalistic expectation of death, soldiers felt like they were 'the walking dead'. A study of American soldiers found that nearly 40 per cent almost continuously expected to be maimed or killed, and only 15 per cent were usually free of the thought. One veteran commented: 'You think you're living on borrowed time after a while' (Stouffer et al. 1965, pp. 88–89).

The psychological response to battle had a number of stages. Swank and Marchand gave an account of an American unit before, during and after D Day in 1944, concentrating particularly on the development of 'Combat Exhaustion'. During the anticipatory phase most men exhibited 'feelings of insecurity and irritability. A number experienced functional physical disorders for which they were hospitalised, others harmed themselves, some quite clearly malingered and a small minority became delinquent. The worst period came soon after they were told that they would be involved in the invasion of France, but most settled and 'adjusted to the role they were going to play'.

The first few days of combat were marked by a constant state of fluctuating fear, with accompanying physical experiences of urinary frequency and urgency, intense thirst, anorexia and increased sweating. This was accompanied by a fear of being left alone or of displaying some form of embarrassing behaviour. Gradually, men adapted to the conditions and became familiar with the noises of battle. The first symptoms of exhaustion appeared after 25 to 30 combat days, when they became increasingly tired, tended to overreact to minor stimuli, and became more and more cautious and increasingly irritable. Hopelessness increased as the casualties mounted up. However, they struggled on until a particular incident acted as the 'last straw'. This could be a 'near miss' or the death of a friend. At this point all self-control would be lost, and the man would run about wildly and aimlessly, heedless of danger, or roll about on the ground crying convulsively. Afterwards he would have lost all memory of the events leading up to his breakdown (Swank and Marchand 1946).

Fear on the battlefield is a frustrating subject for the researcher who has no military experience. It is quite clear that, historically, military discipline, culture and tradition have all combined to repress any association between fear and warfare. The psychologically-minded investigator tends to criticise this approach because of callousness, and yet it has been more or less successful in that soldiers have fought and won battles for centuries without being overtly bothered by such concerns. This attitude tended to prevail during the Second World War, with some chinks opening up in the official armour. The use of the term 'lack of moral fibre' in the Royal Air Force was one method of sustaining this, as it discouraged those people who were experiencing panic and anxiety from reporting it.

Despite the acknowledgement of fear by many soldiers, many found it difficult to accept that it had got the better of them. Few found it easy to report on their personal experiences of breakdown. Even fifty years later this reticence remains. Interviews carried out by this author and colleagues with individuals who were patients at Northfield and other men who were prisoners of war in the Far East demonstrate this. Even in those cases where they were relatively happy to talk about their experiences, most made little mention of their feelings at that time. Usually, the accounts were given in a 'matter of fact' manner. It was only following narco-analysis that a 23–year-old gunner, a veteran of the retreat at Dunkirk, acknowledged: 'I couldn't stick the guns; I'm scared, I shouldn't be yellow; I'm too big for that; all the chaps thought I was tough (Anderson 1942). Some soldiers were able to express their emotions more directly in personal correspondence. Wishart gave some examples from letters written home. Milder cases would write such things as 'I was shaken up a bit by a near one, and have come back to what they call an Exhaustion Centre for a rest, but I'll soon be all right and back with the unit'. Those more severely affected might say: 'My nerves have all gone to pieces and I know I can't stand that hell any more' (Wishart 1944).

Initially, the worries would be over 'letting the side down', or disgracing oneself in front of one's comrades. As the soldier gained in experience the focus would shift. Exhaustion left the individual more vulnerable, but the pre-eminent concern was of death or being crippled (Ellis 1990, pp. 239–242; Holmes 1987, pp.206–210). In addition to the powerful psychological effects of particular weapons, other stresses included frustration at being pinned down by enemy gunfire, fear and anxiety about one's own aggression, distrust of leadership, anger and resentment towards others who appeared to have 'let one down', loneliness, guilt over killing, and the horror and grief of seeing friends killed or maimed (Bartemeier *et al.* 1946). In Palmer's broad experience, 'the most common contributory factor was the death of a close comrade or platoon officer (1945b). A continual concern was the family left at home.

Under these conditions, all soldiers in the front line were under intense emotional stress and would break down sooner or later unless they were relieved. In the United States Army it was calculated that the average soldier would break down after something in the region of 200–240 combat days, although many front-line officers considered that their men were ineffective after 180 or even 140 days. The British Army operated a relief system that gave the men four days rest after twelve days in action. This prolonged the length of time they were able to survive to 400 days (Appel and Beebe 1946). The numbers of men breaking down with nervous disorders at any particular time varied according to the nature of the warfare and the terrain being fought over. Tom Main reported that the rate of breakdown for any particular battle could vary between 2 and 30 per cent of all casualties (1946b). Palmer reported that it was usually about 10 per cent of all medical and surgical casualties (1945b). Swank and Marchand found that emotional exhaustion was evident in most men from the 40th day of combat following D Day. After 55 days they were in a 'vegetative state'. Swank and Marchand also noted how the change in the nature of battle from being 'pinned down' to a fluid advance led a number of soldiers who appeared to be at the end of their tether becoming effective again. However, once the battle line returned to being static the symptoms returned (1946). Similarly, Rosie found that the frequency of psychiatric problems increased when the conditions approximated those of the First World War. Flowing actions in which the British Army was winning, such as in the Western Desert in 1940, produced few casualties. However, 'when men were continually exposed to methods of warfare they dreaded most, when they separated from each other in fierce battle and were without sleep, the incidence rose to 10 per cent or even 20 per cent of the total casualties (Rosie 1952, p. 364).

Hubert was the first specialist in psychological medicine to gain experience of acute war neurosis, working with the British Expeditionary Force before and during the retreat to Dunkirk. He found men suffering from anxiety, hysterical, stuporose and mixed states, as well as a small group of individuals with acute psychotic reactions. He considered that most cases could usefully remain in the army (1941).

Sargant and Slater saw cases from the same campaign and found 'that men of reasonably sound personality may break down if the strain is severe enough'. Although these men responded quickly to treatment, the longer-term outlook was less clear (1940). The men were physically exhausted, with 'thin, fallen in faces, pallid or sallow complexions. The expression and the whole attitude of the body was one either of tension and anxiety, or of a listless apathy'. They were further affected by anxiety, with tremors, sleeplessness, nightmares, internal unrest and a 'tendency to be startled at the least noise but particularly at the sound of an aeroplane going overhead or any sound resembling it'. A number repressed the worst of their experiences. Others showed hysterical symptoms. One individual had repeated fits during which 'he would suddenly shoot up in bed, throw his hands over his head and give a series of loud groans. As these gradually diminished in frequency, their place was taken by persistent air-swallowing and eructation'. A torpedoed seaman had flashbacks of his ship sinking and 'his mates drowning beside him' (Sargent and Slater 1940).

Sutherland found that the two-thirds of the soldiers he saw experienced 'trembling and jumpiness', and one-third suffered hysterical conversion symptoms (1941).

These cases came from the defeat in France early on in the war, when the outlook for treatment was perhaps unavoidably gloomy. Later findings were more optimistic. In 1944, Anderson and his colleagues reported on 100 combatants from the vanguard of the Normandy landings. They had adapted well to the military environment, maintaining high morale and fighting valiantly for up to ten days under intense battle conditions. Most experienced mounting fear and anger, becoming jumpy at the sound of gunfire or other sudden noises. Despite this they fought on, 'trembling, sweating, stammering and weeping till they were overtaken by death or emotional collapse'. When the latter happened 'some panicked and ran around, others could not be persuaded to leave their slit-trenches, and some lost consciousness' (Anderson, Jeffrey and Pai 1944).

Similarly, in the Middle East, men broke down suddenly after days of continuous fighting, as the result of 'blasting by mortar and shell fire and the loss of comrades, brothers and officers'. The sight of disfigured and mutilated bodies, either friend or foe, upset some, whilst others couldn't take the 'whine and explosion of accurate mortar fire'. In one case, a soldier's brother was killed whilst protecting him from a mortar explosion with his own body. He was immediately consumed by grief, fury and panic. Another short-sighted man, who had always concealed this, 'always went into battle wearing the spectacles he secreted on his person'. He gave way when he lost his glasses, because he couldn't see 'the enemy or his missiles' (Anderson *et al.* 1944).

These soldiers were largely aware that their problems resulted from fear, and wished to rejoin their comrades as soon as they could. A few developed conversion symptoms, which disappeared rapidly. In contrast, the men who had broken down during the retreat four years earlier tended to have a prolonged course and an increased frequency of physical symptoms, with bed-wetting, headaches, heartaches and stomach aches. All they wanted to do was to go home. It seemed that the perceived disgrace of defeat made it more difficult to cope with neurotic problems (Anderson *et al.* 1944).

Brooke reviewed 500 cases of 'battle exhaustion' evacuated to England from the Second Front in 1944. Most of those who broke down had either under 18 months or over four years of service. The latter had exhausted their reserves after the accumulated experiences of the North African campaign and the landings in Sicily (Brooke 1946). Palmer told a similar story of 'campaign reactions' in those soldiers who had prolonged stress. He found they withdrew gradually from all contact with everyone except their closest confidants. Relief was sought through alcohol abuse and sexual relationships, and their comrades found that their behaviour had altered. They were 'ill at ease in company, especially with strangers,' strove to avoid 'any stimulus to their emotions,' and showed traits of 'explosive anger or abnormal sexuality' (Palmer 1945b, p. 456).

Of those 109 men in Brooke's study who had earlier battle experience, the reasons for their later breakdowns were various. A third couldn't face the shelling, a sixth complained of the blast from explosives and another sixth broke down when their friends were killed or injured, 16 were exhausted from being in the front line for days on end, 14 could not bear horrible sights, and 10 were trapped in burning vehicles or buried alive. Only three admitted to a fear of being killed or wounded. Only a twentieth were discharged from the army. Of those that remained, nearly a fifth returned to full duties, and the rest took up new roles (Brooke 1946).

In North Africa and Italy, Palmer examined 12,000 military psychiatric casualties. In acute cases seen within a few hours or days of battle he identified a number of syndromes. Two-thirds were panic reactions, induced by the sight of fear, pain or death in others. These usually settled without specific medical treatment. He termed the rest of his cases 'Anguish Reactions', which he considered to be true illnesses only amenable to medical treatment, including continuous narcosis for three days. Most were referred on to the base unit. He saw men who had been wandering aimlessly, completely incapable or screaming, or had lost motor or sensory function. Other cases were immobile and mute, or restless with continual hypersensitivity, tremor, sweating, headaches, anorexia and sleeplessness. Some were individuals of high morale who had become tremulous and stammering, in some cases suffering from tics and paralysis (Palmer 1945b, p. 456).

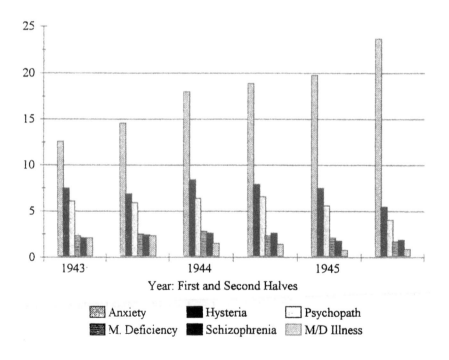

Figure 4.1 Diagnoses of psychiatric discharges from the army 1943–1945
Source: War Office 1948, p. 3

Again in the Middle East, Alfred Torrie, who later worked at Northfield, reviewed 2500 cases referred back to the base unit. Virtually no cases had less than four days of symptoms. A third had been in danger of death from explosion, and some had experienced the wounding or death of a colleague. A particularly potent cause of breakdown was the transfer of a soldier from a unit in which there was a high morale to one in which morale was low. The most common symptom was headache (30 per cent), followed by anxiety (26 per cent), tremulousness and tremor (26 per cent), disturbed sleep (22 per cent) and depression (21 per cent). Some men behaved in an uncontrolled way, 'running around in circles, screaming, jumping out of slit trenches or staying in them long after the danger was over' (Torrie 1944). Non-commissioned officers displayed largely similar characteristics. Nearly 8 per cent had psychopathic features, of whom half were discharged from the army, compared to the 80–90 per cent of those with neurosis who remained on either full or modified duties (Sim 1945). Anxiety states occurred equally frequently in officers and men. The former, however, tended to be depressed, whilst the other ranks suffered more frequently from hysterical symptoms (Sim 1946).

Most papers in the psychiatric press concentrated on neurotic disorders arising from experience of warfare. Whilst individually they often fail to meet even the simplest scientific standards, together they begin to illustrate the uniformity of both aetiology and forms of breakdown, whilst occasionally giving an insight into the individual soldier's experience. A number of soldiers arriving at Northfield had gone through these and similar experiences, particularly during the later part of the war. Their symptoms would usually have become chronic by the time they reached hospital.

Barbed wire syndrome: Prisoners of war

During the latter years of the war Northfield Military Hospital received a significant number of ex-prisoners of war. Those from northern Europe were in the majority, but there are a number of reports of men returning from the Far East. When comparing the conditions in both theatres of war, the horrors of the Holocaust and the Eastern Front in Europe, and the sufferings of non-European prisoners of the Japanese stand out. The white Commonwealth armed forces captured during the war were a small part of the whole, and often tended to be treated rather better than their counterparts from other countries, though at times the difference in the Far East became almost negligable (e.g. Cochrane 1946).

For soldiers, airman and sailors who were captured by the Germans, the conditions were often appalling; for those who were captured by the Japanese they were worse, and for a majority lethal. The slight variations in clinical psychiatric diagnoses of ex-prisoners of war returning from Europe and the Far East disguise very real differences in their physical states, with the latter experiencing profound loss of weight, vitamin deficiencies, malaria, cholera, dysentery and tropical ulcers (see Table 4.1, p.226).

The reports about conditions in both Europe and the Far East are legion. Each contributes new insights and variations on the theme of how human beings can mortify the flesh and spirit of others. Any attempt to generalise the experience is flawed: the different theatres of war produced different consequences, rank affected conditions (officers were usually excused from work activities), and the individual's make-up led to variation in response. Thus the following brief outline can only be a pale reflection of the whole.

Prisoners of war went through a series of phases. Prior to the event most did not consider the consequences of capture, and were usually more preoccupied with the thought of death or mutilation (Cochrane 1946). From the moment of surrender they were dependent on their captors' behaviour. Many were killed, either immediately to avoid the necessity of escorting them behind the lines, or indiscriminately later on (e.g. Ellis 1990, pp. 159–161; Garret 1981, pp.148–149; Newman 1944; Walker 1944). Often there was the expectation that this would happen. They were usually bewildered and tired. The organisation the soldier had belonged to had disintegrated, leading to a sense of being let down and a feeling of resentment towards those he believed allowed it to happen (Walker 1944). This anger continued in one form or another even after release.

Subsequently, prisoners of war tended to neglect their self-care and become apathetic, sullen and withdrawn. Every act and decision required an effort out of all proportion to the circumstances. Nostalgia for home, security, female society and sympathy was profound. Cochrane coined the term 'acute gefangenitis' for this (1946), and Newman used the phrase 'breaking-in period', and felt that this was the most painful period of captivity (1944). Later, the combined effects of poor diet, low morale and nervous tension led to a variety of different behaviours. Some became apathetic to the extent that they died of intercurrent infections. Others lost all sense of proportion in a sort of 'midsummer madness' and acted in disinhibited ways. Neurotic complaints swelled the sick parade, with many men exhibiting hysterical or hypochondriacal problems. Aggression was expressed, most commonly verbally, towards the Germans, other national groups and the prisoners' own officers. Everybody distrusted one another and theft was common.

The next phase was when, having plumbed the depths of their depression, the men gradually recovered their morale and started to organise their lives. For the officer, once he had accommodated himself to his plight, boredom predominated. There were three main constructive approaches to survival: activity that was of value following release, welfare work amongst the prisoners, escape and sabotage (Newman 1944). For those who were expected to work in Germany and Japan the picture was regularly one of struggling to survive. For some, however, for whom the work was not too arduous, it helped to keep away the boredom and depression (Garret 1981). A major distinction between the civil prisoner and the prisoner of war was the latter's uncertainty about when the 'durance vile' would end, which added to the stress (Newman 1944; Walker 1944).

In the Far East the most significant deprivation was that of food. For the majority, by the end of the war the calorific value of what was provided was approximately 600. The rice that they were fed was often dirty and infested with insects. MacCarthy described the preparation of maggot soup from the weevils in the rice, which acted as a source of protein for the sick (1980). There were no vegetables, fruit or meat, except that which could be scavenged whilst working. By the time of release, those who had survived were extremely emaciated. Vitamin deficiency diseases such as beriberi and pellagra were common (Kirman 1946). On top of this was the scourge of infectious diseases such as malaria, dysentery, cholera, jungle sores and dengue (Anon 1980; Gill and Bell 1981; MacCarthy 1980).

In spite of being 'keyed up to a high pitch' in expectation of the pleasures to come, release did not bring an end to suffering (Newman 1944). Indeed, a number of escapees in Italy were reluctant to return to the Allied forces (Jeffrey and Bradford 1946). During a group session at Northfield one commented on how they had been cut off from English society whilst in prison camp. Another retorted immediately that following their return they were still cut off. A third explained: 'It is as if the POW had been caged not only behind barbed wire but also behind a wall he had built to protect himself from the realities of prison life' (Foulkes 1946b).

A common feature in these men was irritability and suspiciousness of others. Aggression was often expressed towards authority figures, especially within the army, but also including parents. The repatriates had difficulties with socialisation and a sense of being lost. They wandered about with deadpan faces, poor concentration and a fear of asking for anything (Bavin 1946). Newman saw these responses as being the effect of trying to come to terms with all the changes that had occurred during the time they were away. He found that in most cases the syndrome would pass off within six to twelve months. A small number had persistent or exaggerated symptoms (Newman

1944). Maxwell Jones treated 829 POWs from Germany and examined 100 in greater detail. He found that in general the group originally had been more stable psychologically than the group of soldiers he had been accustomed to treating. Now they felt that they did not belong, were shy of women, resented the army, were easily tired and had a low tolerance to stress. The emphasis in rehabilitation was on work in local businesses and group activities, including education and entertainment programmes. He was able to follow up 56, of whom 36 had started work soon after leaving the unit, 16 had begun after eight or more weeks rest and only four had done no work whatsoever. Marital infidelity by spouses left at home contributed significantly to psychiatric breakdown (Jones 1946).

A few personal accounts illustrate these findings. Soon after a 26-year-old sapper was captured by the Italians, he and his fellows were lined up against a wall as if to be shot. Later in a POW camp in Benghazi, they were bombed by the Royal Air Force. Conditions there were so poor that prisoners died in large numbers. After being transferred to Italy he had a relapse of malaria and lost a considerable amount of weight. He escaped in 1943, and lived in a shepherd's hut in the mountains until he was recaptured. On release he was emotionally unstable and twice went absent without leave from his unit. He suffered severe frontal headaches, bad fits of depression, nightmares about his experiences, and insomnia. He was irritable, tense, upset by noises that sounded like gunfire and had marked mood swings. Previously a sociable man, he now avoided friends and dreaded going to work. Other symptoms included giddiness, tremors, occasional nausea with loss of appetite; a stammer and facial tics (Edkins 1948, pp. 280–281).

Mr J. was captured at the fall of Singapore and incarcerated in Changi Jail. When one of his comrades began screaming, having 'lost his nerve', a guard shot him dead in cold blood. Later, in Saigon, he was forced to work, unloading cement in the docks and stacking petrol cans. On one occasion he was hit by a Japanese officer for no apparent reason, with the flat of a sword. On another he was mistakenly apprehended for trying to get cigarettes from an Asian worker. He was tied to a post with barbed wire and beaten with a bamboo cane. The marks from this were still visible to his wife four years later. Another colleague was hung for stealing. Mr J. then worked on the notorious Burma Railway, where he was forced to work in appalling conditions. One event still causes nightmares 50 years later. Whilst hauling on a rope a large, poisonous centipede climbed onto his shoulder. He couldn't let go of the rope to knock it off. To his surprise, a Korean guard placed a tissue paper in front of it, and when the creature climbed on, flicked it off.

Many thousands of Mr J.'s fellow captives died of malnutrition, disease and injury. On two occasions he saw individuals returning from other camps, the only survivors of 150 or more. One 'had lost his mind, screaming about all the people who had died'. He himself suffered from dysentery, beriberi and malaria. On one occasion he was placed on the bench in the sick hut reserved for those who were about to die. Deciding he was going to survive, he managed to crawl back to another bed.

On release, he was given no assistance in resettlement, and the only debriefing was an hour's interview in which he was asked about the activities of the officers in the camps rather then his state of mind. Like so many other who underwent similar experiences, fifty years later he still suffers from nightmares, irritability and intrusive memories (Fenton 1990; Gill and Bell 1981; Harrison 1995; Tennant, Goulston and Dent 1986).

Unlike Mr J., many ex-prisoners of war were resettled through the Civil Resettlement units, which because of their close connection with the practice at Hollymoor, will be described in more detail later in this paper. Before these were instituted a number of men were released or escaped from German and Italian camps. Their views significantly influenced the development of the later facilities. One young soldier gave his views on returning to the United Kingdom in 1943 from a German prisoner-of-war camp. Initially, he found that life appeared to be much the same as when he had left. His main plan was to make up for lost time by enjoying himself. He was impressed by the apparent prosperity compared with the prisoner-of-war camp, where even the guards ate poorly, commenting: 'To return to English food was almost unreal'. Entertainment was various and wide-ranging compared to Nazi Europe, where 'dancing is forbidden and feet only march to one time (Directorate of Army Psychiatry 1944). For ex-prisoners of war the sense of having 'missed out' was exacerbated by the fact that whilst in captivity other men who joined the army later had been promoted above them. The fact that others had died was not much consolation (Walker 1944).

Even once the Civil Resettlement Units had been established, some of the facilities for repatriation of prisoners of war were less than satisfactory. Most of the members of Davidson's psychotherapy group of August 1945 had been taken, after their release, to Piper's Wood Selection and Training Battalion. This environment, surrounded by dark woods, where they rarely saw the sun, reminded them of their earlier incarceration. None of the instructors appeared to have the foggiest idea of what they were supposed to be doing. For example, non-commissioned officers were subjected to training aimed normally at new recruits. They showed war films about Japanese atrocities, aimed at instilling hate for that particular enemy, but which in the event tended to provoke fear and revulsion in the audience. The authoritarian attitude of the staff tended to deny any initiative, and was deeply resented. This was despite the fact that in the POW camps the only way of surviving had been by using one's wits and creativity. Because of the lack of medical staff, the ex-prisoners of war were compelled to run five miles uphill before any of them had been examined physically. For men who had been subjected to malnutrition, some of whom had suffered severe infections, this was downright dangerous. Many of the soldiers exposed to this stupid and insensitive treatment broke down, although not all of them sought medical help (Davidson 1946, pp. 93, 99–100).

Effort syndrome and paranoia: Psychosomatic and psychotic disorders

Freud's attachment of phases of psychological development to physical locations within the human organism gave impetus to the exploration of the relationship of mind and body in disease. It also established a strong psychoanalytical predisposition in psychosomatic medicine (Macleod, Wittkower and Margolin 1954). Other contributions came from behavioural psychology, in which Pavlov and his disciples were able to demonstrate changes in physiology as a result of conditioned reflexes; meanwhile others were exploring the behavioural characteristics of those people who had a tendency to particular forms of physical illness, such as migraine, hay fever, eczema and cardiac disease (Wittkower 1949).

The overlap between psychiatric and physical disorder was a subject explored repeatedly throughout the war. Hysterical phenomena were less common than during the First World War, but neurosis frequently presented with physical symptomatology. Eric Wittkower, who worked at Northfield in 1944, was particularly interested in the psychological aspects of injury. He had a strong psychoanalytic bent, and in an early paper of effort syndrome was already recommending psychotherapy as treatment (Wittkower, Rodger and Wilson 1941).

Apart from the evident interrelationship of mind and body in 'combat exhaustion', where tiredness led to psychological disorders, psychosomatic disorders were common (Douglas-Wilson 1944; Moll 1954; Torrie 1944). In these, mental distress expressed itself by causing physical symptoms. Most frequently recorded was headache. Nearly as everyday were cardiac symptoms, often described as 'effort syndrome'. Other disorders included abdominal problems, motor and sensory disturbances, and urinary symptoms (Douglas-Wilson 1944). One man had a painful operation scar in which he believed a nerve was trapped. He also 'complained of a headache that felt as if there was a tight band round the head, defective vision uncorrected by spectacles, and night blindness caused by the strain of driving at night'. Later he began to exhibit pseudo-epileptic attacks. All these symptoms were identified as being hysterical in origin (W. Jones 1942).

Military discipline made soldiers afraid of reporting nervous symptoms, so they complained that they were ill. Consequently, some disorders were treated medically without the real cause of their problems being identified (Cook and Sargant 1942). Douglas-Wilson found that between a quarter and a third of patients he saw presenting with physical illness had underlying psychological problems. Headache was the most frequent, with shortness of breath, precordial pain, palpitations, indigestion, cough, frequency of micturition, hyperidrosis, joint pains and 'blackouts' also being common (Douglas-Wilson 1943; 1944).

'Effort syndrome', which had received a lot of attention from the physicians of the First World War, continued to figure prominently during the earlier stages of the Second. It was often associated with pain over the precordial region and the experience of fear. It almost solely affected individuals who had not been in battle (James 1952). It was quickly established that emotional and psychological causes underlay it. Typically, it was characterised by disproportionate breathlessness and fatigue on exercise, with a varying degree of undue disturbance of the pulse rate. There might also be dizziness or fainting attacks, blurred vision, pain over the heart region, palpitations and a fast heart rate, indigestion and constipation, headaches, sleeplessness and nightmares, 'nervousness', excessive sweating, tremor, cramps and numbness of the limbs. Wittkower and his colleagues considered that most of the affected men would improve with psycho-therapy, but that some would never become useful soldiers (Wittkower et al. 1941). Danson was more colourful in his description, writing that, after minor exercise, 'such patients have a "hang dog" appearance, with cold pale skin, and bluish lips and extremities; yet they sweat copiously on the palms and soles whilst the dorsum of the hands and feet remains dry, and sweat trickles from their axillae' (1942).

The diagnosis was largely abandoned after 1941, largely following the comprehensive demolition of its value as a diagnostic entity by a cardiologist, Paul Wood (1941a; 1941b).

Attention also turned to the mental aspects of physical injury. Wittkower found that emotional problems were prominent in those who had had amputations or been blinded. The reactions of others to their disability could often cause problems, and employment proved a struggle. He was concerned that, although the surgical and financial aspects were often well attended to, insufficient attention was paid to the psychological reactions. As a result a great deal of unhappiness and distress resulted for both of them and those in contact with them (Duke-Elder and Wittkower 1946; Wittkower 1945; 1947; Wittkower and Davenport 1946).

Although hysterical reactions were less common than during the First World War (*Journal of The Royal Army Medical Corps.* 1945; Craigie 1944, p.107; Hadfield 1942; MacKeith 1946a, p.549; Markillie 1993), the inter-reaction of mind and body continued to provide material for those psychiatrists interested in psychosomatic medicine. The conjunction of physicians and psychiatrists in units on active service, as well as at hospitals in the United Kingdom, stimulated a great deal of activity and interest in this area, which was reflected in Northfield (Lewsen 1993).

Psychosis, on the other hand, was largely neglected (Mulinder 1945). This was despite the fact that from the first, some soldiers' breakdown in battle would be accompanied by paranoid delusions and catatonia (Hubert 1941). Brigadier James, in the Middle East, stated that 'true psychosis' occurred in about 10% of all psychiatric casualties (1952). The lack of interest in wartime psychoses is partly explained by Beccle, who emphasised that they differed little from those that affect the population in times of peace. However, he did state that war stress could precipitate the condition where peacetime conditions might not have done so (Beccle 1942). It is evident that there was controversy about the nature of acute psychosis under these conditions. Problems with diagnosis proliferated. Swank and Marchand considered that the final picture of combat exhaustion was very similar to that of schizophrenia, with apathy, lack of response to stimuli, and physical and mental retardation (1946). In the Middle East the term schizophrenia ' was used so frequently that it was clear it served as a convenient label for almost any mental illness occurring in young men' (James 1952).

It was a commonplace that acute psychotic episodes could occur as a result of combat (e.g. Main 1946b; Palmer 1945b). However the evidence supporting this is limited. Mulinder identified 91 cases of acute, transient episodes precipitated by battle stress out of a total of 138 cases of psychoses he reviewed in Normandy after D Day. He admitted that they did not fit readily into any established nosology, but considered that their detachment from reality, confusion, mutism, delusions, hallucinations, psychomotor retardation and catatonic immobility were diagnostic. They occurred in men who were not normally expected to develop this form of illness, with no family history of it and no significant prodrome in their personal history (Mulinder 1945). This conflicts with Beccle's earlier study, which looked at 50 unselected cases. In those men with schizophrenia, the evidence of pre-psychotic symptoms was evident, with many of the men affected being shy, dreamy and socially inept, and exhibiting inertia. Most broke down as a result of recruitment, although some did so following minor wounds or dive bombing (Beccle 1942).

A typical picture was that of an acute paranoid state. The soldier might be terrified, believing that other patients were disguised Germans, his food was poisoned and that he was to be murdered in the night (Hubert 1941). One individual was admitted in a state of extreme terror, 'believing that a Messerschmitt was after him all the time'. He took every sound for some form of weapon and became extremely frightened, at times trying to run away and at others burying 'himself in abject terror beneath the bedclothes'. Gradually, this modified to a condition of acute anxiety, with headaches aggravated by noise (Mulinder 1945). In another instance, a tank driver's vehicle was hit and the commander killed. After several further severe stresses the driver was rescued. On admission he was agitated, hardly speaking, depressed and half asleep. The few words he volunteered indicated that he believed he was responsible for his tank commander's death, and that 'voices' were reiterating this. Over the next week he improved considerably 'but remained mildly depressed. He tended still to blame himself, and lacked self-confidence' (Mulinder 1945).

Perhaps these papers, more than any others, go some way towards justifying the pronouncements of Healy and Trimble about the lack of scientific rigour in wartime psychiatric research, referred to earlier. Strict criteria for the diagnosis of schizophrenia were not used; Schneider's work, which introduced what are now widely accepted diagnostic criteria, was not translated into English until 1959, and Bleuler's vague and more embracing descriptions were current (Bleuler 1902; Schneider 1957). As a result, more patients were so diagnosed than would be today. However, this state of confusion continued to lead to marked differences in diagnosis between the United Kingdom and the United States until the 1970s, and to be overly critical of the earlier practitioners in the field for not having solved this conundrum during the heat of battle is perhaps naïve in itself (Cooper *et al.* 1972).

Psychosis was rare in Northfield. The criteria of potential for recovery would have excluded all known cases. This author, however, had under his care one ex-patient who was diagnosed subsequently as suffering from schizophrenia. It is likely that the breakdown in the army was the prodrome of this illness.

THERAPEUTIC OPTIONS

Up until the Second World War, physical treatments were prevalent in hospital psychiatric practice. The psychodynamic school produced a great deal of literature and debate, but only consisted of a relatively small number of individuals, working in private practice and a few clinics. The total number of psychoanalysts in the British Society was less than 50.

The attraction of these physical measures was twofold: they held out the promise of rapid results and they fitted the illness model. In 1944, Sargant and Slater, two of the foremost practitioners, advocated these methods because they brought psychiatry closer to general medicine. They hoped that through building a coherent body of knowledge related to other sciences through biology, psychiatry would evolve into an 'exact science'. They were sceptical about the effects of concentrating on psychodynamic theory, believing that the result of this had been 'an exaltation of theory at the expense of experiment, and a remoteness and rarefaction of the atmosphere of clinical approach that alienates the ordinary doctor or student' (Sargant and Slater 1944, pp. 3–4).

Other forms of treatment were implemented, but even during the therapeutic community phases at Northfield this was always against the background of the medical approach. This approach was clearly often effective in bringing rapid results in acute cases, and with lack of available expertise in other methods it was difficult to offer alternatives. Pyscho-social treatments thus tended to remain as adjuncts, following on from the implementation of more vigorous therapies. Psychotherapy was widely practised in its various forms, and occupational therapy similarly took many guises.

Pills, potions and shocks: Physical treatments

The physical therapies used can be divided into three categories: restorative and curative measures, and means of expediting other forms of treatment. There is some ambiguity in the terminology used: 'modified insulin' and 'abreaction' could cover a wide variety of practices and techniques (Bartemeier et al. 1946). This section describes the approaches, without encompassing all the multiplicities of procedure.

Good food and 'jungle juice': Restorative measures

These were measures that were intended to support the individual in recuperating from traumatic experiences. They were sometimes associated with other forms of treatment, but for many psychiatrists they were sufficient treatment in themselves. There were the three main forms: Weir Mitchell therapy, modified insulin and continuous narcosis.

Weir Mitchell, after his experiences in the American Civil War, advocated a regime for treating neuroses that continued in practice into the next century. He would withdraw the individual from the stressful situation and enforce absolute rest in bed, in isolation for six weeks. Attention was paid to building up the person's physical strength through feeding them with prodigious amounts of food. This included two quarts of milk and three full meals, with additional meat extracts, soup and fruit juices. The appetite would be stimulated with both massage and electrical stimulation of the muscles. Weir Mitchell maintained that: 'If I succeed in first altering the moral atmosphere which has been to the patient like the very breathing of evil and if I can add largely to the weight and fill the vessels with red blood, I am usually sure of giving relief to a host of aches and pains and varied disabilities' (1885, quoted in Sargant and Slater 1944, pp.41–42). Although Sargant and Slater stated that the experience of the Second World War confirmed his views, there is little evidence of the regime being carried out as he suggested it. It was time-consuming and required careful and intensive nursing.

With acute war neuroses, more common was therapy which was introduced immediately and included a good sleep, hot meals, hot showers and a change of kit. Palmer was surprised to find that a large proportion treated in this way returned to full duty (1945b). The greatest difficulty was ensuring adequate sleep. The majority found little or no difficulty in getting off to sleep, but had problems with the nightmares that disturbed it later. This was treated with sedatives (Sargant and Slater 1940).

Modified insulin therapy was a derivative of this approach. It originated in the insulin coma technique developed by Sakel in 1930 for the treatment of his patients suffering from schizophrenia (Sakel 1959). Sargant and Craske introduced it for war neuroses. Initially, they induced a light coma by giving an intra-muscular injection of insulin, and then fed the person sugar through a naso-gastric tube. This method was later abandoned, as it was time-consuming and needed high nursing input. Less insulin was used, insufficient to induce any coma, and the patient was fed by mouth. As well as this, the sugar also was replaced by potatoes due to the shortages of supplies. The aim was to get the exhausted patient to gain weight. They found that the best results were in 'men of fairly good personality with anxious, hysterical and depressive symptoms of a reactive type'. Weight gain was achieved in most of their 64 patients (Sargant and Craske 1941). Slater, as well as Minski, later found this procedure useful with a wide variety of patients, especially those who had suffered marked loss of weight (Minski 1944; Slater 1943).

It is difficult to be sure how widely this method was used. Bartemeier et al. reported that there were advocates for its regular use in hospitals for treating neurosis, particularly because of the sense of cohesion it brought to the ward staff (1946, p. 498). Whilst it was used at Mill Hill regularly for soldiers and civilians in a 'latent or delayed anxiety state', Charles Lewsen recalled that it was used only very occasionally at Northfield (Bartemeier et al. 1946, p. 498; Lewsen 1993).

In the nineteenth century, Griesinger noted that restless psychotic patients sometimes responded well to drug-induced deep sleep (1867). This was taken up in 1922 by Kläsi, who produced prolonged and profound somnolence in his patients suffering from schizophrenia using Somnifen (Kläsi 1922). During the next two decades the technique evolved, with developments including the use of sodium amytal, with varying success (Bleckwenn 1930a; 1930b; Sargant and Slater 1944; Windholz and Witherspoon 1993). There were strong advocates. In late 1942, reporting on his work with 350 cases of acute war neurosis, Craigie found the use of intravenous barbiturates, in removing hysterical conversion symptoms, of great value (Craigie 1942). In the Navy, Curran and Guttman recommended the use of continuous narcosis for states of prolonged agitation, excitement or tension (1946, pp. 62–64). For Minski, in 1944, it was 'the method of treatment' for anxiety or severe exhaustion resulting from battle stress and fatigue. In his technique the patient was put to bed, preferably in a side room. Various sedatives such as somnifane were given intra-muscularly, alternating with chloral hydrate orally at four-hourly intervals. The doses were spaced so that the patient could be roused for meals and other necessary functions. Additional calories were given in the form of glucose drinks. The aim was that the patient remain asleep for 20 hours out of 24 for between five and twelve days. The patient's condition was assessed when he was emerging from sleep to have his meals or other activities. Occasionally, the patient became confused and restless, in which case the treatment had to be discontinued (Minski 1944).

Others also advocated drug-induced deep sleep strongly for 'mental disturbance accompanied by anguish', where this was related to recent trauma, acute anxiety states, melancholia, catatonia, depression or cases that had not responded to electro-convulsive therapy (ECT) (Palmer 1948, p. 246; Parfitt 1946). Some workers advised that the patient should be kept asleep for between 16 and 20 hours a day for a period of five to ten days, which could be repeated for a second time if necessary (Curran and Guttman 1946, pp. 62–64). The longer periods required very skilled nursing and medical attention, and were viewed as very risky by many physicians (Lewsen 1993; Minski 1947; Palmer 1948; Sargant and Slater 1944).

There were those who were not so convinced. Sargant and Slater considered that for many neurotic patients, modified insulin therapy was more efficacious and safer, and they recommended electro-convulsive treatment for those with depression (1944). Thorner found that continuous narcosis had no lasting effect on psychoneurosis (1946).

Mr L. arrived at Northfield two months after D Day, having been wounded at the Battle of the Falaise Gap in France, and suffering from loss of speech and nightmares. His experience of continuous narcosis was of being given a 'jungle juice' that:

> induced a twilight sleep and you did everything automatically. You went to the toilet automatically and you ate your food automatically for about three weeks…You were in this perpetual twilight world…you know, the thing that amazed me was that you ate your food automatically. (Interview: Mr L. 1998)

Later, in the same hospital, Tom Main was amongst those who used a modified version of continuous narcosis. The regression of the patient to an infantile state was encouraged, even to the extent of singing nursery rhymes to them and feeding them milk from a nursing bottle. The recovery from the narcosis was treated as a period of weaning, through which the patient progressed slowly. The motive behind this form of treatment was specifically to re-enact the process of early mothering, and it was only carried out on carefully selected patients (Bartemeier et al. 1946). This author was once involved treating a patient in this way and found it remarkably effective in a man who had already regressed to a helpless, unhappy, fretful dependence on psychiatric services.

Drastic cures: Convulsive therapy and psychosurgery

The 'organic' approach of many psychiatrists led to a constant search for cures that were quick and effective. In retrospect, some of the treatments that resulted appear to many as at the very least daunting, and to others as barbaric.

Whilst many of the other therapies had been in use for some years, convulsive therapy was relatively new. Cerletti and Bini published their work on the use of electric current to induce fits in 1938, the year before the outbreak of the war (Cerletti and Bini 1938). Meduna initiated convulsive therapy in 1933 using cardiazol, and continued to promote its value up until 1939. Henderson and Gillespie gave a detailed account of the methodology in 1950, indicating its continued use up until then (Meduna 1938; Meduna and Friedman 1939; Henderson and Gillespie 1950, pp. 419–422).

In Northfield the staff used the electrical technique. Its use appears to have increased through the period of the war. Debenham, Sargant, Hill and Slater did not mention it in their article on the treatment of war neurosis in January of 1941, though by November of 1942 Sargant was advocating its use for depression in NCOs with obsessional personalities (Debenham *et al.* 1941; Sargant 1942). Sutherland reported its use in a few cases of depression in September 1941 (Sutherland 1941). In the same year, Good was using cardiazol-induced convulsions for a range of difficulties including hysteria, anxiety neurosis and pyschopathy. He found the results poor, stating that in some cases the treatment was not to blame, as the patients didn't want to get well again. They had a 'negative therapeutic attitude' (Good 1941). In late 1942, working with acute war neurosis, Craigie was becoming increasingly confident of its effectiveness with depressive states and 'certain hysterical cases' (Craigie 1942). Parfitt reported in 1946 on work he had done on 400 cases from 1939 to 1942, comparing prolonged narcosis with convulsion therapy. He emphasised the safety of ECT, finding no serious complications in over 200 cases (Parfitt 1946). By 1944, Sargant and Slater recommended the use of electro-convulsive therapy in a far wider group of conditions than is generally acceptable today. These included schizophrenia, involutional and bi-poplar depression, reactive depression and some forms of neurosis such as depersonalisation and hysteria (Sargant and Slater 1944). Other authors recommended it for conditions as diverse as schizophrenia and 'simple tension syndromes' (Beccle 1942; Palmer 1948).

The treatment technique evolved throughout the 1940s. In 1944, Sargant and Slater described giving a small dose of Sodium Amytal intravenously as pre-medication. They emphasised that the control of the patient's movements was very important in order to avoid fractures. This could be done either by nurses holding the individual down or by means of a specially constructed jacket. This was a modified straitjacket with long sleeves, which encased the body from neck to foot. After being made comfortable with pillows and pads, the patient was strapped to the couch by means of cloth belts. The arms were left with more freedom, strapped across the chest (Sargant and Slater 1944). In 1944, Mr L. saw men having ECT at Northfield:

They got them into this ward, this side ward, and they strapped them. They put a strap across their legs, and across their middle, and across the chest, and they just plugged…the apparatus into the wall, and they switched, did they switch on and you'd see the patient jerk, jerk each time it was pressed…They got a convulsion and this was supposed to reactivate the brain, to do something to the brain to make it jolt into action. It wasn't a very pleasant thing to look at really. (Interview: Mr L 1998)

Palmer used muscle relaxants as early as 1939, and as a result had to maintain artificial respiration during the treatment. By 1948 he was able to reduce the patient's initial anxiety by giving thiopentone. He also described the research that was continuing to find the most suitable voltage and wave form of the electric current to be applied (Palmer 1948). It was clearly still a period of experimentation, though many workers were reporting good results in otherwise untreatable forms of mental disorder.

Psychosurgery was another relatively new form of therapy. Moniz had persuaded his colleague Lima to embark on their series of leucotomies in late 1935, and began to report on their results in 1936 (Moniz and Lima 1936). Sargant and Stewart reported on one case of psychosurgery in a case of 'chronic battle neurosis' in 1947 (Sargant and Stewart 1947). In this paper they stated that over 30 of their civilian patients had had the operation since 1941. The indications for this treatment in this particular case were intractable 'pains in the legs, lethargy, headaches, irritability and poor sleep'. The patient was continually ruminating on his war experiences and was concerned that people were criticising his behaviour. He had been in tanks during the war and, as well as having many friends killed, twice barely escaped with his own life when his tank was destroyed. Interestingly, he was treated in a 'military neurosis centre' in 1944, possibly Northfield. The treatment was reported as having returned him to his previous state of good mental health, and he began work again.

These were early days for a treatment that had its heyday in the 1950's, when over 1000 operations were being carried out each year (Tooth and Newton 1961). There is no clear evidence that it was ever used in Northfield. One literary allusion occurs in the novel by Rayner Heppenstall, who refers to one individual being sent for psychosurgery to another hospital (1953 p.168). He only came to the conclusion that this was a lobotomy in hindsight. The actual description indicates that this individual was a case of the physician, Dr Lewsen, who suffered from a cranial tumour, especially as the character in the novel died afterwards (Lewsen 1993).

The truth drug: Narco-analysis

Narco-analysis was a technique that chemically facilitated the emotional release of suppressed memories in what was described as an abreaction. It had its origins in two sources. The first was the experience of hypnosis and catharsis during the First World War. The second was the observation by Bleckwenn, whilst carrying out continuous narcosis with sodium amytal in the 1930s, that there was a short period of lucidity for the minute or two before the patient went to sleep. During this time the patient could talk his problems clearly and with insight (Bleckwenn 1930a; 1930b). Lindemann developed this in the next year and found that patients wished to communicate and were willing to talk about very personal problems (1932). The term itself was coined by Horsley in 1936, when he described how he combined it with psychotherapy in order to enhance the therapeutic process. He recorded that a wide range of drugs were being used at that time. Of his four examples, one was a case of 'shell shock' from the First World War. The technique was used to enable him to recover his memories of a bayonet attack. 'Persuasion was then effective in promoting a good recovery' (Horsley 1936). Ellis Stungo, later to use the technique in the army and at Northfield, reported on his modified version in 1938. He used Evipan Sodium (Pentothal), at that time injected intravenously, to conduct what he described as a superficial psychological investigation in people who were reticent about revealing their feelings and thoughts (Stungo 1938).

During the war, the use of barbiturates as a method of bringing repressed psychic material to consciousness was widespread (Bartemeier *et al.* 1946; p. 499–502; Patrick and Howells 1990). Lambert and Rees considered that, although they had been increasingly popular since the outbreak of war, their use was controversial (1944).

The more organically-orientated psychiatrists like Sargant and Slater tended to value them as a diagnostic tool, finding that under their influence people slowed down by depression became talkative and even cheerful. Hidden thoughts came to the surface and revealed the person's delusions, suicidal ideas or repressed experiences (Sargant and Slater 1944, p.111). They recommended it for the recovery of memory in acute war neurosis, in combination with persuasion or suggestion to remove symptoms. Horrifying events could come to light through this process, such as one man recalling that he had to shoot his brother to put him out of the misery caused by his injuries. Salvaging these forgotten incidents often elicited immense emotion, and they would use an injectable sedative to damp this down and save the patient from unnecessary misery (Sargant and Slater 1940). They considered that this was kinder to the individual than the psychotherapeutic approach, which took the man repeatedly over the same material (Sargant and Slater 1941).

Later, their colleague, Louis Minski, also emphasised use of barbiturates in reinforcing suggestions for removal of hysterical conversion symptoms, as under the influence of such drugs suggestibility was increased and inhibitions were removed (1944). Wilde used the technique over a period of 13 months for all cases under his care who were resistant to other forms of treatment. He found it particularly effective for hysteria, anxiety states, the after-effects of head and spinal injuries, borderline psychoses, mental deficiency, epilepsy when the diagnosis was in doubt and, finally, malingering. He also stated that Emanuel Miller, later to work in Northfield, also used the same technique (Wilde 1942).

Chemically-mediated abreactive techniques were widely used. The British psychiatrists perceived them as being techniques that relatively inexperienced doctors could use with safety, close to the theatre of war, as long as it was done gently and with the intention of relieving acute symptoms. However, Bartemeier and his colleagues were more cautious, and were concerned that they found some using the methods with 'considerable violence an aggressiveness'. They did not state whether this was in American or British practice, although they did recommend that such methods should only be used by experienced doctors (Bartemeier *et al.* 1946, p. 510, 523).

Barbiturates were so widely used that they became known as the 'truth drug'. Mr M. recalled having them used on him at Northfield:

> The other one was you were given an injection, it was the truth drug…you just lay on the bed, and he injected you, and then he asked questions and he was trying to get into your inner thoughts, the things you couldn't remember. (Interview: Mr M. 1994, p. 6)

Basket weaving and dreams: Psycho-social treatments
The talking cure: Psychotherapy

Psychotherapy was a widely used term with a great deal of variety in its meaning, ranging from didactic techniques, persuasion and encouragement, and discussion through to full-blown psychoanalysis.

Early in the war, Hubert taught patients about their disorders, emphasising, for instance, that anxiety states were normal variations of fear in a sensitive individual. The person was encouraged to discuss the emotional conflicts that underlay his actions. Hubert aimed to make sense of the situation that the person found themselves in and encouraged them to make sensible, realistic decisions about returning to their previous role. As much as possible, exhibitions of 'ill' behaviour were discouraged and ignored. It was assumed that the person could relate in a normal and rational manner. In this he was supported by the 'strong suggestive influences of a trained staff and the practical atmosphere of a war-time hospital' (Hubert 1941).

This approach exemplified the most common use of the term. Practice regularly included discussion of symptoms, explanation and giving of reassurance by the psychiatrist (e.g.Andersen *et al.* 1944; Debenham *et al.* 1941; Tredgold 1944). This was seen as having value even in cases of psychosis (Beccle 1942). Persuasion and suggestion could be used to broaden the armamentarium (Jones and Lewis 1941). Individual therapy could be combined with group therapy (Foulkes 1946a). In general the emphasis was on brief, supportive interventions in an atmosphere 'which inspires feelings of confidence and hope in the patients' (Minski 1941). Later, Minski relegated this role to the social worker or welfare officer (Minski 1944). The psycho-social atmosphere of the treatment unit was of great importance. 'On the whole the atmosphere of the hospital is cheerful, but not at all relaxing' (Thorner 1946) was typical of a number of commentators' views of the ideal milieu.

It was constantly reiterated that it was not possible to do long-term therapy, so different shorter-term approaches were attempted (e.g. Bennet 1941). Thorner reported on the dilemmas facing the psychoanalyst who treated soldiers. His usual practice with civilian outpatients was out of the question. In Thorner's experience, those who applied strict psychoanalytical approaches had the same results as others who were more pragmatic. He did, however, find the theory valuable for diagnosis and exploration, but used whatever means were appropriate and available for treatment (Thorner 1946). Torrie came to similarly pragmatic conclusions. He considered that the aim was to get the man fit for duty within three weeks. Analytic techniques had to be focussed, and use had to be made of dream material. Hypnosis, either using sedatives or suggestion, was useful for removing symptoms, but didn't help the patient gain insight into what had happened to them. Any therapy that could be helpful was used. 'At all times it was borne in mind that the aim was adaptation to warfare and not a radical change of personality' (Torrie 1944).

In exploring the differences between psychotherapy in the First and Second World Wars, Rickman gave an insight into his practice. This did not entail a full psychoanalysis, but a focused therapy that included practical activities and followed unconscious leads that the patients gave about their conditions. In particular, he emphasised the importance of relationships in modern therapy, deriving his argument from the work of Melanie Klein, and rejecting the instinct theories of the First World War (Rickman 1941).

In Bennet's view, the hidden elements in amnesia could only be treated using an abbreviated technique of exploratory psychotherapy such as hypnotherapy. Explanatory methods, such as those described above, were of no use. The dissociation of emotion from the memories had to be remedied by the patient re-experiencing the repressed experience (Bennet 1941). Behavioural techniques were also employed. McLaughlin and Millar exposed individuals who had become hypersensitive to air-raid noises to gramophone records of actual warfare. This, in combination with reassurance and explanation, was intended as a form of 'conditioning; however, it rapidly became clear that it served as a form of abreaction, with patients recalling their experiences as vividly as under hypnosis or drugs. They indicated that the treatment was effective, though there was no control group (McLaughlin and Millar 1941). Torrie also called upon these techniques in his eclectic approach (1944).

Occupational therapy

Occupational therapy was widely promoted from very early on in the war (Snowden 1939). This ranged from what Bion described acidly as 'helping to keep the patients occupied – usually on a kindergarten level' (1946), to specific attempts to prevent 'hospitalisation', which was conceived of as an 'insidious adaptation of the individual to an idle and abnormal existence', through instituting a programme of work activities during normal working hours (Cameron 1940). This was part of a much wider push to maximise the ability of disabled men to contribute. In civilian practice, the Ministry of Labour promoted a scheme for the 'training and resettlement of disabled persons in industry' in 1941. This led to hospitals increasingly employing rehabilitation officers and expanding their facilities to retrain those patients with physical problems (Titmuss 1950, pp. 478–480).

Minski unwittingly confirmed Bion's observations, quoted in the previous paragraph, when he described the services at Mill Hill in 1941. He stated that the hospital was fortunate in having an occupational therapy department with various workshops that included a room where a trained woman occupation officer held 'classes in rug-making, basket and leather work, weaving, painting, embroidery, etc.' (Minski 1941). To this he later added felt toys and pottery (1944). Where there was little expectation of the men making improvements the tendency appeared to be to provide diversional therapy. This was certainly the case in the British Army in Italy, where Sergeant Mills was at pains to explain that the men in his unit were considered by the psychiatrists to be unlikely to benefit from routine measures because of their mental condition. Here, 30–40 patients did embroidery, soft toy making, tinsmithing, rug making, bookbinding, basketry and cabinet making. It was 'designed to give an agreeable and not too exacting employment' (Mills 1945). After having worked in Mill Hill, Trist considered that there 'had to be a better way' (1985, p. 5).

Wilde and Morgan felt that it was necessary to 'get beyond the "arty crafty" stage', although they too, in 1943, were offering clay modelling, woodwork and drawing at their unit. Even so, they were able to demonstrate that such activities were catalysts for individuals to find new skills and then become employed in more appropriate activities within the army (Wilde and Morgan 1943). Snowden revealed that no patients should be idle, and recommended the development of graduated physical activities up to and including military exercises (1939). Thorner reiterated Rickman's recommendations, and was emphatic that the atmosphere in the hospital should be military and that the patient's day should be mapped out for them as it would be in any ordinary army unit. Weapon training was forbidden under the Geneva Convention, and so other activities such as parades, marches, physical training and work around the hospital itself were all used (Thorner 1946).

In the Middle East and Italy, the development of forward psychiatry encouraged the creation of rehabilitation units. In contrast to the experience in the United Kingdom, the institution of a military atmosphere was customary. Units were expected to promote physical well-being through exercise. Welfare and other problems were to be attended to efficiently, in the setting of a framework which would 'combat the tendency to valetudinarian self-justification'. Socialisation was considered important to prevent the depressed soldier from isolating himself. Overall, this form of rehabilitation provided a regime that encouraged the soldier to regain his pride and sense of responsibility and duty in a 'controlled paramedical and paramilitary atmosphere' which would 'discourage the development of invalid reactions but permit the salvaging of missed therapeutic opportunities'. The motto was 'discipline, skill, morale' (Palmer 1945b). The programme had a number of elements: military and physical training, recreation, education, medical and psychiatric supervision, religious support and welfare. It was graduated into three levels: the truly convalescent who had been recently sick; the main training company; and the 'hardening high-grade' company for those about to be moved on. At these centres the personnel selection officer interviewed the men and arranged for their reallocation where necessary (Palmer 1945b).

Rehabilitation was often poorly resourced, there being no specially trained instructors available or materials provided. This led to ad hoc arrangements which relied on the generosity of local civilians and the ingenuity of the commanding officer (Pearce 1945b; Wilde and Morgan 1943). Rickman and his colleague Sergeant Bryant instituted military training as occupational therapy in Wharncliffe partly as a practical response to this lack of equipment. The training for certain groups of partly trained professionals such as masseurs and arts and craft teachers was shortened in order to increase the supply of appropriate personnel (Kersley 1942).

Much emphasis was placed on physical exercise as a supportive rehabilitation measure. It was divided into three grades: convalescent, light and full. At Mill Hill, as elsewhere, it was provided under military instruction (Minski 1944). Its effect on effort syndrome was debatable, some finding in those cases carefully diagnosed that it was not helpful, and others finding that it was (Baker and Tegner 1945; Hill and Dewar 1945).

Outcomes

In military psychiatry the only really relevant measure of effectiveness is the number of capable soldiers returning to some form of service. Relief of symptoms is of secondary significance, a view that is beginning to regain ground in psychiatry today. As remarked on before, follow-up of patients was almost impossible. Crude figures for return to active service do not reflect how long individuals remained with their units subsequently. Thus the following section is inevitably flawed and impressionistic. Furthermore, had the figures been accurate they could never have been sensitive enough to indicate subtleties such as the impact of the returnees on their units. A well-respected sergeant offering 2–3 weeks of effective service at the height of a battle would have had an important impact on improving morale at a crucial time. In contrast, returning unstable men who were unreliable would have had a deleterious effect. Perhaps the most important skill of the psychiatrist was making this judgement and, in liaison with unit officers, ensuring the most effective outcome.

There were three immediate outcomes of treatment: return to full duties, redeployment, or discharge from the army. Which of these was chosen depended very heavily on the specialist's opinion and practice could vary from individual to individual (Hadfield 1942).

Psychiatric disorders made up a third of all discharges from the army on medical grounds in the years 1943–1945, and contributed to an increasing rate of discharge over those years. The next-most-frequent medical conditions were battle casualties, which by 1945 made up one-sixth, and peptic ulceration, which contributed 10 per cent (War Office 1948 p.3). The psychological aspects of the latter were well recognised (Ahrenfeldt 1958, p. 276). In 1943, nearly 0.7 per cent of all ranks were being discharged on psychiatric grounds. By 1945, this had increased to over 1 per cent. Neuroses made up the bulk of these figures.

Anxiety neurosis rose from less than half to nearly two-thirds of all psychiatric discharges between 1943 and 1945. The second-most-frequent diagnosis leading to discharge on psychiatric grounds was hysterical neurosis, which declined in relative importance over the three years. Mental illness in the form of schizophrenia and Manic Depressive disorder was of relatively little significance. Personality disorders contributed a relatively constant sixth of the total psychiatric disorders (see figure 4.1) (War Office 1948, p. 3)

Early in the war, battle casualties received psychiatric treatment in EMS hospitals, often after a significant delay. The results were poor. In Sutherland's 100 cases of soldiers who had seen active service, 72 were discharged from the army, 19 were working on a lower grade of service and only nine returned successfully to full duties (1941). In his study of 2000 cases of neurosis, Slater found similarly poor results. A quarter returned to full duty, half of whom had to be invalided out within twelve months (1943).

The return to 'civvy street' usually left the soldier worse off than before. A small number of studies were carried out, which revealed that they were more likely to be unemployed, be in trouble with the police, have domestic difficulties and have continuing neurotic problems than before the war. The first enquiry was carried out by face-to-face interview, often including the spouse, of ex-soldiers who had been discharged after treatment in a neurosis centre. This was done, on average, six and a half months after their leaving military service. Although it relied on self-report it can still be regarded as giving a relatively accurate picture. Of 120 cases, 11 had never gained employment and 53 were earning less than before enlistment, 44 of whom were carrying out 'light or desultory work' (Lewis 1943). This was at a time when the employment prospects were fairly good (Calder 1994, pp. 322–323). For 39 men there were social problems, mostly as result of violent outbursts of temper or irritability, making them very difficult to live with. Two had become vagrants. In 62 cases their mental health had markedly deteriorated. Lewis concluded that if they had been prevented from joining up through the use of proper selection methods, they would have maintained a better social and employment history, contributing effectively to the war effort rather than detracting from it (Lewis 1943).

Stalker saw 130 ex-servicemen discharged on mental health grounds, as outpatients and found that 103 should never have been accepted into the services on account of their pre-existing difficulties. Few had been exposed to real military stress such as combat or prolonged service. Half the men had been unemployed for six months or more and 29 had committed offences known to the police (Stalker 1944). These studies took place in the United Kingdom after the retreat from Dunkirk. At this time treatment and disposal still relied on the Emergency Medical Service, in which the men were in-patients and subject to long periods of inactivity. Selection procedures still had to be organised, and the Annexure scheme for redeployment had not been instituted. All these factors contributed to the poor outcome, and provided ammunition for those who wished to improve the system. Aftercare was disorganised and caused immense stress to civilian services, whilst failing to prepare the ex-soldier for his new tasks (*Lancet* 1943; Industrial Medical Officer 1943; Lewis 1943).

Despite improvements in army selection and management, a more comprehensive study carried out later revealed similar problems after discharge. This surveyed a sample of 382 cases from both rural and industrial areas, including Birmingham. Again it was found that there was a great deal of maladjustment in the fields of both work and family. The men continued to complain of neurotic problems fifteen months after their discharge. Three-quarters of them had neurotic problems before enlistment. Similarly, three-quarters required medical attention after discharge. Of the 72 who wished for psychiatric advice, only 22 received it because of lack of available services. Only six per cent were still unemployed, but overall, one in ten working days were being lost due to sickness and absenteeism. Again, one in ten had four different jobs within fifteen months. Ten per cent had social problems (Guttman and Thomas 1946).

Following the establishment of forward psychiatry, the picture in the field of combat changed markedly. The acuteness of the cases, the lack of predisposing constitutional factors, the rapidity of treatment and the availability of alternative employment opportunities all combined to give much improved results. In North Africa, nine-tenths returned to duty after treatment, more than half of whom went back to full duties. Only a twentieth were invalided out of the army (Torrie 1944; Palmer 1945b reported similar figures). In northern Europe nearly all were retained in the army, and again just over a twentieth were discharged. However, only 17.6 per cent returned to full duties, and the rest were recategorised or relocated under the Annexure scheme (Brooke 1946).

From these rather sketchy figures it can be seen that early in the war the results of treatment were poor. Men finished up being returned to civilian life as failures, worse off than before they joined the services. The impact of forward psychiatry cannot be measured directly, because no study disentangled the results from the many other confounding variables. However, the outcomes for the survivors of Dunkirk were much less satisfactory than for the men in Italy, northern Europe, the Middle and Far East, and wherever rapid reaction services were established.

Minds the dead have ravished: Summary

Wilfred Owen's poem 'Mental Cases' from the First World War paints a picture of torment and anguish in the romantic tradition, echoing the paintings of Hogarth. The real picture was duller, drearier and drier, men were pushed to the edge of their resources, usually through exhaustion, and became isolated, bewildered and ashamed. Organising a system of care that maximised their abilities as soldiers, whilst releasing those who could no longer achieve a suitable role, was fraught with subtle complexities that could never be entirely satisfied. Clearly, in certain circumstances, people who were unsuited to ordinary soldiering could become heroes. The pioneer corps during the retreat to Dunkirk exemplified this. To devise a system, from a zero base, to account for this was patently impossible. It thus became easy to snipe at the changes once the war was over. Inevitably there would be individual cases, perhaps many hundreds of them, that appeared to demonstrate the failure of the system.

In order to affect morale, forward psychiatrists would have had to be chameleons, blending in with the attitudes of the regiments and units they were attached to so as to avoid outright rejection of their ideas. Wishart describes the hostility that he faced initially in North Africa. Most of these doctors were young and inexperienced, and likely to be opposed to the more rigid ideas of military discipline, which were often held most vigorously by their generalist medical colleagues. For instance, the literature demonstrates that few of them would have been comfortable with the term 'malingering', preferring to frame that which it referred to in psychological terms. To defend this approach against the traditional views of cowardice, 'lack of morale fibre', 'skrim shankers' and 'yellow steak' would have been uphill work. Interestingly, it was civilian psychiatrists who tended to hold a position closer to this than those recruited into the army. In stark contrast, the Royal Air Force psychiatrists largely adopted the traditional value-ridden attitude lock, stock and barrel.

It is against this background of prejudice, shared by politicians as well, that the achievements of army psychiatry have to be seen. Every improvement had to be fought for, and inexperienced personnel had to be trained rapidly. Seen in this light, the results were extraordinary. The effects spread throughout the army, from the United Kingdom to North Africa and the Far East. The burden was carried by less than 400 psychiatrists and psychologists in an army that in 1945 was two and a quarter million strong (Baynes 1972 p. 27).

CHAPTER 5

The Northfield Military Hospital

There once was a psychoneurotic,
Whose behaviour was most idiotic
He preferred doing piquet,
to seeking his ticket,
and his rational moods were spasmodic.
So to Northfield they sent him ...[1]

A HAPPY CONFLUENCE: THE HOSPITAL, ITS STAFF AND THE SOLDIERS

As Foulkes declared, the key to the Northfield Experiments was the company of people who participated (1948, p.18). Each of the leading figures interacted with at least one significant other. Ideas flowed from discussion, some of which has been recorded. To be in the thick of the enthusiasm, enterprise, and intellect reverberating around the building was exciting and stimulating. It also provoked rivalries, jealousies and exaggeration.

The others who contributed were the largely anonymous soldiers who passed through. Once their energies were liberated from the bonds of neurosis, they became a significant force. The most potent source of therapy was the help they gave to each other. A number were, or later became, poets, musicians, artists or writers, and during their stay became involved in the magazines, band or art groups. For others their stay was less creative. At different times therapies were misguided or absent. Even much of the group therapy was amateurish and experimental, particularly the psychodrama. The Northfield Experiments proper only affected a minority. It is important, however, to remember the less visionary but equally compassionate staff who provided thoughtful, sensitive and effective care for many soldiers. The

---

1 Anonymous poem from *Psyche*, a magazine produced by the patients at Northfield, 1943.

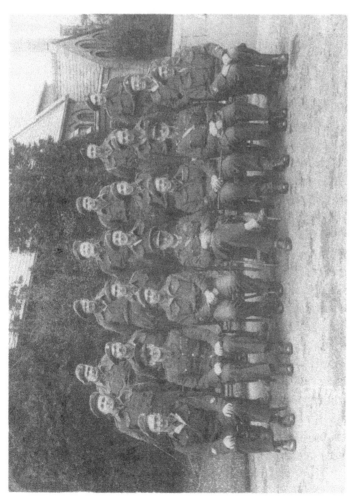

Administration Staff, Northfield Military Hospital, 26 April 1946
From left to right: (back row) Sgt. French (General Office), Sgt. Lilles (Pay clerk); (middle row) Sgt. Humphrey (i/c Charles Ward), Sgt. Bradbury (Art Therapist), Sgt. Tucker (Education Corps), Sgt. Gaskin (i/c Discipline), Sgt. Jones, S/Sgt. Smith, Sgt. Connolly (Hospital Office); (front row) C.Q.M.S. Watson, Major Finlayson (Hospital Registrar), R.S.M. Pickford, Colonel Rowlette (Commanding Officer), Sgt. Maj. Ebdale, Lt. Newton (Company Commander), C.S.M. Howsen.
(Reproduced by kind permission of Irene Gaskin; information about individuals kindly provided by Irene and the late Same Gaskin, and Professor Laurence Bradbury)

anonymous corporal from the medical corps holding the hand of a man crying on VJ day because the World seemed such an impossible place was just such a person (Interview: Mr H. 1994). Equally, there were the local women, fascinated by the strange, stammering, mute men. They took them out for walks, danced with them, brought them cigarettes and chocolates, and last but not least, married a few.

In this section some idea is given of the environment in which the reformers worked. This relies almost entirely on the accounts of people who were there, and their recollections up to half a century later. For the sake of veracity, where possible more than one piece of testimony is given to support a particular observation. However, this was not always possible, and some descriptions are given verbatim, without such confirmatory backing. This is done when the story appears to be supported by circumstantial evidence, or when it was given by someone who has supplied other credible information. It is clearly impossible to ensure absolute accuracy after so much time, and for this reason all the main contributors remain anonymous, although the author is able to identify all the witnesses and many of the staff members described.

The crucible: Hollymoor Hospital and its staff
The red brick wilderness: The building

Hollymoor Hospital was a traditional late-Victorian asylum. It was typical in consisting of a series of large open wards connected by long and seemingly endless corridors, which could accommodate a maximum of 800 patients. It was set in attractive grounds, originally a farm, in close proximity to an older and larger Birmingham asylum, Rubery Hill Hospital. Rayner Heppenstall described Hollymoor as a 'small brick wilderness' engulfed by the red brick rash of Birmingham as it extended southward (1953, pp.86–87). He drew attention to its most famous landmark, regularly referred to by all who know the area: the water tower visible for miles around.

At the beginning of the war, in September 1939, Hollymoor was taken over as an Emergency Medical Service hospital. The previous residents, people suffering from mental illness, had been transferred to other psychiatric hospitals in the Birmingham area six days earlier (Hollymoor Hospital Records 1920–1939). Hollymoor's intended use was to provide treatment facilities in anticipation of the large number of air-raid casualties expected, but in the event it served mainly as a sick bay for nearby military units, and as a convalescent service for local general hospitals. It only once had a role in a major emergency, when over 1000 casualties were admitted in the space of two weeks during the evacuation of Dunkirk in May 1940 (Hollymoor Hospital Records 1939–1942).

The War Office requested that Hollymoor be handed over to them in January 1942. The Mental Hospitals Committee of the Birmingham City Council agreed to this 'after due consideration', and it became a military hospital on 1 April 1942 (Birmingham City Council 1942). Its fundamental task then was to be a rehabilitation unit for soldiers suffering from neurotic problems. They were to be transferred from other units that had not been able to achieve a satisfactory recovery within their resources. Only those for whom there was some possibility of returning to active service in some capacity within the army were supposed to be selected. However, this did not always happen, and men with a great variety of complaints were housed there at different times. Dennis Carroll, the commanding officer, complained regularly in 1944 that many of the patients being accommodated were inappropriate, took up too much of the staff's time, and prevented good work being done with those who could best benefit from it (Carroll 1944a, b and c).

It is unclear why Hollymoor was selected for such work. It had served, in conjunction with the nearby Rubery Hill Hospital, as a military surgical unit during the First World War. Then the advantage had been the location of a railway station nearby (Birmingham Asylums Committee 1915; 1920). Some participants believed that this was still the reason for its selection for the same purpose during the next war, although most accounts describe people arriving by road or via the station in the city centre (e.g. Dewar 1993). However, an interesting alternative was put forward by Haas. He suggested that the hospital was selected because it was in the radar shadow of the nearby Lickey Hills and was thus less vulnerable to German bombing (Haas 1989). Indeed, it did escape all air raids on Birmingham, the only mishap being that a 'friendly' anti-aircraft shell exploded in one of the cellars (Hollymoor Hospital 1956).

Initially the hospital did not run at full capacity. As a consequence it could host a conference on the 'stability factor' in assessment of new recruits in July 1942. Eighty-nine military psychiatrists were resident for one week, which must have represented the majority of those in the army at that time. They included many who later worked at Northfield (MacKeith 1942; Markillie 1993). Lilian Hewitt recalls that initially there were only about 50 patients (1989). By the end of the year the numbers had increased so that the rehabilitation wing contained between 100 and 200 soldiers, although Rickman's ward only held 14 men (Bion and Rickman 1943). Later, as the hospital approached its official capacity, some wards were lined with beds and bunks, including down the centre of the dormitory, and on one

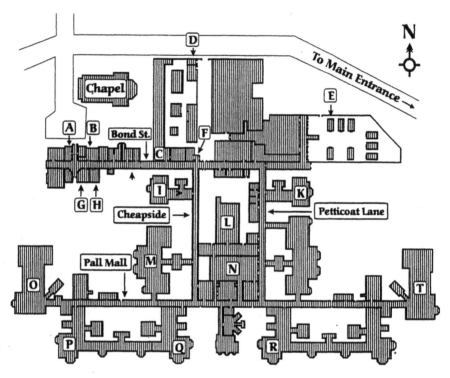

Key:

A - Telephone Office
B - General Office
C - Pathology Laboratory (Sergeant's
Mess Above)
D - Guard Room
E - Art Hut in Activities Yard
F - Admissions Office
G - Registrar's Office
H - Commanding Officer
1 - Henry and Arthur Wards

K - Medical Wards (Anne & Adelaide)
L - Kitchens
M - Officer's (staff) Mess
N - Main Hall and Dining Room
O - Charles Ward
P - Hospital Club and Mercury Office
Q - George and Edward Wards
R - Elizabeth and Caroline Wards
T - Officer's Ward with A.T.S. quarters
above

Pall Mall, Cheapside, Bond St. & Petticoat Lane - Names for the Hospital Corridors.

Plan of Northfield Military Hospital c.1945
With thanks to Laurence Bradbury, Irene and the late Sam Gaskin and others

particular occasion patients were sleeping on blankets in the corridors (Interviews: Mr G. 1995; Mr L. 1998, p.65; Mr N. 1994; Gaskin and Gaskin 1990).

Following the recommendations first put forward by John Rickman, the military authorities split the hospital into two. The eastern wards were named after British queens and acted as a medical and treatment wing, with a nominal 200 beds. The other half, where the wards were named after kings, was the training wing, and had up to 600 beds. Foulkes described the two as being separated by a military guard on duty in the corridor, although no other witnesses have confirmed this (1948, p.45).

A further distinction was that whereas the soldiers in the rehabilitation wing wore normal battle dress with a blue epaulet, those undergoing treatment had to wear 'the blues'. This latter consisted of 'a white flanellette shirt, a red tie, a pair of socks and bright blue jacket, waistcoat and trousers', clothes which meant that they were easily identified by the local population and became the targets for abuse such as 'skrim-shankers' and worse (Foulkes 1948; Heppenstall 1953, p.88; Hewitt 1989). This uniform was not much liked. Mr O. described it as 'the most degrading thing I could think of' (1995, p.9). Some managed to avoid this humiliation. Mr N. managed to convince the authorities that he didn't need to wear it, and he wasn't alone in achieving this (Interview: Mr N. 1994, pt.1, p.40). Because he was in the hospital band, and as part of his rehabilitation was playing in other venues, Mr. O. also used his powers of persuasion so that he could wear his proper battle dress on these occasions (1995, p.40).

In and out of khaki: Military and civilian staff

The hospital was run as a specifically military establishment, with military personnel taking most functions including administration, nursing, pharmacy and catering. There were a number of Queen Alexandra Imperial Militaryl Nursing Service (QAIMNS) nurses, including a matron for the whole establishment and sisters running each treatment ward. Their work was supplemented by Auxillary Territorial Service (ATS) workers and Royal Army Medical Corps (RAMC) orderlies. Many of the latter would have had considerable experience of psychiatric nursing, often in senior positions, before the war. Crew pointed out that it was a source of grievance that their pay and prospects for promotion were markedly inferior to that of the QAIMNS nurses, who were equivalent to commissioned officers in rank and yet were usually much less knowledgeable in this field (Crew 1955, p.472).

There were regimental military police, and a sergeant in charge of discipline (Foulkes 1948; Gaskin and Gaskin 1990). Pay parades were held in the Great Hall, with 10 shillings a week issued to each patient in 1943, along with cigarette coupons (Interviews: Mr M. 1994, p.7; Mrs O. 1995, p.9). This had risen to 14 shillings 18 months later (Anon, undated). This was at a time when it cost 2/6 to go to the cinema and 6d for a pint of beer, and the average wage for a male was between £5 and £6 (Interview: Mr M. 1994, p.7; Calder 1994, p.352).

Weekly parades were held for the military staff. Mr P., then a corporal in administration, remembered someone

> putting their head around the door and saying 'Sam, don't forget the parade', and you're then, you're deep in conversation, and 'I'm sorry, I'll have to go, I've just got to attend the parade', you know, and sure enough, just outside and you're a soldier again, you know, and there we are. He'd done the inspection and 'alright you're dismissed' and you're back to your respective duties. (Interview: Mr P. 1993, p.20)

Drill in the RAMC was very different to the infantry. Sergeant G. having been in the Green Howards, was picked to lead the parades because, he explained, 'I had – well, a better understanding of the way they used to parade' (Interview: Mr G. 1995). Anthony recorded that Foulkes' salute was a 'somewhat bizarre manual gesture that could have meant anything from "stand at ease" to "come and have a cup of coffee"' (1983, p.29).

In 1947 the commanding officer was making weekly parades around the wards. It was expected that the patients would 'be properly dressed and stand to their beds' for this (Harding 1947).

There were still civilian workers in some departments, such as hospital engineering, X-ray, the laundry and the laboratories. The latter were run by Dr Pickworth, who, in conjunction with Dr T.C. Graves, had an international reputation for his theories of focal sepsis as a cause of mental illness (Scull 1996). The conflict between the military and civilian groups is well illustrated by one incident. Sergeant Gaskin, who was in charge of discipline, was parading a miscreant member of the military staff outside the front door, barking orders in true parade-ground style, when an officer beckoned to him from his office. This latter made the recommendation that he should perhaps carry out the punishment elsewhere. When Sergeant Gaskin argued that he should continue where he was, the officer drew his attention to the fact that the hospital engineer's wife had a shotgun trained on him from her house at the entrance to the grounds (Gaskin and Gaskin 1990).

Most of the military staff lived in the hospital. One of the wards, normally used for a maximum of 32 patients, was the residence of 70 ATS workers, who had to sleep in bunks (Gaskin and Gaskin 1990). The doctors lived in the mess, previously the nurses' home. Lewsen described the bedrooms as cell-like (1993). Some of the commanding officers, who had families, resided in the medical superintendent's house in the grounds. Married officers were quartered in local accommodation outside of the hospital because of the lack of room. In 1944, Markillie and his family lived with the widow of Cadbury's chief chemist in West Heath, about three miles away (Markillie 1993). Corporal G. only spent the nights he was on guard duty in the hospital; otherwise, he cycled eight miles from another suburb of Birmingham each day (Interview: Mr G. 1995).

The view from inside: Accounts of the hospital at work

Staggering up the drive: Arrival

Men arrived at the hospital by ambulance, taxi and truck, but most often they came by rail to Birmingham and then took the tram to Longbridge.

> I remember coming along the Bristol Road, the dual carriageway, and looked over the road, sort of thing, and there was those huge iron gates. It looked like a prison gate, wrought iron gates, a long drive behind them and they were locked. We went and they had to wait and send for somebody to come and unlock the gate for you to go in. (Interview: Mr L. 1998, p.15)

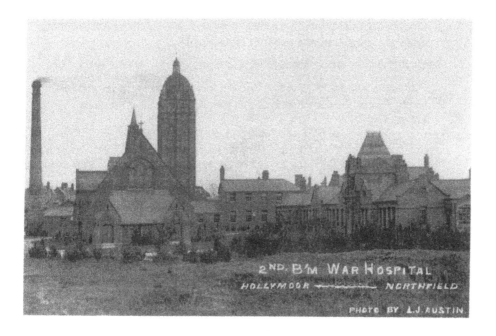

Northfield Military hospital in the First World War. It had changed little by 1945 and presented the same grim outlook to the men arriving there for the first time.
Reproduced by kind permission of Mary Harding.

The drive up to the hospital figures in everyone's memory – ex-staff, visitors and patients. Charles Lewsen, the physician, still had dreams about it fifty years later (1993). Mr A recalls struggling up the hill with his suitcase, feeling hot and sweaty as it was summertime (Interview: Mr A. 1990).

Foulkes gave a graphic account of the patient's arrival at the hospital:

> The patient arriving at the hospital after these inquiries had a five mile journey from Birmingham on a rickety tram before walking nearly a mile uphill with his kit... Standing at the end of the drive it presented a forbidding institutional appearance... The remoteness of the hospital and the length of the drive are very much part of the picture, and were the constant subject of jokes by troops and staff alike (1948, p.43).

This picture is confirmed over and again: 'And then we went up this long drive and then we were received into the place and they took our uniforms off us and issued us with the blue coats and blue trousers and they didn't fit' (Interview: Mr L. 1998, p.16). The only dissenting account is Ronald Markillie's observation that the trams weren't actually that rickety! (1993).

Mr N. arrived on a gloomy day in 1945. At the top of the drive

> there was this brick building. A very large – I've seen bigger – but large brick, and I think brick-tiled roof, red-tiled roof. Very obviously either a jail or a mental asylum... Slightly heavy, I won't say menacing or foreboding or anything imaginative like that, just a damn dreary looking brick building. (Interview: Mr N. 1994, pt.1).

Similar thoughts went through Mr. L's mind:

> I thought you know it really, it looks like a medieval building, sort of thing, where they used to lock the people up for life (Interview: Mr L. 1998, p.19).

Heppenstall's novel, *The Lesser Infortune*, gives an accurate account of life there in 1943, and provides a vivid contemporary account of the environs as Bion and Rickman would have known them. On arrival the new soldier went to the guard room, a small outhouse by the back-entrance of the hospital. Here he was met by an orderly who placed his luggage on a trolley, and then led him down a labyrinth of corridors to the admissions office.

Just ahead of him was a staff-seargent in the Army Catering Corps, who had evidently seen a great deal of active service to judge by the number of medals he was wearing. He had to wait whilst this man underwent questioning by the clerk. Then, whilst he was being interrogated about his own details including his hobbies, the staff-sergeant was led into another room by a young lady in the uniform of the Auxiliary Territorial Service and wearing Royal Army Medical Corps badges. Moments later the other man emerged looking very shame-faced, and he in turn was ushered through the door. After asking him to take his shirt and vest off, the woman minutely examined his arm-pits and then indicated that he should remove his trousers, whereupon she closely inspected his groin.

After being told to dress he then went to the reception ward to await allocation to one of the treatment teams. Here he was physically examined by one of the physicians and interviewed by the senior psychiatrist. This latter he described as being the 'world's greatest authority on bed-wetting'. This was possibly either Backus or Mansell, who later published a paper on their work at Northfield on enuresis in soldiers (Backus and Mansell 1944). After an initial psychiatric interview he was then transferred to one of the psychiatric wards (Heppenstall 1953; Lewsen 1993; Foulkes 1948).

Thorner described this as he saw it occurring in a number of different military hospitals throughout the war, and at Northfield the process would have been similar, with minor variations depending on the individual psychiatrist involved. First, a decision would have been made about whether or not the patient was suicidal. If so, then he was confined to bed. The first psychiatric interview was usually short, the purpose being to get a rough idea of the main complaints. The opportunity would be taken to inform the patient how the hospital functioned, his duties and privileges, and the choices of occupation open to him. The soldier then had to write out an account of his illness with the assistance of typed guidance notes. Thorner employed special tests to examine certain aptitudes and studied the psychiatric social history with the man. All this material helped to build up a complete picture of the patient (Thorner 1946).

Overcoats in summer: The wards, discipline and the clinical staff

The views of the medical wards were varied. One man found that 'the conditions were terrible, with double bunks' (Interview: Mr M. 1994, p.4). Another found in his ward 'of all things a luxury, a real bed. Iron, you know? A little locker, one shelf, top shelf, a hard chair' (Interview: Mr N. 1994, pt.1, p.3).

The conditions were spartan. The

hospital itself was a very bare sort of building. It was a sort of Victorian place where there weren't any sort of easy chairs or settees or anything like that and the floors were all bare, no curtains up at the windows, and of course you'd got these old iron beds and you lay in long rows. The wards held as many as forty or fifty people and they were all side by side down these wards. And each door was locked at night... and the heating was very poor. There wasn't any central heating or anything like that you know it was terrible. And the floors were all stone floors. (Interview: Mr L. 1998, p.36)

On some units, particularly Henry Ward, security was a high priority. 'All the doors were locked'. This made Mr M. angry: 'The windows in the ward, they were up and down windows, and if you raised the bottom it would only raise six inches, and the top only dropped six inches, so therefore you couldn't get out or anything like that, because it was – it had been an asylum' (Interview: Mr M. 1994, p.5).

The sense of being continually watched over could intrude into the most private of areas:

if you went to the loo you didn't get total privacy. There was that gap under the door, and it didn't come any higher than your chest. So if you were sensitive, or you wanted to read or go to sleep or whatever, now and then you might just find an orderly coming just – and all of a sudden there was a face. 'I don't wish to see your face up there. Do you mind kindly removing yourself?' You didn't say that; but you felt 'Oh God!' You know it took a bit of coping with, did that. (Interview: Mr N. 1994, pt.1, p.9)

The half doors on the toilets, 'all polished wood', upset others as well, especially when there was 'someone on duty looking over the place' (Interview: Mr I. 1996).

As one might expect, the officers' ward was more congenial. One resident recalled: 'I mean it was very comfortable, as I remember it, you know. It was very pleasant. It was a nice little holiday', and 'it was quite like a sort of nice sitting room as I remember. Rather like an officers' mess, really' (Interview: Mr K. 1994, p.4).

Another feature was the corridors: 'Well, to start off with there's this incredibly long corridor. That's the thing that sticks in my mind' (Interview: Mr N. 1994, pt.2, p.1). What impressed Foulkes was that 'once inside, the hospital was as uncomfortable as the approach to it and its appearance would suggest – echoing stone corridors and enormous barely furnished wards, many of the doors locking' (1948, p.43). Another man was taken on admission 'into this hideous long corridor, which was tiled' and 'lit by twenty-five watt bulbs every fifty yards' (Interview: Mr F. 1992, pp.1, 11).

The resident staff could be equally unhappy. Mrs O., the telephonist, had to live in the hospital: 'I was quite horrified when I first walked in to this large room with all these bunk beds, rows and rows of bunk beds, and that was our billet' (Interview: Mrs O. 1995, p.8).

A constant feature was confinement to the hospital after 8 o'clock in the evening, which most men found onerous and oppressive. The staff also appear to have largely turned a blind eye to the constant stream of men leaving the hospital through the windows to go to the local pubs to get a drink. Mr L. described how the system operated. The patients

> used to try to get out of the hospital at night because you had to be in by eight o'clock of an evening, and of course you were used to being up till ten or eleven. So they used to get out at night for an hour or two. Two or three would cover for you in the hospital while you were out and let you back in. So all sorts used to go on; because they used to let you go down the grounds of the pub. You could have a drink if you could, you weren't allowed in the pub; but if you could get someone to buy you one to bring you one outside you were alright so you, you could have one. Then you used to get back and...one or two of the lads would let you in, you see, and they'd let you in and close it up after. And they'd cover for you, because there used to be a patrol at night. They used to have these male nurses come in and make sure everyone was in their bed; but they'd cover for you. One would get in your bed while you were out sort of thing, and then move on to the next bed. They'd cover for you so it was a bit of a game. (Interview: Mr L. 1998, pp.85–86)

In 1946, Corporal P. was sometimes the on-duty Fire Piquet Officer overnight. This entailed guard duty as well. Men had to book out their leave passes with him.

> Now on the odd occasion the time limit had expired, and you'd see a furtive figure dart quickly past the guard room, you see. And to combat this what I used to do towards that time – obviously I had a crew with me, you see – and I'd say, 'take over', and I would hide. Yeah, I would hide down the corridor and wait for them to come past, you see, and just step out and nab them. I gave them a caution, you know but. They must be in on time, otherwise they'd forfeit the pass. (Interview: Mr P. 1993, p.10)

Discipline as a whole never really measured up to the standards expected elsewhere in the army. Typically, ex-patients reported along the lines of: 'But they used to close their eyes to a lot of things at Northfield. It was very loose really', or 'Strict? No, they weren't strict. Because we were left to our own devices' (Interview: Mr M. 1994, p.5; Mr O. 1995, p.30). For Mr P., the standards were very low compared with other units: 'it was easy' (Interview: Mr P. 1993, p.20). Mr. F. enjoyed the freedom: 'indeed you could go out whenever you liked actually. Nobody did anything, even you went out on other days. So there wasn't a real feeling of incarceration at all' (Interview: Mr F. 1992, p.2).

The public house was out of bounds, ostensibly because alcohol didn't mix with the medication. If you were wearing the blues 'you weren't supposed to be sold alcohol. So everybody had their greatcoat on, buttoned up to the neck in the middle of summer to go and get a pint' (Interview: Mr

O. 1995, p.3). This was well recognised by all the local landlords and their regulars. Mrs Hewitt saw them as a young woman when she was in the King George V with her husband. The soldiers would come in with their long coats buttoned up so that you couldn't see the uniform underneath, trying to get a drink which the landlord would refuse them (Hewitt 1989).

Serious breaches of discipline were treated more rigorously. Mr B. left the hospital without leave to visit his relatives. He was recaptured after ten days, and had to spend a fortnight in 'Jankers' – the guardroom (Interview: Mr B. 1990).

One of the areas where people congregated was the Navy, Army and Air Force Institute (NAAFI), which sold tobacco and confectionary. Coupons were given for the equivalent of 40 cigarettes a week, and these were exchanged there. Both Mrs Hewitt and one of her successors, Mrs O., would give out extras to patients 'if they were sweet' (Hewitt 1989; Interview: Mrs O. 1995, p.9). Members of staff would go there as well. Laurence Bradbury, the art therapist, was amongst those who would play the piano sometimes (Gaskin and Gaskin 1990; Interview: Mrs O. 1995, p.30).

WEARING THE BLUES: BEING A PATIENT

Most of the patients were 'other ranks', which distinguished them from the doctors, who were all officers. They came to the hospital after having had a number of earlier interviews and treatments in other units. There was a considerable procedure involved in referrals being made, and it was only done if the local psychiatrist felt he couldn't manage the task (Foulkes 1948). There was usually a complete history already prepared before their admission (Dewar 1990).

Different types of patient arrived at the hospital as the war wore on. For the first two years up until D Day they were mainly men who had not seen combat and were preparing for the opening of the Second Front. The second phase was marked by the return of soldiers who had experienced combat in northern Europe, and lasted up until the end of the war there. Next came the prisoners of war from Germany, and finally a varied collection of individuals, including prisoners of war from the Far East, conscripts who joined the army after the cessation of hostilities, and a varied bag of others. This last stage was particularly marked by rapid turnover of staff and patients. The main aim of it all appears to have been to get demobbed, and there was a general sense of purposelessness.

The morale of the soldier arriving at the hospital was usually very low. He had been assessed at a number of other units and was coming to believe that he was to be discharged from the army. He would have seen many like him being invalided out, and might have known that he would achieve the same end if he was regarded as equally ill (Lewis and Slater 1952, p.398). On the other hand, many witnesses describe just being bewildered and confused. Mr A. was interviewed by a number of medical officers before being sent to the hospital. No one explained where he was being sent or why (Interview: Mr A. 1990). This was a common experience: many men were given no explanation about the purpose of their referral or where they were going (Interview: Mr B. 1990; Mr C. 1990; Mr D. 1990). 'It was a kind of uncertain state. You didn't know really whether you were a weekend visitor or there for life' (Interview: Mr N. 1994, pt.1, p.9). 'I didn't feel I had been sent to a hospital. You know I didn't think I needed to go that far' (Interview: Mr L. 1998, p.13). Another man arrived 'very late at night, having got lost in Birmingham, and I thought 'My God, I've made a terrible mistake. I'm going to be incarcerated in this place for the rest of my life', and he believed 'at last I have made a totally disastrous mistake' (Interview: Mr F. 1992, pp.1, 11). At times the attitudes of the staff didn't help: 'Nobody seemed particularly bothered one way or another whether I came or went' (Interview: Mr N. 1994, pt.1, p.1).

There was no systematic collection of data about the patients at the hospital, though a number of papers were published about different therapies. In 1942, however, Hadfield described his experiences in a 'neuropathic' hospital, where he worked with Emanuel Miller, and where conditions were similar to those obtaining during first couple of years at Hollymoor. Their unit, in Bath, was a precursor to Northfield Military Hospital (Ahrenfeldt 1958, p.149). In a ten month period they saw 700 patients. Using the army nomenclature then in use, half were cases marked by anxiety and a quarter had hysterical symptoms. Just under a tenth were men with anti-social personality disorders. A smaller group had psychoses, manic depressive disorders, epilepsy and physical problems. Seven had serious learning difficulties (Hadfield 1942, p.282).

Hadfield and Millar assessed what had precipitated the breakdown for 332 of the soldiers suffering from psychoneurosis. For a third there was no real acute aggravating cause. These men broke down because they could not adapt to army life. Maxwell Jones, in Mill Hill, observed their limited understanding of the world. They rarely read the newspapers and had a very limited conception of the nature and aims of the war. Their home was the centre of their existence, and the rest of the world was vague, ill-defined and threatening (Jones 1942). An example of this, in Northfield, was Mr A. who came in the latter part of 1942, having broken down after being posted away from his home in South Wales. He found the harsh realities of army life difficult to cope with after his strict and loving Presbyterian upbringing, and became tearful, and couldn't eat or sleep (Interview: Mr A. 1990).

In the second group there was some degree of acute strain, 'such as a bomb falling in the neighbourhood', or the evacuation from Dunkirk, without particularly bad conditions affecting them. This group made up about a quarter of the total. In the authors' opinions they were 'of neurotic disposition, some of whom have had previous nervous breakdowns of a mild nature'. As an officer cadet, Mr N. experienced Battle School training before it was reformed into a graduated exercise. This involved strenuous physical training along with thunderflashes (very large fireworks) being thrown near him and rifles being shot over his head, all intended to simulate actual battle conditions. His complaints were of diabolical tensions and a diabolical stomach ache: 'I couldn't relax at all. I've never been able to relax, so I don't think that was anything to do with – I was treating my body harshly.' He also had some evidence of predisposing traits: 'All I was was fussy about the cleanliness. I valued privacy; but I couldn't stand things that were untidy' (Interview: Mr N. 1994, pt.1, p.1).

The third group, about a fifth of the total, had been subjected to more serious conditions such as being wrecked, or evacuated from Dunkirk under persistant machine gun fire, or had been in serious road accidents. There were often predisposing factors in such cases, but they were not always as obvious. They were capable of good work before service and were to be considered as genuine war casualties. The final fifth were those who had experienced severe traumas such as being blown up, being concussed by injury from a bomb or shell fire, or being involved in motor cycle accidents. Occasionally there was evidence of predisposition, but the most important factor was the precipitating cause (Hadfield 1942, pp.282–283). Mr H. was captured by the Germans in North Africa after seeing action outside Tobruk. At times he suffered depression and had considered suicide. On release he started drinking heavily and attacked a company sergeant major (Interview: Mr. H. 1994). After four to five years as a regular soldier in China, Mr M. saw action in North Africa, and narrowly evaded capture on a Greek Island, where a number of his 'mates' were killed. 'I was blown up. A bomb burst in front of me. There was a Stuka, there were a dozen Stukas and they were just floating overhead and one of them broke formation and came down'. He had amnesia for a period of two to three months and also attacked two recruits he was supposed to be training, and was taken to Northfield (Interview: Mr M. 1994, p.2). An early patient at Northfield, Mr B., was 'shot up at point blank range' before being evacuated from Dunkirk. Later, he was driving a target around Catterick when he was shot at with live shells. As a result he attacked a corporal and was knocked out (Interview: Mr B. 1990).

The final diagnostic group was also represented at Hollymoor. Mr F. had 'misused explosives rather gravely' whilst on an officer training course. He was diagnosed as a 'psychopathic personality with emotional instability' at the age of eighteen and a half (Interview: Mr F. 1994, p.1).

Other early patients at Northfield included a German scientist who had escaped from a concentration camp, and a nephew of Lord Balfour who had been the centre of some publicity, probably because he was homosexual (Interview: Mr A. 1990). Though the hospital was mainly for the army and for individuals with neurotic conditions, throughout the war individuals who didn't fit these categories were also admitted. At different times there were RAF personnel and men suffering from physical conditions (Lewsen 1990).

Their behaviour once admitted was varied, but some themes were common. Withdrawal, mutism and shyness were a regular feature, often noted by visitors. 'A lot of the patients were like that. A lot of them were dumb, they couldn't speak' (Interview: Mrs O. 1995, p.5). At the dances, Mrs C.'s friends would 'fool around and laugh and listen to the music; but they didn't talk. They didn't, honestly. They stammered. They stuttered and stammered. They didn't talk' (Interview: Mrs C. 1994, p.4). Sergeant C. was taken prisoner in North Africa and survived 'severe privations' until his camp was bombed in Vienna. Then he became tense, nervy and suffered battle dreams. On return to the United Kingdom he found that his wife was suffering from congenital syphilis. He was admitted to hospital for jaundice and became depressed, wishing that he had never returned home. He became virtually speechless (Davidson 1946, p.90).

The men themselves related the other side of this story: 'I was sort of very anxious and sort of, and I lost my speech, quite a bit of my speech at the time'; 'you didn't relate to anybody hardly. You sort of kept yourself to yourself and you know you got a bit reserved in your manner and your actions and everything. You never bothered with anybody' (Interview: Mr L. 1998, pp.11–12). 'I just got up and didn't bother anybody'; 'I was just wandering about in a sea of other blokes' (Interview: Mr I. 1996). 'I didn't make any friends, most kept themselves to themselves' (Interview: Mr D. 1990).

Many were depressed and anxious. All of the six ex-prisoners of war in Susannah Davidson's group had depression and anxiety symptoms (Davidson 1946, pp.90–92). Another patient was markedly tremulous after the tank he was in was hit and he was wounded in the right knee (Foulkes 1948, p.94). The effects of this could be extreme. The trembling of some patients was so bad that the beds shook (Dewar 1994). One of Foulkes' patients reported that 'his body ached all over' because of it (Foulkes 1943b).

A recurrent problem was nightmares:

you had nightmares. It was alright during the daytime but at night as soon as you dropped off to sleep all these things re-occurred in your mind and you got these, these hot sweats. You got very hot and sort of clammy. (Interview: Mr L. 1998, p.12)

Mr N. walked about the hospital at night, and wandered into one of the wards where

there was this chap, and it gave me no joy at all, because he suddenly started to moan, in a great sort of shuddering, and he was tossing and turning, throwing himself about in his bed, and obviously he was reliving something…all of the other patients who were sleeping, of course they kept waking up, because he kept waking them up. And he no sooner got to sleep, and after about five minutes, six minutes, it varied, the dream, the nightmare came back and he started again. (Interview: Mr N. 1994, pt.1, pp.8–9)

Many were extremely tense. Some would react out of all proportion to sudden noises:

a number of the officers, and it happened to the men too, they were so ashamed of themselves; because if there was a noise they jumped on the floor in an inkling… And the noise of the trolleys on the wires [of the trams] was unbearable. It was very much like the noise of mortar coming over and they found it agony. In fact some of them just couldn't face it and going on the tram was really quite a nightmare. (Markillie 1993, p.19)

One of the non-commissioned officers in Susannah Davidson's group in August 1945 had been a prisoner of war in Italy and Germany. During this time many of his comrades had died from starvation; he himself had suffered from dysentery and coughed up blood. On arrival at Northfield he was emaciated. He couldn't settle down or mix with people. He was also restless and agitated, and he couldn't stand noise. During his first few days in the hospital he had to be nursed in a side room on his own and given sedatives (Davidson 1946, pp.90, 92).

Similarly, Mr E. tried to work at the Austin Motor Company as part of his rehabilitation, but 'the noise of the pneumatic wrench sounded like machine guns', and he had to request a transfer to another form of work (Interview: Mr E. 1990).

Eccentric or violent behaviour was much less common, but memorable when it happened. In Mr N.'s ward, one man was behaving oddly:

I think he was doing this on purpose, really, rather as though he was facing television cameras. Who he thought was going to applaud or lap it up I don't know; but he would do all sorts of things. He spoke with a very exaggerated...Wooster kind of accent, and actually his origins were not quite that sort of standard. But he shot this terrible line and sort of when he was going about anybody would have thought he was a demoted brigadier... one morning in the NAAFI [he] suddenly decided that was enough. And he got hold of a lemon cheesetart, crammed it on his head and rubbed it into his hair. Well I think that's a bit offbeat. But he did it only to get attention. (Interview: Mr N. 1994, pt.1, pp.7–8)

Another patient (an Irish paratrooper) 'used to rush across the ward and bang his head on the wall' (Interview: Mr C. 1990, p.2).

Mrs Gaskin was called in to help Dr Lewsen manage a tall airman who had become violent and whom no one could approach. She, being female and small and consequently unthreatening, went in. After reassuring himself that she was British, he told her that all the people outside were German. As she agreed with this he became more trusting of her, and was persuaded to take some medication. She continued to visit him occasionally, and later on, once he had recovered, he came to her and thanked her (Gaskin and Gaskin 1990). Other patients stayed a long while in Charles ward, which was specifically allocated to the difficult cases:

> They'd been shell-shocked for months and months and months and they could be very difficult. A lot of them never recuperated sort of thing. They were violent when they came in and they stayed violent and in the end they had to go to a mental home. (Interview: Mr L. 1998, p.64)

The distress of the men was reflected by the suicides, of which there was a steady trickle. There was always 'a sense of failure in the hospital' after one. In one case, Dr Sutton 'attempted comfort by explaining to the bereaved that complete avoidance of the death might have been more cruel, since the patient would have had to be locked up under constant surveillance to suffer a seemingly unending misery of dreadful memories' (Bradbury 1990b). A young pathology technician, Mrs Clayton, recorded four in the winter of 1947 alone (Clayton 1991). One body she recalled seeing had been rescued from a stream. Mrs Gaskin was greeted by the unpleasant sight of a naked man hanging from a tree outside her office one morning (Gaskin and Gaskin 1990). Most of the suicides appear to have occurred outside of the hospital; one particular oak tree, in 'Hanging Lane', was used more than once. Ronald Markillie's introduction to his ward was particularly traumatic. He was called on his first day to one of his patients, whom he had not even met, who 'had cut his throat in the toilets and was dead' (Markillie 1993; p.19). Eighteen months later another officer-patient of his shot himself (p.20).

Most of the men were young, sometimes only just past their eighteenth birthday. One case at least was only fourteen years old (Backus and Mansell 1944). They were also inexperienced in life. Their shyness in front of women was remarked upon by many visitors, and Tom Main found that they often had no idea how to approach them (1984). It is worth noting that many had been exceptional soldiers. At least one had won the Victoria Cross, another the Military Cross, and a third had the Military Medal (Interview: Mr E. 1998; Mr K. 1994; Discussion Group No.4, 1945, p.1). Edkins, in another unit, treated army officers who had psychoneurosis. Of a total of 21, six had the military cross, and one other was recommended for the Victoria Cross and received the Distinguished Conduct Medal (Edkins 1948, p.266). In order to counteract the discrimination from local civilians in Birmingham, Bridger gained permission from the hospital authorities to allow the patients to wear their medals outside. This demonstrated that many of them had distinguished themselves in their service (Bridger 1990b).

'NON-COMBATANT GUILT': THE PRACTITIONERS

The organisation of the clinical staff was rife with potential tensions. There were doctors, nurses from the Queen Alexandra Imperial Military Nursing Service (QAIMNS), Royal Army Medical Corps (RAMC) mental nursing orderlies, Voluntary Aid Detachment (VAD) workers and Auxiliary Territorial Service (ATS) nursing assistants. These were supplemented at different times by a Sergeant Art Therapist, occupational therapists, mental nursing orderlies trained as instructors, and two social workers.

The work was often hard. Carroll was at pains to emphasise the stress that staff underwent when the admissions were high or the patients inappropriate (Carroll 1994a, b and c). Strain also developed from a number of other areas. Amongst the nurses were two groups. The female Queen Alexandra's nurses were officers, the matron being a major and the sisters being lieutenants (War Office 1943b, p.85). They tended to have a general nursing training, there being insufficient dually-qualified nurses available (Ahrenfeldt 1958, p.145). The mental nurses (RMN) could only join as mental nursing orderlies, and were non-commissioned officers despite their greater psychiatric experience. This split could also be repeated between the medical staff. For example, the commanding officer at the time of the Second Northfield Experiment was a pathologist rather than a psychiatrist.

The ward nurses were usually perceived positively by the patients. Mr A. found that he was 'charmingly received' on the ward, and the nurses were 'extremely gracious cultured women' (Interview: Mr A. 1990). After coming round from his continuous narcosis, Mr H. sung praises of some of the nurses: 'They were absolutely first rate you know' (Interview: Mr H. 1994, p.14). However, one senior nurse was an entirely different kettle of fish:

you had the old matron who was a right terror. She used to be like Hitler and she used to stand at the end of the ward and make her inspections each morning and of course you had to abide. And she would tell you if the bed space wasn't right. (Interview: Mr L. 1998, pp.58–59)

Working with psychiatric casualties of war produced mixed feelings. The caring professional approach of ensuring the patient's recovery conflicted sharply with the idea of returning them to war. In addition, the safe and relatively adequate working environment of the male staff, contrasted with the dangers and appalling conditions which the patients had had to endure. In an effort to both explain and contain these anxieties, the term 'non-combatant guilt' was coined. Pat de Maré recalled this being employed at Northfield in 1942, where it formed the focus for discussion groups (1994, p.2).

The psychiatrist had to face the fact that successful therapy could mean providing able men prepared for fighting. This meant that the outcome of assessment, management and treatment was that the patient was exposed to the lethal danger of battle. The pre-eminent role of psychiatry was to assist in defeating the enemy. To this end, short-term objectives became paramount, as Tom Main explained:

If a sergeant can recover his poise for one month, it can be regarded as a satisfactory therapeutic result in an army fighting for its very life, though such a result would not be worth having in civilian life. (quoted in MacKeith 1946a)

Many found this unpalatable. Bion described the dilemma:

One of the difficulties facing a psychiatrist who is treating combatant soldiers is his feeling of guilt that he is trying to bring them to a state of mind in which they will have to face dangers, not excluding loss of life, that he himself is not called upon to face. (Bion 1946)

This ambivalence would have been deepened by the recognition that the soldier's task is also to kill and maim others. For male staff there would have been the temptation to compensate for any sense of inferiority, or even shame, engendered by exposure to those who had been involved in the fighting. But in general this reflective approach, including recognition of counter-transference issues, promoted by the psychodynamic approach became a way of thinking that influenced even those who were not psychoanalytically-orientated (MacKeith 1994; Snowden 1939; Tregold et al. 1946).

All psychiatrists and, indeed, other doctors entering the army had to re-examine their role: 'the psychiatrist's preoccupation with the needs of the individual has to be modified... Time and military needs are pressing'

(Lewis 1940). Hunter insisted that 'The Army psychiatrist must first know his Army, for his patient is the Army rather than the individual. Next he must have a clear picture in his mind of what the ordinary soldier has to face and how he contrives to face it' (Hunter 1946).

Few had previous experience that prepared them for this role. Many were 'young and inexperienced both in Life and their special subject' (*Journal of the Royal Army Medical Corps* 1945). This became increasingly true as the war progressed, the need for specialists outstripped the supply of older, more experienced, individuals and the net had to be cast wider (Crew 1953, p.150). Most junior medical officers early on in the war were ignorant of anxiety states, hysteria and other neurotic conditions (L'Etang 1951, p.193; Lewis and Slater 1952, p.391).

Thorner pointed out that the process worked both ways. The soldier himself would approach all officers with a degree of suspicion, including the doctors (Thorner 1946). This reticence is noticeable in the patients' recollections:

> Yeah, we had to accept what the psychiatrists said, because they were the learned people, sort of thing, and we were sent there for treatment; but we often thought to ourselves actually they hadn't experienced what we'd experienced; but they'd, they'd got the ideas and they were, they knew what they had to do and we accepted that. We had to accept it because you were in the army and you had to do as you were told; but they were, they did a good job in the finish. It worked out. (Interview: Mr L. 1998, pp.44–45)

Another man listened patiently to inappropriate advice from his psychiatrist, but didn't answer back: 'I mean you can't insult a man who's genuine and trying to help, and in any case, if he outranks you it's foolish to start throwing your weight about' (Interview: Mr N. 1994, pt.1, p.17).

However, it is noticeable from interviewing ex-Northfield patients that many of them liked, respected and even felt some ownership of their ('my') psychiatrist. Often this was the only name that they could remember of all the individuals they met during their stay. Stungo, Casson, Foulkes, Mclean, Miller, Captain Day, all have been recalled with affection 50 years later. Mr L. was enthusiastic: 'you got this star treatment and it was a great help. It improved it considerably'; and 'They gave us this therapy stuff and that sort of thing. It helped quite a bit, improved it' (Interview: Mr L. 1998, pp.44–45). Despite ambivalence about his therapeutic aims and treatment methods, one soldier still found that his psychiatrist 'was kind' (Interview: Mr L. 1998, p.12). Others reported, just as simply, that 'he was kind and understanding', or 'Can't remember his name, no, but we seemed to get on reasonably together' (Interview: Mr C. 1990, p.1; Mr K. 1994, p.2).

ZOMBIES AND EMBROIDERY: VIEWS OF TREATMENT

The most common perception was that there was no treatment, apart from the occasional interviews with the doctor. Otherwise, life consisted of going to the NAAFI, Jones' cafe, attending dances, smoking and skiving off to the pub at night. It is difficult to be clear how accurate these perceptions were, given that most of the men were quite unclear about why they were there, what psychiatry was and how their behaviour appeared to others.

On the locked ward, Charles Ward, and during the early days of treatment, a close watch was kept on the patients. 'If you went to the toilet you more or less asked to go sort of thing…and now and again somebody followed you to see you were all right' (Interview: Mr L. 1998, p.35). Another man found it particularly irksome:

> If you went through one door to go into the next ward, a nurse used to come, or an orderly used to come, unlock the door. You went through the door, and it closed behind you, and it was locked. It was automatic…it was only an asylum. I mean to say at the bottom of the ward there was – what do you call it? There was a – where they used to put violent – padded cell. (Interview: Mr M. 1994, p.5)

The supervision in the toilet area has already been mentioned. This rigour relaxed as the patient improved. 'Of course as you progressed in the hospital itself, in the treatment, as you got better things got less stringent. You weren't so controlled as you were when you went in and that was all sort of helping towards your rehabilitation.' (Interview: Mr I. 1996).

All of the men had interviews with the psychiatrist. Some of these would have been deliberately psychotherapeutic, whilst others collected material for diagnostic reasons. As stated earlier, psychotherapy was a mixed bag of psychodynamic techniques ranging from suggestion and persuasion through didactic approaches to more traditional psychoanalytic approaches. Sometimes this was daily, at other times much less frequent (Interview: Mr I. 1996). Vernon Scannell bitterly recalled not being seen for a fortnight, after the end of the war (Scannell 1983, p.59).

Some sessions were advisory. They were not always thought to be helpful: 'He came out with an awful lot of what I suppose he thought were helpful things. I thought, "Well, look, I haven't got a waste disposal human type problem that worries me. You're off course, if I may say so "' (Interview: Mr N. 1994, pt.1, p.17). Two or three weeks after his arrival, Mr F. had a first interview. In this he received a lecture, and a recommendation to read a novel on suicide (Interview: Mr F. 1994, p.11).

Commonly, the approach would have been a form of basic psychotherapy, enabling the individual to talk about the circumstances that led them to come into hospital and their hopes and plans for the future. In January 1944, Mr K. saw his psychiatrist a few times: 'I didn't have much to say except to tell the story of how I got into this traumatic condition. And I think that was – he accepted it' (Interview: Mr K. 1990, p.2). Around about the same time, once he had finished a course of continuous narcosis, Mr L. had a daily session. He

> went into a room like an annexe and you'd see a psychiatrist and he spoke to you for about an hour or two hours, and talked about all sorts of things, and put you at your ease, and asked you all about, you know, what you'd done before as a child and all this sort of thing, and where you'd lived, and what you'd done, and what your expectations in life were. And he sort of brought it forward. He brought your, all your past up in front of you kind of thing and tried to explain what it was all about... Well I think what he was trying to find out was what you actually were or what you wanted to do in life, sort of thing, because the idea was to get you back in the forces again, you see, as quickly as possible. (Interview: Mr L. 1998, pp.29–30)

Early on, this form of therapy was carried out over many months. Markillie remembered working in Dumfries, where he had the time to carry out individual sessions in some depth, before he came to Northfield (1993). After arriving in the summer of 1942, Mr A. reported being a patient in the hospital for at least six months and probably longer (Interview: Mr A. 1990). Later this luxury was not permitted. Men were expected to spend no longer than six weeks in the hospital before being placed elsewhere or discharged from the army. Any form of psychotherapy had to be focused on the main symptoms and the recent trauma that caused them.

Hypnosis was sometimes used in an attempt to hasten the process. One specialist put Mr C. 'to sleep – sort of with a pencil', saying 'I'm going to put my hand into your head and bring out all the badness, all the things worrying you.' Mr C. came out of the session feeling exhilarated, but the improvement didn't last (Interview: Mr C. 1990). Pentothal and other barbiturates were used to induce a sense of disinhibition, in order to allow forgotten memories to come to the surface. The doctor who carried this out with Mr M. ignored the traumatic incidents that led to his breakdown, and was described as asking 'leading questions about your childhood, who your mother was, who your father was, what your sex life was... They dwelt mostly on sex, and I can't understand why' (Interview: Mr M. 1994, p.6). The patient's implied criticism would have been shared by most other contemporary military psychiatrists.

Continuous narcosis was established early on as a treatment, probably in 1943. Mrs Gaskin, who was at that time a nursing assistant, remembered

Anne Ward being converted into a darkened unit, with one small light bulb. People would be brought in in wheelchairs, 'shocked' and shaking. They would then be given somnifane or paraldehyde and kept semi-conscious for at least ten days. They would not be able to control their bladders or bowels and consequently did not wear pyjama bottoms during that time (Gaskin and Gaskin 1990, p.2). When Mr H. came round he 'was on this mattress, no blankets or anything like that...the front of my pyjamas was all ripped out, either ripped out or wide open as it were' (Interview: Mr H. 1994, p.13).

On cessation of the treatment patients were transferred to Adelaide Ward upstairs, where they would have a blanket bath and shave. They would spend a convalescent period there (Gaskin and Gaskin 1990, p.2). Although the therapy was prescribed by the psychiatrists, the physician, Dr Lewsen, was in charge of this unit. This was in spite of the fact that, as reported earlier, he was unhappy about this form of treatment.

As described earlier, Mr L. underwent a course of this therapy. When he came round he recalled seeing 'about fourteen people I think, and they all lay on the bed...they were all like sort of zombies laying in their beds and all laying there, nobody spoke and looked at you' (Interview: Mr L. 1998, pp. 14, 24). After refusing an injection Mr H. was offered seven capsules, following which he sat in the waiting room for what seemed hours waiting for them to work.

> And I thought, well, I must be tired now, you know. And of course I recall no more until I woke up in a darkened ward on a mattress underneath a window shaking a blind that was – raining outside, and shaking the raindrops on me. Sitting by my side is a nurse. She can't understand what I'm saying because I'm talking German all the time, and I don't even know the German language. Only smatterings. So – she tells me it's a week hence from when I thought it was and I'd been there a week. And I do recall that in that sedation period I can remember being fed from a long spouted feeding mug. There are snatches of it. I know I insisted on going to the loo on my own two feet. Which I did, and apparently, I don't know, but apparently I was too violent to go the full sedation course of two weeks. (Interview: Mr H. 1994, p.13)

Dr Markillie outlined some of the dangers of this treatment, in particular those associated with the use of sodium amytal. He had awful results 'because you got such hallucinosis when you stopped, and the poor normal man was seeing things going around the ceiling and just couldn't control it' (Markillie 1993, p.2). When Mr H. regained consciousness, he was quite happy:

> there's this nurse sitting beside of me... And I do recall that in that closed, little closed ward of mine – big, brass doorlocks, solid wooden doors. I

recall it clearly. And the parquet floor with the wood blocks coming up out of the floor and running round and round the bed. Now it's quite a fantastic experience. And I always used to say that I've had the most gorgeous 'up' – if you like. If you know what I mean. Because that is – probably, I don't know – probably as good a description of that little ward as one could have. I mean to see these blocks of wood come up absolutely symmetrically and go round the bed, run round the bed, and then come back – bearing in mind that I'm on a mattress on the floor – and then going back into the floor, seeing these lovely oil paintings, on the ceiling, which was an ordinary whitewashed ceiling, nothing on it whatsoever. Having someone pull your legs off, pull your head off, your body fold inwards and then outwards – it's indescribable – well, I can describe it, but you can't imagine it, you know. (Interview: Mr H. 1994, p.12)

The treatment seems to have had its successes:

Well the relief of coming out of this sedation they called it, sedation period, when you came out you felt more relaxed sort of thing and you were able to talk to people. Before you had the treatment you were all tensed up. Your body was tensed up like a coil, like a spring, and you hadn't got any more or less control of what you wanted to say. But having come out of this it completely rested you and gave you a rest period and that helped it I suppose...you're feeling more relaxed, you're feeling calmer. (Interview: Mr L. 1998, pp.28–29)

Electro-convulsive therapy was a rather different experience. Mr M. reported: 'There was one electrical treatment, and you've heard about it. Electrodes on your head and you went out. We won't go into that' (Interview: Mr M. 1994, p.5). This was carried out in a specialised unit. At this time there was no use of sedation or muscle relaxants. As described earlier, the patient was strapped to the bed and the shock was given directly to the temples. The experience would have been frightening for the recipient, even though they would have remembered little of it.

Sometimes individual therapies were dictated by expediency, with the aim of achieving rapid results. This could lead to some unusual, ad hoc treatments. Main instituted a form of 'compulsory mourning' for tank commanders who had repeatedly lost their crews. In explaining this therapy it is important to emphasise the respect that he had for these men. He described their situation:

There was a particular lot of people I paid attention to. This was the depression that hit some tank commanders who refused to fight. They'd say I don't mind if you shoot me, I'm not going back...the story was always the same. They'd been quite decent soldiers. I don't want to make them heroic; but they were ordinary tank commanders, high quality people, selected by a now extremely efficient personnel selection service. Computerised high IQ, high stability... They were good human material: sergeants, young lieutenants. And they had lived with their crews in intense group loyalty, they depended on each other for their lives. The tank would get hit and when a tank gets hit the metal that's just been struck by a shell blows in at once, white hot, and the ammunition inside starts to burn – the shells aren't timed, so they don't explode. It's the gunpowder burns and shock! A great flash of flame envelops the tank. And the tank commander has time to get out. But he hears the people, cries, screaming, he gazes at them, covered in flame, burning, probably die at once. But these were people he'd lived with intensely, slept with nights, enormous crew loyalty... He'd be given another tank the next day and then he'd go into battle three or four weeks later. He's a bit more cautious about getting to know this lot. Didn't want to get too close to them this time. And the same thing would happen. He'd hear the screams. By the third time he wasn't friends with these people. He couldn't afford to be. (Main 1984)

In the hospital they were remote, stand-offish and dismissive of 'base wallahs'. The treatment consisted of being confined alone in a darkened room for three days, with one hour of daylight, one hour of electric light and a diet of bread and water. This was with the instructions to 'bloody well cry mate!' – an attempt to sanction the grief that the army wouldn't. This draconian measure was aimed at counteracting the numbing sense of loss that afflicted them, and inevitably inspired anger and bitterness against the man who instituted it. This would have been a successful result compared to keeping the feelings pent up and locked in (Dewar 1993; Main 1984). Main explained his rationale to Bartemeier *et al.* in 1945. The patient, in his opinion, had difficulty in accepting his feelings of bereavement, so he instituted a mechanism by which the individual's own conscience was reinforced and their unspoken self-accusations were made more articulate. The latter was achieved by Main actually calling them insensitive to their faces. The whole approach was comparable to the relief of profound grief experienced in military units when the men were allowed to express that emotion 'in formal burial rites with appropriate ceremonies and muffled drums' (Bartemeier *et al.* 1946, pp.502–503). Fifty years later, Vernon Scannell, after reading about these events in a previous paper, responded as Main hoped the men would. In a paeon of anger, Scannell verbalised the fury of the tank commander who was subjected to such apparently brutal behaviour and grieved for the men whom he had lost (Harrison and Clarke 1992; Scannell 1992).

Another paradoxical tactic was used in the treatment of a man complaining of homicidal feelings. He was told to go off and kill the hospital cats. He was found later on feeding and looking after them rather than carrying out the prescribed treatment (Dewar 1993).

Other therapies, such as the use of insulin for promoting the appetite, were used; but none of the survivors interviewed recalled either having these treatments themselves, or others having them. The use of group therapy was widespread at certain times. This will be described and discussed in a later section, as it is germane to the main theme of this book.

As the person recovered they were expected to carry out chores. 'You had to help clean out sometimes, that was all part of your therapy as well, to help clean the place up.' (Interview: Mr L. 1998, p.37).

> You had to look after, you know, make your own beds and do your own area, keep your space clean. And then when of course in this place, as in all military hospitals, when you were, you were recuperating you were expected to do and of course we used to have to polish these sort of tiled floors and scrub the skirting boards and helped in the kitchen. It was all part of bringing you back into the public way of life sort of thing, you know. (Interview: Mr L. 1998, pp.55–56)

It was well recognised by many patients that the task was to recover in order to return to some form of service. However, in common with, many other units, the occupational therapy was not always the most appropriate. Many soldiers report either doing embroidery themselves, or seeing others do it. This was precisely the sort of work that Bion considered was more therapeutic for the staff than the patients.

SKRIM-SHANKERS, CHOCOLATES AND THE DANCES: THE ATTITUDES OF LOCALS

According to Scott, a psychoanalyst, the attitude of the public to psychiatric war casualties had changed by the time of the Second World War. Before the First World War the courageous soldier had been considered to be fearless. Any acknowledgement of apprehension was thought of as cowardice. At the beginning of that war men who didn't wish to join the army were handed white feathers as a mark of shame (Partridge 1981; Taylor 1970, p.67). In 1941, Scott's opinion was that the public accepted that abnormal fear was understandable in a war casualty (Scott 1941). Unfortunately, not everyone in Birmingham was aware of this change, and the blue uniform could still attract derogatory remarks such as 'skrim-shanker' and worse, or refusal to board a tram because there were 'six on board already' (Discussion Group 3, p.3; Foulkes 1992, p.52; Hewitt 1989). One reason for this vilification, apart from prejudice about nervous disorder, was the fact that the patients were not subject to the same rationing restrictions as the civilians, and thus had good food including regular meat (Markillie 1993).

The shame of the hospital uniform was felt far more keenly by the patients themselves; this provided a stimulus to improve and get transferred to the training wing, where the khaki was worn (Foulkes 1948, p.52). Bridger's response was to get permission for the men to wear their medals (Bridger 1990b).

Mr L. mused philosophically on these issues 50 years later:

there used to be a certain amount of resentment to anyone who was in there, sort of thing, initially but as time went on people got used to it; because it must have been a bit of a shock to the people living in the area to find all these men being moved in who were shell-shocked and all that sort of thing... But after a while it went alright. We found it alright. They used to welcome us into their homes and that sort of thing, you know, get an armchair, cup of tea and a sandwich so it wasn't too bad. (Interview: Mr L. 1998, p.77–78)

Despite the prejudice of some, it is clear that this was not widespread. Many soldiers found eventually that if locals knew that they were from the hospital 'people would tend to treat you very kindly and generously' (Interview: Mr O. 1995, p.3). The hospitality could extend even further: 'Some people used to take us into the pub and buy us a drink' (p.3). This generosity was expressed on a regular basis. Men and women in the local factories made collections on behalf of the soldiers. Mr O. is one of many who recalled that 'the workers from the Austin factory...used to come down just about every week with cartons of cigarettes that their workers had collected and brought us all down cigarettes' (p.3). Mrs B. worked at Nettlefolds, and the factory girls there adopted Margaret Ward. They would put on concerts to raise money, which would be spent on cigarettes, biscuits and confectionary. Eight or nine of the girls would then take these to the hospital every Saturday, and arrange to accompany the soldiers for walks, picnics or visits to the cinema (Interview: Mrs B. 1990). On another ward the soldier would find 40 cigarettes thrown onto the bed every Tuesday, either from the Red Cross or from the Austin Motor Company workers (Interview: Mr E. 1990).

Whilst collecting material for this survey, a number of advertisements were placed in the local paper and in the national press for people to come forward to talk about their memories of Northfield Military Hospital. What came as a surprise was the number of replies from women who had very fond memories of the dances held there.

Mrs C.'s enthusiasm was very evident: 'you know, it was something you looked forward to, you were that excited' (Interview: Mrs C. 1994, p.9). The large number of men had its attractions: 'So there we would go, you see, and you'd arrive and there would not be many girls. There were millions of men! And so you were always having to dance. You just had one dance after another. And it was brilliant' (Interview: Mrs D. 1994, p.1). The music was sometimes just from a gramophone, but at other times was performed by the patients or professional dance bands.

Bridger recognised the contribution of these women when he stated that his social therapy department was providing a service 'together with the whole of the neighbouring population' (1946, p.75).

GRIPPED IN THE MACHINE: MILITARY PATIENTS AT NORTHFIELD

When the soldier arrived at the top of the hospital drive and compassed the large Victorian asylum that was about to embrace him, he would have felt that he had reached the nadir of his army life. Escape would have seemed to be the only way of alleviating sense of isolation, humiliation and failure. It was no longer a question of 'working one's ticket', but just an urgent need to run home.

They were like fish out of water. Either they had never adjusted to life in the army or they had been removed from the camaraderie of their unit. After this they floundered through a succession of interviews, confinements, and transfers from one place to another. They were rarely given any explanation of what was happening, and many were in awe of authority anyway. Impotent, frightened and bewildered, they were then engulfed by the hospital, and often given treatments that further unmanned them.

This process was not deliberate; it was the outcome of a system that could not cope with the humanity of its constituent parts. All along the way, people could be caring, thoughtful and considerate, but that did not make up for the organisation's need to excrete those it couldn't absorb. The difficulty was that the army had never really faced up to these realities. Whilst the psychiatrists and their colleagues had brought a rational recognition of the fact that fear and fatigue are part of the soldier's experience, the organisation itself hadn't moved an inch to accommodate itself to this fact. Certainly, all over the world some concessions had been made, but the machine itself had not changed at all. So the individual soldier whose personal traumas so dramatically threw up challenges to this Victorian mentality had to be eliminated. The process remained an embarrassing secret, locked away behind the privy door. Despite its huge impact on the lives of soldiers and its effects on the efficiency of the army, military medical histories of the army, training manuals, and doctors' accounts nearly all relegate mental health to a few paragraphs, if they mention it at all (e.g. Cotrell undated; Lovesgrove 1953; Mackintosh 1940; War Office 1944).

All human beings, subjected to continual strains of battle, will break down at one point or another. At a fundamental level, the British Army in the Second World War denied this fact. Ad hoc arrangements were made to cope with mental health problems, but the basic changes needed to adapt to the fact that the core material of the organisation was human were never made.

For some of its time, the hospital played its part in sustaining the soldiers' sense of failure and humiliation. It continued the same process. However, another set of traditional ideals also came into play: those of the 'caring profession'. Once in Northfield, the soldier became a 'patient', and his troubles could be reified into 'illness'. This prevented him, and the staff, from criticising a system that managed its resources so ineffectively. It also changed the rules. Now the soldier had to be grateful for the care he received and the protection that was provided. Some treatments took this process so far that he could become literally infantilised, requiring toiletting, washing and feeding.

Tom Main tartly expressed it:

> By tradition a hospital is a place wherein sick people may receive shelter from the stormy blasts of life, the care and attention of nursing and medical auxiliaries, and the individual attention of a skilled doctor. The concept of a hospital as a refuge too often means, however, that patients are robbed of their status as responsible human beings. Too often they are called 'good' or 'bad' only according to the degree of their passivity in the face of the hospital demand for their obedience, dependency and gratitude. The fine traditional mixture of charity and discipline they receive is a practised technique for removing their initiative as adult beings, and making them 'patients'. They are less trouble thus to the staff... So, isolated and dominated, the patient tends to remain gripped by the hospital machine even in the games or prescribed occupations which occupy his time between treatments. (1946a)

How could a few staff in a hospital, a military one at that, challenge such ingrained processes? Sisyphus himself would have been daunted by the thought of pushing this particular stone uphill.

CHAPTER 6

Strange Meetings at Hollymoor

It seemed that out of battle I escaped

Down some profound dull tunnel (From 'Strange Meeting', Wilfred Owen 1973, p.102)

DEFORMING THE RUBBER BALL: REFORMING THE HOSPITAL SYSTEM

The Northfield Experiments can be said to have failed. Foulkes, Bion, Rickman, Main and Bridger showed how the enemy could be defeated, but failed to convince their superiors. The bridgeheads established by reorganising whole systems to tackle coherently the social effects of neurosis were always fragile. This was largely because the commanding officers could not shake off their bureaucratic mindset and failed to rally the necessary support. They acted as administrators rather than leaders. It was always subordinates who championed the innovations, never them. In this the unit reflected the army as a whole, in which the psychiatrists pressed reform onto a reluctant organisation. Like tennis balls, both structures sprang back into their preformed shapes as soon as they were released, despite the fact that the new systems were demonstrably more effective.

The natural state of the hospital emphasised form over content. The traditional structure of individually based medicine was maintained, ignoring the wider social issue. Doctors and other staff carried out what they considered to be the task entirely independently of one another and the system as a whole. The only tissue holding the framework together was the military system and the ethos of each profession. At Northfield, the former tended to be a caricature of the real thing, and the therapeutic staff persistently undermined its importance and value. The commanding officer tended to feel that his role was to maintain cooperation between the two sides as best he could (Bridger 1985, p.97).

In their different ways, the reformers tried to manipulate the key forces operating within these fields. The success – and failure – of Rickman and

Bion was that their attempt went deepest. However, they moved so quickly, without anticipating the reactions that would ensue, that the recoil ejected them. The Second Experiment lasted longer, developed gradually and accomplished more. This was achieved by attempting to resolve the conflicts between the administration, which was wedded to military protocol, and the clinical sphere which was experimental and chaotic. Main and Bridger made attempts, more or less successfully, to inform and explain to the commanding officer what they were trying to achieve (Main 1989, p.135). However, despite the contemporary and subsequent fame of the Northfield Experiments, relatively few organisations have followed down the same path.

The events are recounted here in historical sequence, except for the evolution of group therapies during the second phase, which is described in the next chapter. This is because they developed at a different pace to the changes in the hospital as a whole. The work of Bion and Rickman, carried out early on, was so curtailed and integrated as to render any such disassociation unnecessary.

PRELUDE: THE EARLY DAYS

The British Army took over the hospital in April 1942. There is little evidence of the activities of the first few months at Hollymoor. There were few soldiers, perhaps around 50 (Hewitt 1989). Treatment, carried out on an individual basis, could last many months, and life, it would seem, was leisurely, if restricted (Interview: Mr A. 1990).

The first major event at Northfield was a conference in July 1942 to discuss the stability factor in the Canadian PULHEEMS assessment of new recruits (MacKeith 1994).[1] Eighty-nine psychiatrists attended, including J.R. Rees, the senior psychiatrist in the army, John Rickman, and American and Canadian representatives.

During this time Major Wittkower wrote a paper on the Special Transfer Scheme that had recently been instituted (Wittkower and Lebeaux 1943). Although he and his co-author were at Northfield when the paper was published, it is not clear whether the patients referred to were from there. Half of the 50 soldiers with neurotic difficulties suffered from anxiety

---

[1] PULHEEMS was a Canadian introduction that was eventually taken up by the British Army in 1947 (War Office 1946b). It provided a systematic assessment of the physical and mental capaci-ties of the recruit with a view to his or her appropriate placement subsequently. It was an attempt to avoid inappropriate mismatches between the individual and the job they were assigned to. P = physical capacity, U = upper limb, L = lower limb, H = hearing, EE = eyesight, M = mental ca-pacity, and S = emotional stability (Richardson 1978, p.165).

neurosis, 15 had hysterical symptoms, and ten had either personality problems or obsessional difficulties. Twelve had broken down within a year of joining up and found it difficult to adjust to military life; another half had been in the army for up to three and a half years, but similarly, found army conditions too difficult to cope with. The twelve regulars, who had been in the army for longer, had seen combat experience, and their breakdown was a consequence of that.

The Special Transfer Scheme, or 'Annexure system', was instituted in 1941 after Lewis had demonstrated the necessity for some method of reallocating men with mental health problems once they had been treated. The intention was to avoid having to discharge them by ensuring that they found posts which suited their skills and prevented them having further relapses (Lewis and Slater 1952, p.397). Wittkower's paper was the first demonstration of its effectiveness. All 50 men were found suitable placements, though these were predominantly non-combatant posts. Unfortunately, there was no follow-up to clarify how long the positions were retained (Wittkower and Lebeaux 1943). The scheme was central to the reallocation of patients after their treatment at Northfield, and apart from discharge from the army formed the main conduit for disposal of patients.

Bion castigated the hospital organisation at this time, pointing out the 'huge gulf that yawned' between the soldier's army life and that in the wards. The pace was somnolent, the medication appeared to be as much for the benefit of the medical staff's peace of mind as the patients', and the occupational therapy was just that: keeping the patients occupied at a 'kindergarten level' (Bion 1946). He believed that things just had to change.

INTRA-GROUP TENSIONS: THE FIRST NORTHFIELD EXPERIMENT

Early in 1942, Rickman was commissioned as a major in the British Army. He spent a few months at Bishop's Lydeard before transferring to Northfield in July 1942 (Baruch 1998). Little is known of his activities there during 1942 until Bion arrived, except that he looked after an acute psychiatric ward of 14 to 16 beds. Here the patients would remain for about six to eight weeks before moving on to the Training Wing (Bion and Rickman 1943).

The patients at this time were largely non-combatants whose problems stemmed largely from their difficulties with managing army life. Casson wrote later of the 'chronic neurotics, psychopaths and defective unstable Pioneer Corps fellows', which, whilst it is unlikely that Rickman would have found the terminology acceptable, emphasised the long-standing nature of the problems that they had (Casson 1945). This contemptuous attitude, echoing Slater's negative stance described earlier, exemplified the unofficial categorisation of soldier patients into two classes: those whose problems stemmed from their previous heredity and nurture, and those whose basic personality was seen as 'good', but who had been subjected to extreme experiences. Rickman and Bion did not subscribe to this view. Indeed, the latter went as far as to suggest that difficulties were not always confined to the so-called patients, and that members of staff, '*ex officio* stable personalities', were not immune from behavioural problems (1948).

Rickman, besides working in groups, also treated patients individually, and he gave an account of his approach in 1941, probably while he was at Wharncliffe. A soldier wounded in northern France had been treated successfully for his physical trauma. However, once he returned to his unit his arm became paralysed. This affliction was resistant to all normal forms of medical treatment, such as rest, electrical stimulation and massage.

It was only after some months that he came to see Rickman, during which he had become evidently 'morose and dejected'. During the brief discussions that were possible he was punctiliously correct in his attitude, but unforthcoming, nursing his arm to try to keep it warm. He was preoccupied with his affected limb, but he also referred to the death of a companion. This friend, for whom he 'would have given his right arm', was killed in the action in which he himself was wounded. Rickman divined intuitively that the loss of his comrade had not been sufficiently mourned, and put it to him that the arm represented this loss. Despite rejecting this interpretation the man was encouraged to talk about his bereavement. As he spoke he became increasingly tremulous and depressed, in contrast to 'his earlier suspicious and impervious politeness'. Gradually he became more emotional, whilst at the same time gaining sensation in his limb. Eventually he recovered enough to enjoy taking up rifle drill again. In Rickman's view, he had needed to release the emotions of the bereavement in order to allow the hysterical symptoms to recede. This procedure was very brief in terms of time actually spent in therapy, less than an hour all told, and was carried out in conjunction with 'para-military training' (Rickman 1941).

In the individual interviews that Rickman carried out at Northfield he discussed the difficulties of placing membership of a team before the needs of the individual. Because of the nature of army life, into which men were in the process of being rehabilitated, the therapeutic task was clearly identified as developing 'group membership' skills, which would enable the man to adapt to any community afterwards. The focus was on what actions strengthen the group, not on the person's emotional status. Therapy was embedded in the men's real situation, which was consistently underlined by statements such as: 'Although you are a patient you are, remember, a soldier as well'. Other 'here and now' realities were examined, including the transient nature of the ward care, the implications of the soldier's rank and file status, and the doctor's officer role (Rickman 1943). Through these discussions, Rickman aimed to halt the man's flight away from the perceived terrors of the army into the imagined safety of home life. It is worth recalling, at this point, Lewis' findings that men returning to 'civvy street' because of mental health difficulties faced long-term unemployment and social disablement (*see* chapter 4; Lewis and Slater 1942; Guttman and Thomas 1946). In the group setting, constant themes were those of entering and leaving, as well as who should be members. Rickman encouraged a sense of belonging by referring to the unit as 'our ward' (Bion and Rickman 1943; Rickman 1943a).

It is likely that Rickman would have been frustrated by the cloying atmosphere of Northfield during these first few months, but it is not evident what attempts he made himself to change things, except to work in isolation on his unit as everyone else was doing. Foulkes made it clear that early on the sphere of influence of the therapist was strictly limited to his own ward (1964, p.188). Another of Rickman's roles was that of training officer for psychiatric trainees (Payne 1957). He was certainly warmly remembered in this role by ex-students. One later wrote: 'Now that Major Bion and yourself have left we really feel that the course has finished, but that which you have taught us is not likely to finish so easily' (Armson 1943). Pat de Maré was also impressed, and recalled that the seminars were run along group lines (1993, p.3).

Bion joined Rickman in the cusp of 1942 and 1943 to take over the training wing. This housed more than half the soldiers receiving care at the hospital, between 100 and 200 men. There are few witnesses able to confirm or deny the reports of Bion and Rickman, and so this account has to rely heavily on their own necessarily partial view.

Bion immediately felt that changes were needed to bring the milieu of the hospital into line with its function as a military unit (1946). From the beginning he approached the whole unit as one community, which he described as being similar to 'a rather scallywag battallion' (Bion and Rickman 1943). As the officer in charge of this organisation he deliberately assessed the situation in military terms, identifying a foe and determining the strategy and tactics with which to fight it. This unsung battle of the Second World War was against neurosis. It then became necessary to assist the men in identifying this enemy and halt the retreat in which, as he saw it, all patients and staff up to that point had been engaged.

First he determined 'to rally those patients who are not already to far gone to be steadied' through the use of small groups. His only contemporary elucidation of the technique he employed was a comment that they were similar to the leaderless discussion groups in the WOSBs (Bion 1946). However, Rickman was able to observe how they differed from those run by other therapists. There were two particular unique characteristics. First, Bion did 'not steer the discourse when handling the groups', and second, he drew the attention of everyone present to 'what is happening at the moment in the group'. Rickman provided an example of this from his own observations at Northfield:

> For instance, a group of Bion's more or less agreed to meet at 6.30 for 1½ hour sessions, after about half past eight while the discussion rambled and dragged on Bion said: 'Let us see what has been happening lately. We agreed to go on for an hour and a half and yet no one has suggested that we get up and go.' He paused, one person who had been trying to take the lead accused Bion of looking at the clock ever since eight, another accused the last speaker of talking too much, all agreed that the discourse had been fitful, hot and then cold, no one connected this behaviour with the time-element. Bion here made what I think may fairly be called an interpretation, that is to say what he said added no new topic to the events covered by the interpretation but synthesized those events so that what was before subliminal...became clear and events which though everyone was aware of them before seemed much more connected. Bion's interpretation was that though everyone was restless no one was willing to bring the ill will of the group on himself by ending the session. (Rickman 1945)

This is the first eyewitness account of Bion's method of working in a group, and the only one that describes his approach at Northfield. Before turning to Bions's own explanations of his work, it is important to recognise that most of his writings on groups refer to his experiences at the Tavistock Clinic after the war. His explanations and understandings are drawn from this time rather than five years earlier. However, it is evident that his practice was largely similar, although the conclusions that he drew from his observations had evolved.

He described the quiescent role he took:

> When a group starts I usually wait until I become aware of a complexity of feelings which sooner or later are aroused in myself. I find it usual to verbalise these feelings in terms which purport to describe the group's attitude to myself. The mere fact of my doing so causes a change in the emotional situation within the group, and I then wait until I can describe this changed situation. (Bion 1948, p.107)

This passivity was central to Bion's approach. He allowed the group to evolve, and would then comment only when it became clear to him what might be happening. This approach usually left the group feeling perplexed and wondering what the relevance of his contributions was. He would then remain silent again until a number of members of the group had expressed their views. Similarly to Rickman, he conned the clues in the non-verbal communications, which could highlight hidden motives and emotions. After reviewing his own emotional response – his counter-transference – he would then give a further opinion. This might have concerned the fact that the group expected him to 'do something' in the role that they expected him to play as a leader (Bion 1961, p.30). Further discomfort would follow as members digested or rejected this. Gradually they would become more aware of their roles in the dynamics of the relationships. Bion emphasised that the only useful interpretations were related to the individual's relationship with the common unconscious themes of all those present, which he called the 'group mentality' (1948, p.109). It was important to elucidate 'one aspect or another of these three things – the group mentality, the attempts of the individual to achieve a full life in the group, and the culture of the group – and, if possible, to demonstrate their interplay.' Furthermore, it was essential to give evidence to support the exegesis. The purpose was not to provide the person with a solution to his or her problems, but to develop the ability to seek for it (p.110). This echoed Rickman's concept that maturity meant being engaged in constant exploration for more realistic and satisfactory solutions to infantile tensions rather than remaining stuck in rigid neurotic defences.

By this method Bion collected a 'sufficient number of patients' in the training wing, who were willing to face the newly identified enemy. A daily parade was arranged, which lasted half an hour for the whole unit. Ostensibly, the purpose was to make announcements and conduct the business of the unit. Regulations were laid down that outlined the duties of each man, which included participation in physical exercise and study sessions. They were also provided with the opportunity for developing new groups if appropriate, and there were rules for those who were not able to attend such activities. This structure laid the framework for work on the true task of the unit: the development of physically and mentally fit individuals prepared to act as full members of the British Army at war. Those men who did not feel that they could participate were able to go to the rest room. This was an area in which the men could read, play games like draughts, write, or lie on the couches provided if they felt too unwell. There was a nursing orderly present to ensure that they stayed quiet and didn't disturb the other patients.

The less overt intention was for the daily meeting to evolve into a therapeutic seminar, the purpose of which was to examine the progress of the members of the unit towards the goal. As Bion stated: 'Lost tools in the handicraft section, defective cinema apparatus, permission to use the local swimming baths, the finding of a football pitch, all these matters came back to the same thing, the manipulation and harmonization of personal relationships' (Bion 1946). The daily meetings developed rapidly, with a great deal of endeavour and discussion occurring outside of them. Activity groups multiplied, and organisational attempts to co-ordinate them were made through the formation of a programme group. It was clear that a flurry of creativity had been released.

In order to explore and share the experience of reviewing the situation from outside, Bion would take one or two men to go round the groups, 'to see how the rest of the world lives'. This led to him presenting an initial therapeutic interpretation of what was happening in the whole environment to the daily parade. On one occasion he asked the patients to consider what he had observed that day. Numerous groups were running. Each soldier had the opportunity to do whatever he wanted as long as the proposals were practical, and yet virtually no real activity took place. One or two men only attended each venture. Bion declared that the whole affair appeared to be a 'facade', similar to the 'eyewash' that men had previously rebuked the army for. Again, as in the group described above, this elucidation of what was occurring 'here and now' led to the audience feeling uncomfortable and 'got at'.

The outcome was that the men in the training wing gradually became more self-critical. Attention was turned to practical and necessary tasks that contributed to the health and welfare of the community as a whole. An example of this process was the 'orderly group' formed to keep the wards clean, resulting in an improvement which even impressed the commanding officer, Lt. Col. Pearce (Bion and Rickman 1943; Bion 1946).

The role of the rest room, or 'smoking room', is not referred to by Bion. However, de Maré stressed that it became an uncomfortable experience to escape to it, as anyone doing so would be 'frozen out' by the others (1993, p.5). It had become the symbolic dumping ground for projected 'bad bits' of the group.

This process of reflective interpretation of activity enabled the individual to direct his energy and creativity towards the service of his community, and through this actually gain a sense of personal self-esteem and value. It elaborated on Rickman's individual and small group therapy, and brought it into the public arena. They both aimed for a 'good group spirit', which incorporated a common purpose, mutual recognition of group boundaries, the capacity to absorb changes in membership and the ability to manage discontent. Each member was to be valued and have freedom within generally accepted conditions devised by the group, and any sub-groups that formed were to be flexible and contribute to the whole (Bion and Rickman 1943). These became the key attributes of what Bion later defined as the sophisticated or work group as opposed to the basic assumption group (1961, p.136).

He summarised the guiding principles of the whole experiment:

1) The objective of the wing was the study of its own internal tensions, in a real life situation, with a view to laying bare the influence of neurotic behaviour in producing frustration, waste of energy, and unhappiness in a group.

2) No problem was tackled until its nature and extent had become clear at least to the greater part of the group.

3) The remedy for any problem thus classified was only applied when the remedy itself had been scrutinized and understood by the group.

4) Study of the problem of intra-group tensions never ceased – the day consisted of 24 hours.

5) It was more important that the method should be grasped, and its rationale, than that some solution of the problem of the wing should be achieved for all time. It was not our object to produce an ideal training wing. It was our object to send men out with at least some understanding of the nature of intra-group tensions and, if possible, with some idea of how to set about harmonizing them.

6) As in all group activities the study had to commend itself to the majority of the group as worth while and for this reason it had to be the study of a real life situation. (Bion and Rickman 1943)

By the end Bion was able to report that a sea change had occurred in the spirit of the wing. The relationship of men to officers had become friendly and cooperative, and it was felt that both groups were engaged in a worthwhile and important task. Bion wrote: 'The atmosphere was not unlike that seen in a unit of an army under the command of a general in whom they have confidence, even though they cannot know his plans' (Bion and Rickman 1943).

Perhaps the most remarkable change was the fact that a group of men characterised by other psychiatrists as psychopaths, or referred to by other opprobrious terms, were interacting in an effective manner. As Lewin would have pointed out, they operated not as independent atoms, but with an understanding of the forces engendered within their social field. Psychoanalysis was the instrument to examine these unconscious impulses, and by making them explicit it allowed the men to see what was happening more clearly. Rickman and Bion's expectation was that, in a time of war, these soldiers would eventually wish to regain their dignity and sense of self-worth by contributing to the defeat of the Axis powers.

The commanding officer was Lt. Col. J.D.W. Pearce. A sensitive and considerate person, he also had a tendency to rigidity of thinking. De Maré described him as 'a terribly conventional little man' (1994). As a small, youngish-looking man, he could look quite ridiculous when he was flanked by his two older and much larger juniors during tours of inspection around the unit (Interview: Mrs R. 1998). He quite clearly did not fully understand what these two officers were doing with their group therapy, and in this he was not alone. The other psychiatrists were also unable to grasp what was actually occurring. Lewsen reported that they believed Bion and Rickman to be 'too concerned with pursuing their Freudian, slow analysis, and were not prepared to make any concessions to the pressures and expediency' (1993). This perception was confirmed by Bion when he reported that 'one critic expostulated that surely such a system of patient observation would be exceedingly slow in producing results, if indeed it produced results at all' (Bion and Rickman 1943). As a consequence, there was a great deal of animosity between many of the psychiatrists and these two.

The experiment terminated suddenly, with all three senior officers being transferred to other units. What actually occurred is difficult to disentangle. Different stories abound, including one that emphasises Pearce's dissatisfaction with the mess in the Great Hall, and another that argues that Bion had discovered someone taking money from the social club. Whatever the truth regarding the particular circumstances, a more important lesson remained to be learnt. This was that although Rickman and Bion had understood the importance of their role in moving the unit towards an orientation that served the army at war, they ignored and were actually contemptuous of the hospital system and the bureaucracy of the military administration (Bridger 1985, p.97). Bridger blamed this on Bion, but although he was likely to have been the moving force there is no evidence that Rickman tried to convince him otherwise.

This viewpoint is confirmed by Lewsen's account of his brief encounter with Bion and Rickman. He arrived in January 1943, and remembers the rather insular and arrogant approach of the two of them to the rest of the staff, in particular to the commanding officer. It was with a sense of relief that the general body of psychiatrists saw them leave (Lewsen 1993).

ENURESIS AND SMALL GROUPS:
BETWEEN EXPERIMENTS

Throughout the next two years there was a steady throughput of patients, with 1635 admissions between 15 January and 15 July 1943, and 1209 during the next six months (War Office 1943/1944a). Table 6.1 records the gradual increase in numbers:

An officer's ward of about 50 beds was opened on 12 May 1944. This had its own medical staff and tended to be run separately from the rest of the hospital (Markillie 1993).

At the start of this period most patients came from units serving in England, and thus few had seen active service. In December 1943 there was a review of army policy with regard to disposal of soldiers suffering from psychoneurosis. Subsequently, only soldiers with the probability of return to high-grade military duties were to be treated at military hospitals. This was in order to conserve medical resources, and because the army was now employing as many men in the lower grades as were necessary (Ahrenfeldt 1958, p.150).

Table 6.1 Patients in Northfield military hospital 1943–44			
Date	No. of men	No. of officers	Total
20th July 1943			614
April 1943			417
25th May 1944	579	44	623
25th June 1944	639	46	685
25th July 1944			703

Source: War Office 1943/1944b

Surprisingly, there were also some prisoners of war who had been released from Germany. These were repatriated protected personnel, mainly medical and nursing staff, 1200 of whom had been returned in October 1943 (Ahrenfeldt 1948, p.230). Major Whiles had 100 of them under his care at Northfield between January and May 1944. These were men who had failed to adjust to life outside of the Stalag. The majority were irritable, restless, depressed and hated confinement. They were apathetic, with poor concentration, and had problems forming relationships. Often they were markedly resentful of everyone and everything. Many felt guilty about being captured, as if it had been a failing of theirs. This was exacerbated by a number of girlfriends who wrote letters saying that they had now got 'a real man' rather than someone who was cowardly enough to get captured. Some felt that everyone was against them, but this soon subsided once they began to trust the staff.

The key problem for these men was settling back into ordinary lives. During their captivity they had spent many idle hours fantasising about what they would do when they got home. However, the reality they found was entirely different to what they had dreamed of. This was described as the 'Rip Van Winkle' syndrome (Collie 1943). Everyday life in the United Kingdom had changed. Their womenfolk were working long hours away from home, and they had no idea about coupons or what was available in the shops. Their relatives expected them to take up roles they did not feel ready for. As one man expressed it, 'I found myself transplanted from a place of quietness to a busy town. I seemed to be trying to grasp so much all at once. I couldn't absorb it all' (Whiles 1945). Alfred Torrie, who was also working at Northfield, took up a theme that affected a quarter of these returnees: the broken marriage. Like Odysseus, they found that their partners had taken up with a rival. Others took the part of Othello. The fear that many prisoners of war had about the physical effects of their captivity, particularly that of impotence, together with their inevitably highly-coloured expectations of homecoming, led to them and their wives completely failing to understand each other's needs. They rapidly became suspicious of their spouses' activities, and disharmony swiftly ensued (Torrie 1945). These men used Northfield to reorientate themselves to their changed circumstances, work that prefigured the later Civil Resettlement Units.

Two doctors at the hospital, Backus and Mansell, investigated and treated nearly 300 cases of nocturnal enuresis between January and September 1943, which made up about a tenth of all admissions (Backus and Mansell 1944). These men ranged in age from 14 to 45 years old. Three-quarters had been incontinent in bed since childhood, and a tenth developed it after enlistment. Just under half were described as having no gross emotional cause but showing evidence of 'lack of proper care and training in their difficulties'. Otherwise common contributing factors included 'broken homes', with separation or death of parents, sexual traumata or anxiety, and air raids during childhood. About a tenth had some form of physical disease.

Backus and Mansell described half the cases as being of

a timid, immature, dependent, often frustrated type. Some of these showed schizoid trends. They came from the so-called 'broken home' situations, or from homes where there had been much emotional stress in early life. On the whole, this group revealed marked evidence of 'love deprivation' in childhood; a considerable number, however, showed a strong 'mother fixation' (1944, p.464)

Another quarter of the sample 'were of quite an average type of personality', the majority being notable for their marked indifference to the problem, 'having slept in wet diapers for most of their life'! A further tenth were men who were 'a reaction type showing compensatory aggression', and a further 6 per cent were 'what might be called pure aggressives'. The meanings of these descriptions can only be guessed at, and indicate the tendency to value ridden judgements underlying much 'scientific' psychiatry of the time. The remaining groups had personality difficulties or were obsessional in type.

Of relevance here is the rarity of battle experience, and the young age of at least one case at 14 years. The investigations included a battery of physical tests, including a detailed examination of the bladder. The diagnoses tend to reflect the critical caricaturisation of Casson's letter to John Rickman quoted above, which was written, incidently, whilst he was working with Backus in northern France (Casson 1945).

One patient would have agreed with these negative assessments. After having been through traumatic experiences in North Africa and the Mediterranean, where he had seen many of his friends and companions killed, he was particularly angry about the behaviour of these non-combatants:

> I would say it was 95% of the patients in the hospital when I was there in 1943 – in December 1943 – were scroungers. There was nothing wrong with them. They were trying to work their tickets. There wasn't any of them – there was hardly any of them time servers – soldiers. They'd never been in action, they'd never left England… A lot of them – I've got to be honest – a lot of them were married, and their wives were, apparently, from what I can remember now, were playing up a little bit, because they were posted away from home. (Interview: Mr M. 1994, p.4)

As described earlier, although the hospital continued to be run as a military establishment, discipline could be very lax. A particular recreation of this time was visiting Jones' Cafe in nearby Northfield instead of carrying out the rather minimal duties that were expected (Interview: Mr A. 1989; Mr C. 1990; Foulkes 1948, p.44). Mr C. reported: 'I never saw anyone get in real trouble', despite the fact that 'some men used to pop into the pub', which was out of bounds (Interview: Mr C. 1990).

The more lenient environment of the treatment wing, with its hospital beds, contrasted with the spartan conditions of the training area, where the soldiers slept on palliasses and blankets in wards furnished as barrack rooms (Foulkes 1948, p.45). They were expected to participate in regular physical, paramilitary and diversified occupational training (Backus and Mansell 1944). At this time the psychiatrists were discouraged from continuing to look after their patients there and there were no nursing staff.

At the end of April 1943, Major Warren wrote to Rickman and reported that Lt. Col. Rosie had replaced J.D.W. Pearce as commanding officer, describing him as a 'pleasant fellow'. He also recorded the arrival of Foulkes and Whiles as majors (Warren 1943). Major Alfred Torrie came in October, and Emanuel Miller a little later, to take command of the two medical divisions that now existed on the acute side of the hospital.

Foulkes joined the army from his civilian psychiatric practice in Exeter. He arrived in the hospital on April 26, having been commissioned as a Major on joining the army (Foulkes 1943a). He apparently had no idea of the earlier events with Bion and Rickman, although when he did become aware there was some rivalry between him and his two predecessors about whose account of group work should be published first.

Foulkes was inclined at this time to side with the patients' complaints about the army, finding that the hospital atmosphere 'was not always helpful for psychotherapy'. As he adapted to army life, 'such criticisms appeared less frequently and could be dealt with even more easily' (Foulkes 1964, pp.187–188). However, the ambivalence remained, as revealed by James Anthony's description of his salute in the previous chapter.

The immediate impact of the First Experiment on the practice of the hospital appears to have been negligible, except that it perhaps contributed to the sense, that Foulkes reports, of his group work being 'tolerated' rather than actively encouraged (1964, p.189). He had to obtain 'special permission' for group therapy, which was confined to his own wards, 'only on the patients' and my own free afternoons' (Foulkes 1948, p.53). Lt. Col. Rosie, as commanding officer, did not appear to encourage him. However, his view is unclear; in 1952 he wrote, apparently approvingly, that

> Bion and Rickman in 1943 endeavoured to bring the atmosphere of the hospital into closer relationship with the functions it ought to fill, and regarded training in the management of inter-personal relationships as valuable as a therapeutic approach (Rosie 1952, p.368).

One patient under Foulkes' care in 1943 recalled his experience in glowing terms. He spent about six months in the hospital before being discharged to civilian life. The therapy he received included two individual sessions with Foulkes and one 'closed' psychotherapy group per week. In the latter work, Foulkes gave few instructions, sitting quietly most of the time. He talked to the group as a whole rather than to individuals, and encouraged discussion about early childhood and dreams. At the same time, Mr A. considered the therapy to be a waste of time, though subsequently he realised that he had benefited greatly from what he had learnt (Interview: Mr A. 1989).

The series of lectures Foulkes gave to the nurses in March and April of 1944 concentrated on the psychoanalytic mechanisms of symptom formation, and appear to have been almost entirely academic. There is no evidence of their applicability to everyday nursing practice, unlike Rickman's teaching at Haymeads. The subjects centred around Freudian mechanisms such as the unconscious, preconscious and consciousness, repression and allied defence mechanisms, and dreams (Foulkes 1944a).

Contemporaneously, Backus and Mansell were treating their enuretic patients rather differently. After a didactic session on bladder mechanisms, anatomy and control, the patient was placed on a programme. This included stopping all drinks after 6 pm, exercises in retaining urine and relaxing the bladder and abdominal wall, and auto-suggestion about control. All this was carried out in a supportive regime of praise for successes and reiteration of encouragement, using such analogies as how learning to skate is about concentrating on how to remain on one's feet rather than worrying about falling. In a few cases individual in-depth psychotherapy was used. They used hypnosis initially but soon abandoned it, as it achieved nothing that could not be done without it. De Maré made a scathing attack on this particular aspect of their treatment:

> Major Backus…had all these people in hypnosis, you see, in which they'd be told that their bladder was getting larger and larger. And so it became a wonder, a miraculous treatment. They all got cured, and they all went back to their units, and after a fortnight it all started up again. (1994, p.3)

Once some bladder control had been established the cases were then referred on to the training wing. Out of the total of 277 cases, 113 went directly back to duty, and a nearly 100 were discharged from the army as medically unfit. Of the rest, over half were transferred to special postings. The remainder stayed in hospital, apart from one who died in an accidental drowning (Backus and Mansell 1944). It should be remembered that Northfield was a 'last port of call' for cases that could not be managed elsewhere, so to have retained over 50 per cent for military service can be counted as success. Of those followed up for up to six months, three-quarters were still carrying out full duties (Backus and Mansell 1944).

Backus and Mansell appear to have achieved good results. These results, although they cannot be directly related, they compare well with those of Slater at the Millhill Emergency Medical Service a year earlier. He found that about a quarter of those with neurotic disorders returned to duty, and that 2.5 per cent were transferred to other duties between 1941 and 1942. Approximately three-quarters were discharged as unfit (Slater 1943).

In the hospital, every activity remained compartmentalised. The training wing stayed separate from the medical unit. The physical examinations were carried out independently of the psychiatric interviews. Physiotherapy was strictly the domain of the physicians. These attitudes were supported by the hospital administration, who considered that the psychiatrists had to be left alone to do their job in the hospital wing (Foulkes 1948, pp.45–46). There was always pressure to take new patients into the wards and move others on into the training wing, which, in Foulkes' opinion, was then a badly run paramilitary unit with anti-psychiatric attitudes. Men were sent there as if they were cured, and prevented from seeing the psychiatrist any more. The soldiers were reluctant to make this move back to army life from the comforts of the wards (Foulkes' contribution to Discussion Group 21, 1945, p.1).

Many anti-therapeutic practices were instituted to satisfy the bureaucracy. The sisters were moved from ward to ward, and were thereby prevented from becoming part of a therapeutic team and gaining any specific expertise. Those soldiers due to be discharged from the army were notified in a publicly displayed list of names, thus advertising their 'success' (Foulkes 1948, p.46–47).

In May 1943, the first signs of patient activity on a hospital-wide basis began. This was signalled by the production of the first edition of *Psyche*. Previously, there had been a hospital bulletin posted up in the NAAFI. The later publication, however, was a cyclostyled magazine containing pictures, poems, stories, critiques of films and descriptions of events in the hospital, running to 20 or 30 pages (*see* Figure 6.1). Although it is not clear how the magazine started, a number of relatively well-known authors were involved, including Rayner Heppenstall, Dewi Davies and Francis Newbold.

The enterprise was enthusiastically supported by Lt. Col. Rosie, who contributed the following:

> I welcome this, the first edition of the magazine. This is not the first occasion on which a publication of this kind has been produced in the hospital, but the previous issues have been in the form of wall newspapers pinned up in the N.A.A.F.I. While this method is economical of paper it fails to afford a reasonable opportunity to everyone concerned to read at leisure the numerous and varied contributions which have been submitted. Accordingly when it was suggested that a magazine in book form should be produced, I had no hesitation in agreeing whole-heartedly with the suggestion, since it seemed to me that the paper and time would be well spent.
>
> We are fortunate in having here a large number of people with unique experience and ability of one kind or another, and feel that the chance of pooling our resources in this way is too good to be missed.

I hope to use this 'open letter' to make known such items of general interest as may arise from time to time and which I think should be passed on without the formality of publication in Part 1 Orders.

In conclusion I hope the magazine will be as successful as it deserves, and shall do all I can to help make it so. (*Psyche* 1943, Issue 1, p.2)

The magazine ran to at least nine issues, the last of which was in the Autumn of 1943 (Psyche 1943, Issue 9). This was perhaps the first evidence of the 'hospital-as-a-whole' approach that Bridger, Foulkes and Main were to develop in the Second Northfield Experiment.

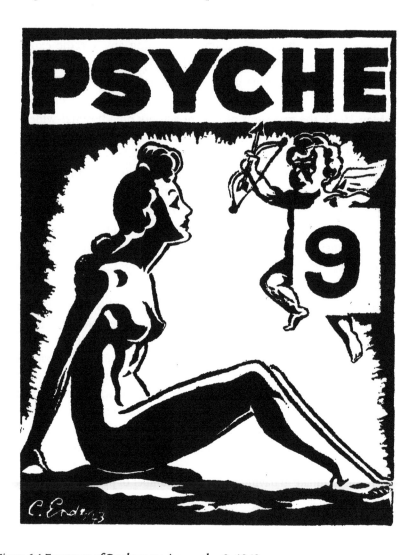

Figure 6.1 Front page of Psyche magazine, number 9, 1943
Reproduced by kind permission of the Wellcome Contemporary Medical Archives Centre

BRIDGING THE GAPS: THE SECOND
EXPERIMENT BEGINS

The appointment of Dennis Carroll as the commanding officer, replacing Lt. Col. Rosie in March 1944, heralded new beginnings. At the end of the same year, Harold Bridger arrived as officer in command of the Training Wing. The experience of the patients was changing as well, with the arrival of men who had been in battle. This brought a new sense of reality to the hospital – a realisation that there was real work to be done and that the unit needed to change its way of operating to achieve this (Foulkes 1948, p.46).

As can be seen in Table 6.1, the numbers of patients were increasing. In July the figures were made up of 422 in Hospital Division and 281 in Rehabilitation Division (War Office 1943/1944a). In the month of October there were 1730 admissions, 200 of whom arrived in one day. The bed numbers in the admission area, Charles Ward, increased to 90. Mrs B., a hospital visitor during the summer, recalls that Margaret Ward was 'absolutely crammed', with beds down the middle (Interview: Mrs B. 1990). It was during this period that a tent was erected in the grounds of the hospital to accommodate the overspill (Gaskin and Gaskin 1990; War Office 1943/1944a). When this blew down, the soldiers had to sleep in the hospital corridors (Gaskin and Gaskin 1990; Interview: Mr L. 1998, p.65).

In June, the opening of the Second Front in northern France brought cases of soldiers who had broken down in battle. Initially, before the setting up of psychiatric facilities out there, men with acute reactions were admitted directly from the front, including during the D Day landings (Carroll 1944a; Foulkes 1948, p.46). The first arrived on June 11, five days after the opening of the offensive (Carroll 1944a).

Emanuel Miller was working in the hospital at this time and saw officers and men returning from France. He attempted to distinguish between the reactions of each group, and his paper suffers from some rather prejudicial underlying assumptions. It is possible, however, to disentangle some characteristics of the disorders affecting the 57 men and officers, all between 20 and 35 years old. On arriving at the hospital they were tremulous and unsteady in their gait, and complained of the incessant mortaring and shelling. Typically, they reported that 'the noise got me down', 'I couldn't stick it any longer', and 'You never knew where they were going to land'. The officers found that the physical exhaustion made them confused: 'I couldn't seem to lead any more', 'I couldn't keep in touch', and 'Very often you didn't quite know whether you were going forward or back' (Miller 1945). At Mill Hill hospital, Anderson and his colleagues were seeing a similar group. Their paper was a little less partial, but under the heading 'First Thoughts' they allowed themselves some latitude in expressing their biases. Their patients came from the Normandy beachhead, and had broken down in the first ten days after D Day. Andersen, Jeffrey and Pai's paper has already been referred to (*see* chapter 4). The pattern of trembling, sweating and weeping, with brief hysterical symptoms of amnesia, muteness, blindness and deafness, was also seen at Hollymoor. Most of the sufferers recovered quickly and well (Anderson *et al.* 1944).

Foulkes kept notes on 20 cases he saw in August and September, though he did not record the diagnoses of all of them. Of these, seven had experienced severe traumas such as being pinned down under a tank, dive-bombed, mortared, shelled or wounded by shrapnel, or having their best friend killed beside them. A 27–year-old had suffered from nerves in a trench 'with bombs and shells falling all round – I lost all sense of feeling, wandering all around' (Foulkes 1943b). Two had been in West Africa, and their disorders appeared to be associated with physical illness and the tropical climate. Another six had had lifelong problems and it was not clear what had caused the problems of three more. One of those with long-term difficulties was described as disgruntled, impulsive and wishing to avoid responsibility, another possibly had epilepsy, and a third wished he had registered as a conscientious objector.

One reason for the erection of the tent was the arrival of the 'Chindits', who contributed to the great influx of soldiers in the late autumn (Dewar 1994; Gaskin and Gaskin 1990). It is not known how many of them there were altogether, but Mr and Mrs Gaskin remember a convoy of about 90 arriving in trucks. 'Chindits' were soldiers who had fought with Orde Wingate behind Japanese lines in Burma, and had suffered extreme food and sleep deprivation and physical disease (Bidwell 1979). The 400 who arrived in a general hospital in the Far East conformed to a particular pattern of appearance and behaviour which Morris and his colleagues described as 'Chindit Syndrome'. This was the association of long hair and long and dirty fingernails with exhaustion, hunger, pallor, loss of weight, skin infections, diarrhoea and malaria in well-mannered men of high intelligence and good morale. They were suffering from a range of infections of the skin and bowels, malaria and anaemia. Over 1000 disorders were found in these 400 men, each individual suffering from two or three conditions requiring hospital treatment (Morris 1945). Dr Millicent Dewar was still emotionally moved half a century later when she recalled seeing them in Northfield. They arrived at all times of the day and night, and the doctors had to work shifts in order to admit them. They were in terrible physical shape, as described by Morris. One man looked over 50 because of his cadaverous appearance and loss of teeth, was in fact in his mid-twenties. All he wanted was his slippers. They were 'all he cared and loved for'. In their ward 'the beds rattled, they rattled with fear. You could hear them'. She did not think that many of them would survive long as they were 'all but impossible to treat'. There was one day when as she walked on the ward one of them gave a wolf-whistle. She was able to retort: 'You're getting better' (Dewar 1993; 1994, p.4).

Despite these changes there still remained the men who were 'browned off' and trying to avoid military service. Mr O. met some:

> Some of them were fed up with the army and they wanted home, and if they could get a discharge fine, they would get a discharge...all sorts of funny little tricks they would get up to... All sorts of stories went round about what you should do to get your ticket, as they called it to be discharged (Interview: Mr O. 1995, p.32)

Mr L. was also aware of them:

> There was one I knew in particular, sort of thing. He was always playing up, and acting up all the while, and saying he was ill when he really wasn't, you know, because it was a way of escape, you see. Because once they said they were ill like that, they said they had a noise in their head and that kind of thing they would put them in hospital so (Interview: Mr L. 1998, p.76)

The new commanding officer, Lt. Col. Dennis Carroll, shared with Foulkes a psychoanalytic approach orientated towards that of Anna Freud. He was also sympathetic to the other psychoanalytically-orientated therapists. The atmosphere with regards to group therapy began to become more supportive, and other psychiatrists were also showing an interest in group work. Amongst these was Martin James, who joined in 1944. Carroll, as has already been noted, was very active in assisting of the work of D.W. Wills in the Hawkspur Experiment, a therapeutic community for young men (*see* chapter 2). It is thus surprising to find that he seems to have made no effort to stimulate such an approach at Northfield apart from giving tacit support to Foulkes and others.

Joshua Bierer is remembered by many participants as being on the sidelines, looking after his own ward in some isolation. Many people recall that as part of the therapeutic activities he organised for his patients he invited his wife, an opera singer, to sing to them (Dewar 1993; Lewsen 1993; Main 1984). He was treated as very lightweight, and received little sympathy from the other psychiatrists, although he was warm-hearted (Lewsen 1993). At this time he had responsibility for the recreational therapy department, the task of which he considered was 'to make the patients physically active' and to 'make them more ready to take responsibility and increase their desire for social relationship' (Bierer 1944). This was attempted largely through sports activities.

In preparation for the Normandy landings, 32 General Hospital assembled at Northfield between January and March, preparing for its mobilisation in the field. This was a unit that was formed to treat the expected psychiatric casualties of the forthcoming battles in northern France. However, it didn't leave until the invasion was well underway, with the result that many of the patients had to be transferred to England, as noted above (Markillie 1993; War Office 1943/1944b). The difficulties of establishing general hospitals in northern France were detailed by Colonel Mitchell, who was evidently very dissatisfied with how the process was handled. As he stated, some hospitals were running active units in France and had little or no training in military matters, whilst others, presumably like 32 General Hospital, 'found themselves unemployed and 'buried' in the heart of the country [England] for several months' (Mitchell 1945).

Foulkes was now able to expand his group work on the ward into the Training Wing. There his patients would be kept together, thus enabling him to follow up the work done on the ward. In this he was supported by Martin James.[2] The range of small groups, one of which was kept together as a team throughout the hospital stay of its members, was supported by a ward meeting where all the patients under one psychiatrist came together (Foulkes 1945a, p.1; 1948, pp.91–102). However, in the early stages it was difficult for new doctors to gain training. Day spent five months in the hospital before he went into a group. Three or four individuals were working in this way and it was a 'very closed and secret matter'. Consequently, Day had to start on his own, somewhat apprehensively (Discussion Group 17, 1945, p.3).

From April 1945, Foulkes organised a weekly peer-group discussion of techniques and aims for all the psychiatrists (Discussion Groups 1945). As a result, this technology of group therapy spread throughout many of the wards in the hospital. Foulkes became known for his expertise in this area, and this, combined with his status as a trained psychoanalyst, enabled him to exert a great influence amongst the medical staff.

Other therapeutic endeavours were encouraged, including allocating Nissen Huts for woodwork, toy-making and modelling. Laurence Bradbury was able to move in to his own hut for art in November 1944. Up until that point he had been employed as an occupational therapist on the wards,

2   Many of the details of when individuals were present at Northfield are based on evidence derived
from their recorded attendance at meetings, or other similar information.

running quiz sessions, giving lectures, and assisting patients to make toys for local schools and nurseries (Bradbury 1990b).

Sergeant Bradbury, as he was then, is significant in the origin of Art Therapy in the United Kingdom. He was visited by Cunningham Dax, a psychiatrist, and some colleagues, who were all impressed by what they saw, in particular 'a painting group conducted by a sergeant with an interest in art'. As a result, they decided 'to introduce such a group to Netherne' (Waller 1991, p.30). Dr Cunningham Dax wrote some years later that he had been 'very impressed with the opportunity given to patients to express themselves freely' (1998). The work that his department then carried out under the leadership of Edward Adamson became a particularly influential stream of art therapy (Waller 1991, pp.52–59). Dr Cunningham Dax believes that in retrospect, this activity at Northfield was the beginning of art therapy in England, and that his subsequent work built on and popularised it (1998).

Laurence Bradbury, later a professor of art and lecturer at the Tate Gallery in London, prefers not to use the phrase 'Art Therapy', stressing that art *is* therapy. Describing the events later he wrote:

> In the hut we worked as individuals, or in groups, just as the fancy took the continually changing 'class'. There was never any organised pattern – just a gang of personalities, sometimes sombre, dejected, miserable and more often uproarious, even 'high', patients reacting one against another or falling in with current fads and styles. On several occasions a group project was mounted but with no compulsion to join in, though most did eventually if only to trounce those already engaged.
>
> We painted an Island on a huge roll of paper, each participant adding his desired bit, be it an imagined Cythera or a monster's cave. And there was a running Theme and Variations, one painter taking over from another. (1990b)

This spontaneity, so warmly advocated by Moreno, took other forms. On a wet day Bradbury might lay a piece of paper just inside the door, where the soldiers had to step on it. When they sat down and started to bemoan the fact that they couldn't think of anything to paint, he would place the paper, with its muddy footprints, in front of them, announcing 'you've already started' (Bradbury 1990a).

> The door was open for anyone to join in, or leave, or simply 'witness', and with painted efforts carried away into the wards by their originators, the interest, ribaldry, enthusiastic if amateur art criticism, and of course all the ingenious attempts by patients to interpret the symbols discovered in their colleagues' works, meant that the goings-on in the art hut acted as a catalyst for expressions to be voiced throughout the whole hospital and thus, I thought a good communal therapy. (Bradbury 1990c).

Bradbury's advocacy of art as therapy in itself was warmly approved of by Cunningham Dax, who wrote after his visit: 'I am sure that avoidance of any previous knowledge of the patient or attempted psychological interpret- ations is an extremely wise approach. I am sure there are tremendous possibilities in the future of the work and I have numerous plans as to what we could do with it in the future' (Cunningham Dax 1945). What did happen in the very immediate future was that the art hut became one of the epicentres of the full-blown 'therapeutic community' for precisely the reasons that Bradbury believed it should. His provision of a freely creative environment acted as an emotional barometer, an opportunity for experimentation and a point of release. It allowed for a discharge of entropic activity, without fear or favour. Many of the men would never have had such an opportunity to use their creativity and have it valued in a non-pejorative environment. This enhanced their esteem both in their own and others' eyes. Of course, all sorts of unconscious forces were operating; but, entirely congruently with Rickman's conceptions of work, this was an arena in which childish conflicts were being explored and new methods of understanding them forged. For Bradbury it was an entirely intuitive process. He himself claimed that he was unaware of any conscious 'wisdom': 'I was completely ignorant so far as psycho-therapy was concerned, but within such a marvellously concentrated institution learning was absorbed every minute' (1990c).

A second focus of activity in the hospital formed around Harold Bridger, an artillery officer. He arrived at the end of 1944 from the War Office Selection Boards to take charge of the Training Wing. Prior to his arrival he had been primed by Ronald Hargreaves, and it is clear from the discussion that they had that the Tavistock Group were interested in and aware of what was happening at Northfield. He was informed that there were a lot of 'groupy things' going on there, and asked if he would he take a look.[3] A little apprehensive about what to expect, he prepared himself by visiting Wilfred Bion and reading up on the Peckham Experiment. The discussion with the former encouraged him to use his own resources rather than ape the previous episode. The latter gave him the idea of creating a central arena, a development of the swimming pool in Pearce and Crocker's enterprise (*see* chapter 2). In a similar manner, this would become a process that reflected and informed the community, and the wider environment, as a whole. He also visited a number of other psychiatric hospitals, including Maxwell

---

3   Bridger 1985, p. 98; 1990a. The whole of the following section is reliant on Bridger's accounts, which, although partial, are supported by the other evidence available from Foulkes, the Discus- sion Groups and Bradbury.

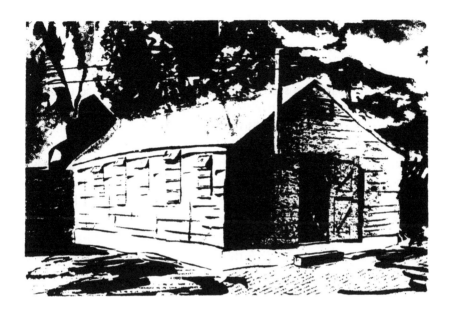

'The Art Hut', a collage by an anonymous artist at Northfield Military Hospital
From a colour original – reproduced with the kind permission of Professor Laurence
Bradbury

Jones' unit at Mill Hill. He was unhappy with what he found there. The
patients seemed peripheral, operating in a closed system centred on Jones
himself (Bridger 1985, pp.98–100). The wartime work of Maxwell Jones
will be discussed in greater depth in the section on group therapy.

As well from his knowledge of the 'leaderless group' selection procedure,
Bridger brought with him another skill. This was the result his experience as
a mathematics teacher at a school in Coventry before the war. Pupils tended
to lose interest in the traditional methods of teaching that subject, and so
Bridger looked around for other methods. Influenced by the work of John
Dewey, the American educator, he always tried to find 'growing points' on
which to build experience. He involved the children in real-life situations
that would have mathematical thinking inherent in them, such as a school
stock exchange. By engaging them in actually modelling the real process, he
taught them both the methods of arithmetic and their value. Similarly, in the
Battery Command he had just left, he found that the men had difficulty in
understanding the orders passed down to them. To overcome this, he

published a set of 'Battery Disorders' alongside them, which illustrated them in cartoon form (Bridger 1990a, p.76).

One of the issues Bridger discussed with Bion was his concern that he was not a psychiatrist. He felt that this might be a handicap (Discussion Group 3, 1945, p.3). It would have been daunting to realise that the radical innovations he wanted to introduce were being critically observed by older and senior psychoanalysts such as Foulkes. Bridger also realised that as an artillery officer the expectation of the staff was that he was going to work in a traditional military manner (Bridger 1990a, p.76). The ground was prepared for him, to some extent, by John Rickman and Ronald Hargreaves, who were both in correspondence with Foulkes. In October, Hargreaves recommended to the latter the papers by Moreno referred to in chapter 2, as they had recently been discussing the use of psychodrama. Rickman had visited late in 1944, about which he wrote: 'It was kind of you to give me so much of your time during my visit to Northfield from which I have learnt a lot' (1944). According to de Maré, this was when Foulkes first learnt about Bion and his previous experiment (1983, p.232). Rickman later penned a long and crucial letter, which laid out the importance of what was

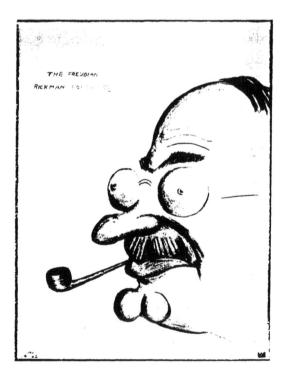

Major John Rickman, drawn 28th September 1942 by an unknown artist at Northfield Military Hospital .
Reproduced by kind permission of the Wellcome Institute Library, London.

happening. In this he spoke 'as a proud Northfieldian', stating Northfield's primacy as a pioneering and expensive psycho-social experiment, and warning that 'if the level falls to less than this answer not to me, but to your conscience and the body of army' (1944). In his view, Northfield was too remote from the work on the psychology of groups that was developing in the WOSBs. He proposed as a remedy that Foulkes pay attention to Bridger's methods, as he was

> an experienced WOSB military testing officer and has handled group discussions and drawn inferences from them over many months, and with considerable benefit to himself and his colleagues including psychiatrists. I do not suggest that you ask him to take discussions or to be a psychotherapist; but I do suggest that you ask him to be present and pick his brains afterwards as to the dynamics of the group interventions... Bridger can tell you a lot more about that sort of thing. It is 'a-historical' data, i.e. the result of forces operating in the present, that came from group movements and not 'genetic-psychology' or historical data, so it needs interpreting (by yourself, to yourself for yourself, i.e. clues only), but what useful clues once you've got the hang of it (Rickman 1944).

Rickman was at pains to make the points he made in previous papers and discussions. The task was to use all available clues, especially those derived from a psychoanalytic analysis, to understand what is going on in the 'here and now'. There was little or no value in interpreting these in the classical psychoanalytic sense by referring back to the patient's history. Apart from anything else, there was no time for this. More importantly, the soldier was having to learn how to manage the dynamics of groups in the army and his impact on them.

It is at this time that the influence of the members of the 'invisible college' is most evident. There is an increasingly active correspondence between Hargreaves, Rickman and Main, with the former two visiting every so often. Hargreaves, as mentioned earlier, briefed Bridger and later Main, and made them both aware of Bion and Rickman's earlier effort.

One lesson that Bridger learnt from this previous experience was the importance of taking on board the wider social system. As a consequence, on arrival, he spent some time discussing his ideas with the commanding officer, now Lt. Col. Rowlette, and other senior members of staff, Foulkes, Emanuel Miller and Alfred Torrie. These latter two were in charge of the two medical divisions of the hospital. Bridger discussed the ideas further with the external organisation as represented by Ronald Hargreaves (Bridger 1985, p.101). Having ensured that these individuals were clear about what he intended to do, he was confident that he could embark on his mission with their support.

Bridger took command of the Training Wing, which gave him control over the military rehabilitation aspect of the hospital. He also established another role, that of social therapist, which gave him the hospital-wide remit he needed to establish a cohesive 'hospital-as-a-whole' ethos. Even though some of the barriers between the different departments had begun to break down, they still largely maintained separate identities, and therapists continued to work independently. In order to establish a coherent system in which all the parts cooperated to achieve the primary goal of returning soldiers to some form of military service, the whole unit needed to work as one. Bridger's strategy contained an implicit criticism of the sequence of commanding officers, who through their role as leader could have established this.

The strategy being established, Bridger now turned to tactics. How to face the whole hospital with its role? Typically, he went a step further than providing a fully functioning swimming pool, as in the Peckham Experiments. His answer was to pose the key question 'what are we here for?' with the means of its solution. He commandeered an empty ward and placed a sign outside saying 'The Hospital Club', thus creating a vacuum at the heart of the establishment. There was no furniture, equipment or rules. His only other action was to organise a meeting of representatives from the other hospital wards in which to discuss equipment and organisation. This emptiness acted like a silence in group therapy, leading the whole establishment to question its existence. What was everybody's role in this? Bradbury had been asking the same question every day in his art hut, when the soldiers sat down to fill in their blank pieces of paper. Bridger now interrogated the whole system.

Bridger met with his social therapy team and explained his intention that all the activities of the organisation were to be integrated into one 'hospital-as-a-whole-with-its-mission'. In order to do this, the whole workforce, including professionals, had to meet together to discuss what it implied. In order to proselytise, the social therapy staff attended ward meetings when invited, where they introduced the new ideas. They themselves had to change their methods and roles. No longer were they to hand out tasks to be carried out. As we have seen, these tended to consist of education, or embroidery and suchlike. Instead, they were to try and leave the initiative with the patients, not just demanding to know what they wanted to do, but, as Rickman would have suggested, watching for clues as to the real needs of the individuals.

It took some time for the empty ward to take on its character. Many meetings were held and gradually the recognition dawned in the various areas that each was going to have to make a contribution. There was a table-tennis table in one ward and a snooker table in another, and no one was keen to give up 'their' property. Consequently, the first representative meeting took some time to arrange, and in the event was a bit of a damp squib. There was no appointed chairperson – indeed, it was a leaderless group! Bridger refused to take this role, and the hole in the middle of the hospital suddenly became a live 'here and now' issue. This led to a lot of discomfort as those at the meeting suddenly grasped that they were in an entirely unpredicted and unpredictable situation. It is easy to imagine the shuffling of feet, furtive looks and general shifting around as the implications began to take shape in their minds. They were going to have to take responsibility themselves; but quite what for? The next task was to find out (Bridger 1985, pp.101–103; 1990b). They thus started on the road that Bion had mapped out in the First Northfield Experiment and explained later in 1946. What was the neurosis that disturbed the group, as a whole rather than its individual members, and how was it going to be tackled (Bion 1946)?

The challenge was taken up only cautiously. Little gaggles of soldiers would pop their heads round the door of the club and ask the social staff questions about when it was to open and when the furniture and fittings were going to arrive. Each time they were reminded that it would start as soon as they organised it. Concurrently, there were discussions with men who were coming forward to find out what they might do in the way of leisure or work activities. All occupational therapy for solely time-consuming purposes was halted. People's previous interests and skills were resurrected, leading to the formation of teams of individuals taking up different activities.

The saga of the social club culminated in a meeting of patients to which Bridger was summoned. Here he was confronted by a group of soldiers wanting to know why he was wasting time and money in wartime. They were especially concerned about the waste of space, which was so much at a premium in the hospital. Bridger calmly agreed, and wondered what should be done about it. After the debate, the men began to realise that they could take responsibility and power, and organise things in the way that they wanted. The first Committee was thus formed as a result of the protest group. Once this energy had been released the patients' creativity knew no bounds. It was not a smooth path: at times the social club was vandalised, and even on occasion smashed up completely. However, progress was made. The Hospital Club acted as a therapeutic test bed. It enabled individuals to place the insights gained from their personal treatment into a social context and test out the consequences in a 'here and now' community. It made it possible for them to ally their personal energy with a social purpose and come up with the organisational structures required to achieve it. This self-evidently paralleled their role in the army and society as a whole (Bridger 1985, p.104).

A particularly important step was the realisation that the 'old hands' could contribute to the care and support of recent admissions. From this sprang the idea of a mentoring system, and an information booklet prepared 'by a patient' for the new arrivals (Anon, undated, see Appendix 2 to this book). This latter outlined the reasons why the person was in the hospital. As has already been explained, most had been told little or nothing about why they were being taken to Northfield. The booklet also gave information about activities, the purpose of the hospital, and leave arrangements. One was handed to the new man by a reception group made up entirely of patients within three days of their arrival on the admission ward. They were encouraged to discuss its contents and make sure that they understood all of the implications. They were then taken on a tour of the hospital to introduce them to all the facilities (Bridger 1946).

The activities of the social club blossomed. A newspaper was established, which went through a number of incarnations as the *Mercury*, the *Weekly Bulletin* and the *Blues Flash*. It began with a duplicating machine, accessories, paper and a debt of £260: 00d (Bridger 1946). One of the earliest volunteers working on the newspaper was Mr N. He recalled Bridger as 'being in charge of occupational therapy or something', and having possibly 'appointed' him to the newspaper role (Interview: Mr N. 1994, pt.1, p.6). There were a number of people working there already. One was a cartoonist, 'about half a stop short of being brilliant' (p.18). They produced several hundred copies in a run, 'dished them out left, right and centre, and gave them to little shops in the area to circulate' (p.20). One campaign backfired. This was against the food, which in the opinion of Mr N. was 'atrocious'. The crisis came about because 'somebody had found a large sized grub sitting on their cabbage threatening them with bodily harm or something'. Publishing this provoked the administration into closing the magazine down. However, 'Bridger said his piece', the administration eventually backed down, and the food did apparently improve a little (p.20). Mr N.'s admiration for Bridger is very clear. He describes the letter as 'full of enthusiasm, but not slap you on the back and jolly hockey sticks. But a nice chap. Plenty to do. Didn't always remember everything you said or what have you, but fair enough' (p.19).

Other activities followed, including theatre, sculpture, pottery, radio construction, gardening, building construction and other handicrafts. For Mr I., the 'radio electronic gear' was the only good thing about the hospital (Interview: Mr. I. 1996). People went out to work, this being the first instance of supported placements in industry for people with mental ill-health in this country. As well as working at the Austin Motor Company, which then was making military vehicles, they also went to the Avoncroft agricultural college and to shops in town. Toys were being made for Child Guidance Clinics and local nurseries. Men were redecorating the play rooms and 'incidentally helping the nurses to bath the babies!' (Bridger 1946).

One of the first groups to get off the ground was a band (Bridger 1985, p.103). As Mr O. started to recover, in late 1944, he was asked by his doctor what he wanted to do. After some exploration of whether he liked basket weaving, which he didn't, he was asked whether he enjoyed playing music. 'Well I play drums', he replied. So he and some others formed the hospital band, playing every Saturday night in the main hall, and sometimes in other units in Birmingham. They were allowed to rehearse in a side ward 'with padded doors'. Mrs O., the telephonist, was aware that it was 'all part of the therapy' (Interview: Mr and Mrs O. 1995, pp.4–5). Mr O. didn't take part in the group therapy; instead he 'talked to the drums' (p.35).

The opportunity to work at the Austin Motor Company, just down the road, had to be negotiated with the unions and management (Bridger 1985, p.103). Once it was established, the patients came into contact with local girls like Mrs E. She enjoyed having the young men to talk to: 'Well it was really a surprise for us, young girls, seeing a lot of young fellows working there. And when they were told that they had dances as well that made it more smashing, you know' (Interview: Mrs E. 1998, p.11). The work that they did at that time was 'on the track': 'it was a very mundane job on the roller track. It was different operations going round you know and each one had done the particular one... There would be about twenty... It was one of the very boring jobs. I suppose you wondered why it helped them when they had such a boring job' (p.23).

However, that wasn't the only type of work available. Mr L. went with a party of five men to the factory where they would strip engines. 'We worked on the strip and rebuild for four months and that was very interesting.' The team members took it in turns to act as foreman (Interview: Mr L. 1998, pp.18, 60–61). This rotation enabled each of them to take responsibility and practice leadership skills. Another group built cold frames for tomatoes and mushrooms, which involved a range of skills: 'some members built the brick foundations, others made the glazed tops and so on' (Foulkes 1945a, p.7).

At this time, six to eight new arrivals often immediately formed a team under one doctor on admission. Initially, this was a therapy group, run by the psychiatrist; but it was not allowed to stay isolated from the wider social system for long. A member of the social therapy staff, often Bridger himself, would attend the second or third meeting to discuss what project the team might embark on. This was consciously derived from the WOSB leaderless groups, and allowed for the development of cooperation and integration, enabling the members to share in the creation of something for others.

Bridger characterised this process as a transitional one, prefiguring the concept of the transitional object later developed by Winnicott (Bridger 1990b). This is an object that acts as a psychological bridge between the individual baby and others. Through loving, cuddling and playing with the object the child is enabled to move from the self-centred, narcissistic love and dependency of infancy to independence and selfless love of others (Winnicott 1971, pp.1–5). Bridger described the move from the initial closed group to the external world. Initially, patients would be confined to a psychiatrist-based therapy group on the ward; finally, there would be a member of an open group in the social therapy unit and all the groups would interact with one another within the hospital field (Discussion Group 7, 24 May 1945, p.1; Discussion Group 9, 21 June 1945, p.20).

Few of the other members of staff fully grasped this framework. More often than not the wards remained the doctors' castles, isolated and operating independently from the rest of the hospital (Bridger 1990b). Bierer's practice was characteristic. He did not participate in any of the discussion groups, and kept himself aloof from the other doctors. Rickman observed that:

> Psychiatry is up against something about as big as itself. It puts the psychiatrists on their toes to discover something which is better than they themselves have concept of. Bridger's department is a challenge to the psychiatrist. (Discussion Group 13, 29 August 1945, p.6)

Another doctor, Lieutenant Martin, concurred with him, arguing that: 'This hospital will have to realise that the most important contribution being made to the patients is Major Bridger's department.' His complaint that 'this much more realistic psychiatry' was not taught in the text books elucidated the steep learning curve that many of his colleagues were faced with (Discussion Group 13, 29 August 1945, p.6).

Ward meetings, in which all the staff and soldiers met together, also began to spread around the hospital. Foulkes and Bierer were the first to implement these. By July 1945 Creak was able to report that on her ward the meeting was presided over by a patient and had a detailed agenda. In the example she gave, 15 subjects were covered including food, the Hospital Club, passes, hospital discipline and the psychiatrist (Discussion Group 10, 1945, p.6). There was some debate about the role of psychiatrists, on whether they should attend or even chair meetings. These gatherings did not always run easily. In one meeting one of the men stated that he did not like the sister. As a result the nurse left, despite attempts to persuade her to stay (Discussion Group 10, 1945, p.1).

The process of change in the hospital was organic. Different projects were developing all over, at different speeds and different intensities. Each individual had to face his own 'vacuum' and find out how to overcome it; consequently, different tactics for avoiding this would be invented and some groups, including staff, would overlook it altogether. However, by the spring of 1945 a whole range of activities were in place, and more were accumulating.

Foulkes began to expand the expertise in group therapy within the hospital. Although still only working clinically with his own patients, he set up a discussion group for the medical staff. These ran weekly and were attended by between four and eight doctors. This began to spread the practice around the hospital as individuals gained confidence. The work of these seminars is examined in more detail later, in the section on group therapy.

'THE THERAPEUTIC INSTITUTION': THE SECOND NORTHFIELD EXPERIMENT, PART II

After VE day, 8 May 1945, more changes began to take place. First, the types of patient and their expectations were different. Increased numbers of ex-prisoners of war were arriving from Germany. Now, with the war over, the expectation was that of going back to 'civvy street'. The sense of an overall 'mission' had gone, and everyone was looking to the end of their time in the army, including the staff.

The initiation of new admissions to the hospital was now well co-ordinated between patients and staff. First, the patient was examined by a psychiatrist on the morning following his arrival (Anon, undated). Then, after the introductions to the 'old hands' described earlier, he was advised on the range of activities that he might join in. These could be taken up immediately, rather than on transfer to the now defunct Training Wing. Often, the patient would deny interest in what was happening in the hospital, and state a preference for other pursuits. Ways of carrying these out would then be discussed. Whilst awaiting allocation to a treatment ward, the person would be given psychological tests and requested to complete questionnaires. At other times he might be invited to a dance, a party, the theatre, or another form of entertainment, and would meet local women who were out to have fun. For many of the soldiers this was the first taste of an England they had left three to four years previously. There was no 'free' time, but the individual was at liberty to make up his own programme without the supervision that the army would normally require (Bridger 1946).

On the third day the new man would be allocated to a treatment ward. A 'ward workers group', whose task it was to look after domestic affairs, would introduce him to the unit and inform him about everything that was going on. He was seen every day by his psychiatrist in the morning ward round, and every week the commanding officer visited to hear complaints or requests (Bridger 1946). In August of 1945 Mildred Creak was admitting two patients a day to her ward (Discussion Group 11, 1945, p.6).

As a result of the increasing range of 'work' activities, the Training Wing was dissolved. Its role became the promotion of the new projects. The hospital was now treated as one unit. The weekly ward meetings now took on a role of self-governance. They were attended by all the staff of the unit as well as the soldiers, and were chaired by the men (Anon, undated; Bridger 1946). Delegates from these formed a central hospital committee, which had evolved from the original meeting that Bridger initiated. This partly advised on and partly took responsibility for the running of the hospital (Foulkes 1948, p.48). It was attended by the senior social therapy staff and the commanding officer. These were responsible for liaising with other parts of the hospital when it was necessary (Bridger 1946; Discussion Group 10, 1945). Bridger was evidently proud of how this group, despite the rapid turnover of personnel, grew in maturity and responsibility. Initially, it had been a talking shop for airing grievances; eight months later it had a constitution and discussed projects such as how to assist the Birmingham Children's Hospital. It had spawned several sub-committees, which organised dances, sports, socials and competitions (Bridger 1946).

Emanuel Miller and Alfred Torrie left, to be replaced by Lt. Col. Sutton and Tom Main. The former was quite out of sympathy with the reforms, and clearly did not really understand them. Tom Freeman, who was under his command, wrote: 'He was an orthodox, conservative psychiatrist and his division was run accordingly'; as a result Freeman 'had little contact with the work which Main and Foulkes were doing' (Freeman 1989).

Main arrived in May, and enthusiastically gave his backing to the changes.[4] He soon became concerned about his and Bridger's relationship with the commanding officer. Previously, Torrie in his gentle way had negotiated an understanding between Bridger and Rowlette; now the latter had to face two of his officers working in tandem. This evidently led to tension, usually signalled by Rowlette looking out of his office window rather than at his two subordinates (Bridger 1990b). Main realised that

4   As over many details, he and Bridger appear to be in conflict about when each of them was at Northfield; but the evidence from the group sessions suggests that Main came about five months after Bridger.

unless he started to understand the CO's position he would suffer the same fate as Bion. He then took time to consider the strains that Rowlette was affected by. Rowlette's task was to balance the requirements of the regular military administration, which was appalled at the apparent mayhem, with the demands of the clinical side. The latter group, of course, considered the former to be archaic and reactionary. It became clear to Main that the anger and resentment was not about individual dissensions, but was the result of dynamics within the system, and it was these that had to be resolved. Each individual had become the repository of the hopes, fantasies, ambitions and dissatisfactions of their staff, and was thus championing these causes rather than dispassionately examining what was behind them. How could they be resolved at the lower levels of the system rather than being amplified and distorted through the senior officers? (Main 1989, p.136). Foulkes was clear about the need for the commanding officer to represent the military administration, as it forced the community as a whole to remain firmly attached to reality. He observed that Rowlette even began to adopt some of the new ideas himself (Foulkes 1948, p.48).

It was as a result of this debate that it occurred to Main that the entire system had to be engineered so that the whole unit became orientated towards the healthy socialisation of the patients. A week after having spoken to John Rickman at Northfield, he was of the opinion that the unit was not a hospital, but 'a therapeutic institute' (Discussion Group 14, 1945, p.6). He later coined the term 'therapeutic institution' (Main 1946a). In his later writings he claimed to have invented the term 'therapeutic community'; however, Harry Stack Sullivan pre-empted him with the phrase 'therapeutic camp or community' in 1939, in his essay on therapeutic conceptions (Sullivan 1955, p.232; first published 1939).[5] Main's previous experience of hospital work enabled him to see the far-reaching effects such an approach would have. The transition of the patient from a passive recipient of care, regarded as 'good' as long as they conformed to dictates of the institution, into an active partner in therapy, making decisions about what form it was to take, challenging previous ideas, and taking power and responsibility in the process of their recovery, was revolutionary (Main 1946a). It is difficult to

---

5   My thanks goes to Craig Fees, Archivist, Planned Environment Therapy Archive, for bringing my attention to this, and also to the work of Wills and others before the war. Whilst the concept may have been new to Main, the evidence for similar approaches, albeit on a smaller scale, has already been adumbrated (*see* chapter 2). Bridger's vision of the 'hospital-as-a-whole-with-its-mission' was also identical in its embrace. There remains the suspicion that Main, in order to accept a new idea, had to reinvent it for himself, like many other pioneers.

improve on his passionate expression of these ideas in the *Bulletin of the Menninger Clinic* after the war. The Northfield Experiments had

> been conceived as a therapeutic setting with a spontaneous and emotionally structured (rather than medically dictated) organisation in which all staff and patients engage... The daily life of the community must be related to real tasks, truly relevant to the needs and aspirations of the small society of the hospital, and the larger society in which it is set; there must be no barriers between the hospital and the rest of society; full opportunities must be available for identifying and analysing the interpersonal barriers which stand in the way of full participation in a full community life. (Main 1946a)

It proved difficult to bring on board the administrative staff and this aim was not achieved by the time Main left in early 1946. However, he had more time to implement these ideas at the Cassell Hospital, where he remained for the best part of 30 years.

Other members of staff also had to come to terms with these new approaches. General nurses had to get to grips with the fact that for much of the day their patients were not even on the ward, and especially not in bed. If the nurses were to keep in contact, they had to become peripatetic themselves. As a consequence, their strictly defined roles began to change as they supported social therapy staff in other venues (Bridger 1985, p.105).

Echoing Bion, Main questioned the standard assumption that the doctors and nurses were well people treating the sick. The traditional healer's role was to step in at times of crisis and 'cure' the patient using his or her specialist skills. The new role meant that the psychiatrist was no longer the sole expert, and had to share the sense of chaos and encourage the men themselves to find the solutions. It was their learning of these skills through practice in real situations that was going to prepare them for their return to military or civilian life.

Bridger left the hospital around September 1945.[6] This coincided with a gradual deterioration in morale, as the consequences of peace manifested themselves. As a solution, Main then invited Foulkes to extend his role into that of a hospital group therapy co-ordinator and ad hoc trouble-shooting consultant. The latter interpreted this role as providing him with the opportunity to become a roving group therapist, intervening in art groups, work teams and other gangs of patients all over the hospital to help them to examine conflicts and disagreements. He also founded the Co-ordination

6   He was present at Susannah Davidson's therapy group of 30/8/45 (Davidson 1946, p.93). This is the last recorded evidence of his presence at the hospital.

Group (Foulkes 1964, p.193). In his own idiosyncratic style he inaugurated this on one ward as a closed group, presumably with the intention of nursing it in its early stages. Later it accumulated representatives from other wards (Foulkes 1945d, nos. 1 and 4). This organisation promoted intra-hospital activities such as a 'Brains Trust' involving psychiatrists and patients, and inter-ward quizzes (Foulkes 1945d, nos. 1 and 4). In Foulkes' view this was significant in improving the life in the hospital, and he praised its rapid effect on everyone from the office girl to the commanding officer (Foulkes 1964, p.193).

As part of his role, Foulkes issued communiqués. These could be somewhat browbeating in style, admonishing wards for failing to attend the committee meetings punctually, complaining that patients were abusing the public houses, requesting people to return paintings to the art hut and encouraging the psychiatrists to get in 'closer contact with the patients' (Foulkes 1945d, no.4). There is no evidence that these many difficulties were interpreted as symptoms of system problems requiring strategic interventions in the manner of Bion, Rickman or Bridger.

In the background there remained Rickman and Hargreaves. The former visited on at least one more occasion on 29 August 1945, having done so in late 1944 and most probably at the end of the previous year (Discussion Group 13, 1945, p.3).[7] The latter had spoken to Main before he came, saying 'there are a lot of groupie things going on there, we're going to send all the group people there we can possibly get hold of' (Main 1984).

At the time, Main was extremely pleased to have such allies. He was disconcerted about the role of Foulkes, and was perhaps expressing his grief at the loss of Bridger when he wrote to Rickman in September:

> Since your visit, which came most appropriately at a time when several of us, who had watched groups with increasing scepticism, were wondering just what the hell we and others were doing... This is at once an apology for Northfield and an explanation of our present state of development. The only alternative was a leader and disciples for the particular cult about which you felt such dismay, a set, in fact of Foulkes worshippers. (Main 1945)

It is not clear precisely what Foulkes was doing to so upset Main. However, the records of group discussions reported in the next chapter certainly hint at marked tensions between Foulkes' approach, and that of Bridger and Main.

---

7   Abrahams wrote in January 1944: 'While you were here you were a very welcome member of the mess – wish you could have stayed longer and provided some more explosive ideas. Yours sincerely Sidney Abrahams (Northfield Military Hospital)' (Abrahams 1944).

It is also clear that the former had trained a number of the other psychiatrists at the hospital in his techniques. Certainly, Main's effusive eulogy to Foulkes later in life, in which he called him 'the outstanding therapist and teacher in my division' (Main 1984, p.132), would seem to indicate that the issue was resolved.

Hargreaves wrote at least four letters to Foulkes. Most of these were concerned with latter's articles for the *Bulletin of the Menninger Clinic*. However, one indicates his sharp awareness about what was happening at Northfield, and also his keenness to keep Foulkes on target!

> The Northfield Experiment to my mind is not limited to group psychotherapy; it is the fundamental integration of group psychotherapy with an attempt to structure the hospital field in a purposeful and therapeutic manner. Your own work in the field of group *psychotherapy* is, of course, in no way derived from Bion's concepts... But the *total pattern* of the Northfield Experiment as I have summarised above, is part of a long chain of developments in the army which originated from Bion's work with the leaderless group tests. (Hargreaves 1945)

These two letters support the contention that despite later declarations of cooperation and mutual confidence, underneath the surface there were dissensions. Others also noted the tensions between members of the medical staff (Dewar 1993; 1994; Lewsen 1993; Markillie 1993).

All this was kept well under wraps for the visit of a prestigious group of Americans in June 1945. Arranged by Hargreaves, this consisted of Drs Laurence Kubie, John Romano, John Whitehorn, Leo Bartemeier and Karl Menninger. A two-day programme of papers and visits around the hospital ensued. One of them interviewed Mr N., who was working on the newspaper. It was with some pride that Mr N. recalled that he wasn't completely overawed: 'I was level pegging in conversation'. However, he was somewhat taken aback, after having expressed an interest in writing, to be asked to describe an English shilling. Apparently, this was supposed to be a good exercise to develop such skills (Interview: Mr N. 1994, p.18).

The visit was not without its lighter side. Whilst the convoy of Americans and their hosts straggled around the hospital, one of them noticed some tomato plants and, impressed by them, asked how they were grown to such high quality. This crop was actually the work of Charles Lewsen, the physician, and the question gradually filtered back down the column to him. On a whim, Lewsen decided to claim that the magic ingredient was blood. The answer, having passed up the line, provoked another query: where did he get it? The response to this was 'I do the Wasserman's on all the patients.' That this seems to have been taken seriously is indicated by the vehement way in which the questioner refused the tomatoes offered him at lunch (Lewsen 1993, p.15).

Karl Menninger was fulsome in his praise of what he saw. Besides devoting a complete issue of the *Bulletin of the Menninger Clinic*, the prestigious medical journal run from the American Clinic, to papers by hospital staff, he wrote in his editorial:

> One of the things which impressed us was the skillful use of the principle of group psychology and group dependency in therapeutic programmes of various types. It seemed to us somewhat paradoxical that the British psychiatrists so generally give the credit for the original stimulus and the development of basic principles of their work to American scientists but have carried the application of these principles much further than is common in American psychiatric practice. (1946)

Menninger followed this up later in 1948, when commenting on American therapeutic communities, by stating that none of them had developed as far as the system at Northfield, 'where the patients all become part of a community, each with his own job' (1948, p.303).

There were other visitors. The Civil Resettlement Units were being established to assist men being repatriated following their time as prisoners of war. Groups of eight officers, both ex-prisoners of war and others, visited Northfield to gain experience of the group work that was taking place. They included medical officers, general physicians, who appeared to be the most 'sticky' in failing to understand what was going on. They were unprepared for, and suspicious of, the radical changes in medical practice that their psychiatric colleagues had introduced into the hospital. The flow of visitors caused quite a lot of disruption to the work of the hospital, and was earnestly debated in the psychiatrists' discussion groups. However, the staff began to recognise their own therapeutic effect on these visitors. The training that the latter had hitherto received was often chaotic, whereas at Northfield they took part in a structured and well-organised programme, which they found reassuring (Discussion Group 13, 1945).

The year finished on a despondent note. The failure of co-ordination between the wards and the activity department reminded Foulkes of the 'bad old days' of 1943. The doctors were overwhelmed with work, with frequent convoys arriving. There were 60 to 70 men on each ward. One doctor reported that he was expected to provide five reports on new patients in less than an hour. Many of the doctors were new and had no experience of group therapy (Harris, in Discussion Group 21, 1945, p.3). Just before Christmas 1945, Foulkes was angry and disappointed about what he considered to be lack of support for the new form of group therapy. The discussion seminars had stopped, and few psychiatrists attended them anyway. Foulkes fell back on the method he knew best, which was to start off a seminar group with the psychiatrists with a ten-minute diatribe on all that was wrong. He was evidently in conflict with Tom Main, disagreeing with the latter's 'liberal' attitudes (Foulkes, in Discussion Group 21, 1945, pp.1–3).

It is clear that the influx of prisoners of war from Germany and elsewhere had led to a general pressure on beds in the army. Selection procedures to ensure that only treatable cases were taken to Northfield were blatantly ignored. One transfer of men from Netley should have had only five appropriate candidates; instead, 27 uncategorised cases turned up. In these circumstances, Foulkes argued, seeing people individually was inefficient and time-wasting, and caused the immense pressure that the doctors were feeling (Foulkes, in Discussion Group 21, 1945, p.4). The 'group spirit' was lacking in the hospital and amongst the psychiatrists (de Maré, in Discussion Group 21, 1945, p.5).

The conflicts still remained with the non-therapeutic military staff. Indeed, the commanding officer was running out of patience with the apparent chaos. The administration felt ignored. Having recognised this ongoing concern, Main was unable to take up the challenge because he was posted away (Main 1989, p.135).

DISINTEGRATION: THE LAST TWO YEARS

Slowly but inevitably, the key participants left Northfield as they were demobbed from the army. Foulkes went in the spring of 1946, and Bradbury on 23 May 1946. The personnel was changing rapidly, and the new staff stayed for only short periods of time. The Reverend Corbin, who at the time was a clerk in the RAMC, stayed for about six months in a job that he was unfamiliar with. He spent so little time at Northfield that he got to know little about workings of the hospital and very few of the other members of staff (Corbin 1990). The few who were there appeared to be overwhelmed with work. The officer in charge of Vernon Scannell's ward in 1947 was young, and clearly felt that the little could be done for the patients under his care. After carrying out the admission, he did not return for two weeks to see his patient (Scannell 1983, p.59). Consequently, the enthusiasm, energy and innovation evaporated, and the 'tennis ball' sprang back into shape.

Whilst inevitably coloured by his own misery and anger, Vernon Scannell's description of the hospital is dismal. He could not read or write because 'that sour air, the feeling of squirming fears, delusions, and sick torments that were being endured all around me' made concentration impossible.

Mr Q. felt much the same about his eight months as a mental nursing orderly on Charles Ward in 1947. He was the only qualified mental nurse on the ward, apart from one other who worked nights. All the patients were categorised as intractable, with little hope of improvement. There were few activities, little treatment and less documentation. The patients were bored and had little to do except vent their anger on the staff. There were no therapeutic groups, the only group activity being 'when they got together to threaten you' (Interview: Mr Q. 1990, p.2). Mr Q. was isolated, not knowing of any other activities that were occurring in the hospital. The QAIMNS sister visited once a week on behalf of the matron. When confronted about why she came, she replied: 'The matron's sent me to see that everything's alright'. She had no reply when he said that it wasn't and that he needed more staff (p.3). The medical officer in charge of the ward appeared to have little therapeutic enthusiasm. When conducting an interview he came out with 'the most foul language', explaining to the shocked Mr Q. that 'it's the only language these lads understand' (p.4). It was the 'end of hostilities attitude': everyone wanted to get out of the army, and 'that was that' (p.5).

Not everyone felt the same. Mr F., after experiencing, like Vernon Scannell, a sense of morbid dread that he was locked up and would never get out, found that Northfield 'was very, very free and decent' (Interview: Mr F. 1992). Even he, however, found little evidence of organised activities.

The hospital was finally vacated by the army in 1948. The condition it was left in was described by the Officer of Works for the civilian hospital division that took it over afterwards:

There is only one adjective which can describe its present condition – that is FILTHY. During the six years of military occupation, no real attempt at cleanliness has been made. Whilst there has been some pretence, such as polishing door handles and electric switch covers, the grime on floors and elsewhere has persisted although moved from place to place with buckets of water by disgruntled fatigue parties.

Soldiers' hobnailed boots and other equipment have all contributed to the deterioration of the property, whilst the noticeable lack of discipline has had the same effect...

...it will be abundantly clear that with few possible exceptions, such as the Commanding Officer's Office and the Dispensary, the whole of the building is in such an UNHYGIENIC state that it is imperative that it must be scrubbed, disinfected, cleaned and redecorated from top to bottom before it can reach that HYGIENIC state which is necessary for the well-being of other patients and staff who will occupy the Hospital. (Officer of Works 1948)

LEWINFILTRATION AND SPONTANEITY: THE PROCESS OF THE NORTHFIELD EXPERIMENTS

Rickman's characterisation of democracy as a continuing resolution of infantile conflicts was central to Northfield. The core aim of Bion, Rickman, Bridger, Bradbury and Main was to bring to the surface the unconscious mechanisms occurring in group situations. By doing so the vectors in the social field were made explicit rather than covert. Using psychoanalytic understanding, they were ever on the alert for hints as to what was occurring underneath the surface for both individuals and the community. Enabling spontaneity both brought these issues to the surface and allowed new solutions to be considered. The task was not to provide answers for specific questions or disorders, but to enable individuals to develop their own tools of enquiry to examine these issues and to develop their own solutions.

Foulkes chiselled away at understanding the therapeutic methods and mechanisms of groups, and only gradually became able to stand back from individual therapy to look at the overall context. This handicapped his style and process of learning. He talked about broader issues, but his practice was curtailed by the limitations of his aims. Constantly, there were contradictions between his ambitions and his achievements.

There is little evidence to support Main's claim that Northfield was a new kind of hospital in 1946. The administrative staff were entirely unaffected by the changes. Sutton's medical division related only peripherally. There were innovations, based on a quite radical concept of what could be achieved; but few staff were entirely committed to these ambitions. The discussion groups demonstrate the uncertainty of most of the participants, the reliance on the key figures and the conflicts between different perceptions. The dawn was false.

CHAPTER 7

ABCA to Psychodrama

The Development of Group
Therapy at Northfield

Soldiers have endless occasions for talk. (Montague 1929, p.47)

ALL ALONE IN A SEA OF EXPECTATIONS: DOCTORS AND GROUP PSYCHOTHERAPY

Doctors are by training, and usually by temperament, people who prefer to be active therapists. They may express this through surgery, most romantically by saving someone's life on an aeroplane using only a penknife and a coat-hanger, or, less dramatically, by giving medication. Even in the field of mental health, for most it is preferable to give advice, education, or training. The psychotherapeutic stance gainsays this predisposition. Instead of talking and overtly taking control, the therapist has to listen and follow the lead of others. Where this happens in a group, the sense of impending chaos can be overwhelming.

The work at Northfield was only one of a number of initiatives that focused on the reliance of the soldier on his comrades. Maxwell Jones inaugurated his lifelong involvement with therapeutic communities at Mill Hill, and group therapies were used widely both in the British and American armies. The Army Bureau for Current Affairs (ABCA) took a lead in developing seminars throughout all military units on topics of general interest, informing the soldiers of the reasons for the war and their role within it.

This chapter outlines these innovations before embarking on a more detailed description of those at Northfield. The evolution of group therapy is illustrated with examples taken from a number of therapists at different stages. This is supplemented with a summary of the remarkable records of the doctor's peer-group discussions held throughout 1945. These relay their anxieties and preoccupations as they struggled with this new form of therapy. The discussion groups were the first testing ground for the rival theories of Foulkes and Bion, and although the arguments were rarely confronted directly, the participants clearly had to judge which approach suited them.

THE REASONS WHY: THE ARMY BUREAU OF CURRENT AFFAIRS

The reforms in the British Army during 1942 were marked by a recognition that the heart and mind of the soldier were as important as their physical presence. Field Marshall Lord Slim expressed this attitude most coherently when preparing for the campaign against the Japanese in Burma. He stressed that each man had to understand that the overall task was achievable, relevant and important, and also had to be clear about his role within the strategy (Slim 1956, p.182). As part of this campaign for commitment, General Adam inaugurated weekly current-affairs discussion groups in all units in the United Kingdom. This tactic was based on the idea that if the men knew why they were fighting and had some opportunity to discuss the war aims, they would be more prepared to sustain the will to do so. The scheme was promoted by the Army Bureau of Current Affairs, known as ABCA, and such discussion groups became wide spread throughout the Army (White 1963, pp.95–103).

It became the responsibility of junior officers to run them, and 4500 were trained in the methodology, supported by specialist majors in the education units of each command (White 1963, p.98). A large amount of training materials were produced, including pamphlets on a wide range of topics. In the first part of 1942 these current affairs bulletins included 'Blitzkreig in the Pacific', 'Russia's Hidden Strength', 'Paying for the War' and 'America in Total War' (Wilson 1948, p.56). These could be supplemented with films, theatre groups and lectures. The way each officer ran his group depended largely on that individual's personality and inclinations. The intention, however, was to provoke discussion and questions; the format was that of a seminar rather than a lecture. It was thus possible to begin to break down the barriers between the junior officer and his men. It was certainly noticed in some areas that the groups did bring them closer together (MacKenzie 1992, p.113).

Although Main referred to these disparagingly in his correspondence with Rickman, they formed a basic training for officers in managing groups. His criticism was based on their value as compared to therapy, and he acknowledged that they could provide a safe introduction to group functioning for the junior psychiatrists (Main 1945). They were implemented in Northfield, but it is unclear for how long. Later on they were superceded by other activities. Foulkes identified his approach as being similar in his paper 'Notes on group therapy', and advocated their value in stimulating interest, discussion and mutual exchange between the participants (1945b, p.2).

FRANK DISCUSSIONS: DIDACTIC GROUP METHODS

Other psychiatrists used group techniques. Over the winter of 1942–1943, whilst a contemporary of Bion and Rickman at Hollymoor, Blair[1] employed a design similar to the 'Class Method' used by Pratt in the United States (Blair 1943). It was characteristic of the period that he worked entirely in isolation on his unit, apparently without either party being aware of the other's activities.

Blair gave a course of 10 lectures, 'frankly discussing mental conditions'. These included an outline of the interrelationship of the body and mind. In support of the lectures he provided written summaries to each student on the day after their arrival in the hospital. Reminiscently of Schilder's practice, he then requested that they write out their life histories, which he used as the basis for long individual interviews. The men found this process valuable in itself, as it was the first time that they had reviewed their difficulties in such detail. When Blair first presented his sessions he was nervous that his audience wouldn't understand them, but was pleasantly surprised by their success. He believed that the change of attitude from telling the men to 'pull themselves together', combined with evidence of his concern for their situations, was crucial in improving their health. It allowed them to move away from a position of self-condemnation to one in which they could be more objective and learn that their experiences had a perfectly reasonable explanation. Blair considered that this was an effective way of giving psychotherapy, which enabled the men to realise that they were not on their own. As was typical of this kind of work, he couldn't back up this perception with objective evidence of improved outcomes.

This form of educational technique was commonly used in the American army, either in the form of a lecture and discussion or through question-and-answer sessions (Robinson 1948, p.69).

---

[1] Internal evidence from the paper suggests that at least some of the work was carried out at Northfield. Two of the officers he gives thanks to for allowing him to publish were Lt. Col. J.D.W. Pearce and Lt. Col. Rosie, both commanding officers of the unit. Robinson, in another paper, also alluded to the use of these techniques at Northfield, although he didn't refer to this particular author (Robinson 1948, p.69).

NERVY NED AND THE DOCTORS:
MAXWELL JONES AT MILL HILL

Maxwell Jones started out using very similar didactic methods in 1942, although he was more explicit about the value of the community (Jones 1942). At this time he was working alongside the Maudsley psychiatrists, whose treatment approaches were largely based on physical treatments, and whose implicit attitude to patients has already been referred to in chapter 4. At this juncture his own language tended to reflect theirs, for instance when he described one group of individuals as 'chronic constitutionally poorly endowed material' (Jones 1944, p.292).

The unit he was responsible for catered for 90 men in eight wards. Two of these were allocated to strictly physical treatments, modified insulin therapy and continuous narcosis. The other six were for 'mixed neurotic material' (Jones 1944, p.295). There were eight probationer and two qualified nurses, divided equally between the two daily working shifts. Each of the students looked after two wards whilst they were on duty, and also had responsibility for knowing the treatment aims of the 20 or so patients under their care. They were expected to spend all the time that they could in the clinical area, and were only allowed to mother their charges to a small degree, for instance, purchasing cakes to go with their tea. The natural loyalty to the ward group was tempered by a primary and explicit accountability to the doctor and the hospital. As an example to illustrate this, Jones explained that patients were expected to attend the teaching round when their case was discussed, and they never refused.

Initially Jones tried out his group therapy technique on men suffering from 'effort syndrome'. Most of these men viewed their symptoms as physical, and as their 'ticket out' of the army. By explaining their disorders to them in a group, using simplified physiological concepts, he encouraged them to recognise that their problems were psychological rather than organic. The communal atmosphere imbued them with a sense of mutual responsibility, and built up morale through a general feeling of support. He found that this approach was more successful than previous practices had been in encouraging men to return to active service (Jones 1942).

Later, Jones elaborated on this technique (1944). Taking a wider range of disorders, he enhanced the traditional therapeutic treatments in three ways. First, he gave group talks about neurosis, psychology and the central nervous system. Then he modified the general organisation of the unit, and finally he incorporated social projection methods.

The didactic component consisted of a course of twelve sessions of an hour each over a period of four weeks, which provided a general education in normal and abnormal psychology. Through explaining how the mind could affect the body he aimed to teach patients with somatic symptoms stemming from emotional conflicts how to evaluate their problems more objectively. He intended specifically to inculcate normal standards of everyday living, and did this by employing examples of common problems. The underlying purpose was to equip the patients with enough knowledge to enable them to play a more active part in treatment than expected in the traditional sick role.

Topics included the parasympathetic and sympathetic nervous systems and their internal harmony, the physiological basis of fear and its 'normality', and psychosomatic disorders. The room in which the classes were given had been redecorated by a patient and two nurses. Jones described it as 'the most attractive room in the unit'. The educational message was reinforced by twelve paintings of 'Nervy Ned' on the wall. One of these showed this poor unfortunate illustrating nervous tension with his muscles tensed and eyes staring, sitting anxiously on the edge of his chair facing a relaxed composed confident doctor (Jones 1944, p.293).

Each week the patients and staff from different wards would present prepared playlets, which would form the basis for discussions between the patients and the staff. The doctor would then sum up, bringing together the various views expressed 'to illustrate the advantages of intelligent assessment of a problem'. Two hours per week were taken up with this activity, one hour for the nurses to present and the other for the patients. There were no stage props, and the sketch could be acted in front of the audience or transmitted via a microphone from another room. Usually, the sketches illustrated aspects of previous, anonymous, successful cases. One serial, performed by the staff, concerned a family in which a hysterical mother had three daughters, all suffering from different disorders, schizoid personality, psychopathy and hysteria. The father, played by the doctor, represented sanity, but was unable to cope with the vagaries of the family. This was apparently enjoyed by all the patients; however, what it taught them about family life is open to question. The other shift of nurses enacted scenes from an outpatient clinic, which were thought to be more successful in bringing real cases to life (Jones 1944, p.294).

The first inklings of the therapeutic-community approach that Jones developed later were evident in the weekly ward meetings, in which both staff and patients participated. These considered issues such as improvements, decorations, and criticisms of both the ward and the organisation. Wherever possible, suggestions and difficulties were acted upon immediately to emphasise the sense of accomplishment (Jones 1944, pp.295–296). Three years later this had progressed to daily meetings in a ward of 70 patients (Jones 1947, p.109).

Despite the almost risible perpetuation of traditional gender roles, and the distinction between the 'well' professional and the disordered patient, there was a significant attempt to modify traditional hospital methods. The intent was clearly similar to that of Northfield in that efforts were made to encourage the men to take an active part in their treatment rather than remain passive recipients of medical and nursing care.

By the end of 1946, Jones' approach had modified significantly, allowing free expression and more opportunity for the patients to take the lead (Jones 1947). There was a small group in which the initial sessions were taken up by open discussion of any problems raised by the men. Once they had gained a degree of mutual trust, the sessions turned into role-play. This had a twofold task: first, re-education, and second, emotional catharsis. The former was achieved by recreating social situations which had caused some minor psychological discomforts for the individual. This would lead to discussion of how such behaviours might be modified to improve the outcome. The latter would involve the re-enactment of traumatic events, with the soldier reliving the experience as much as possible. In a number of cases this led to quite marked distress as the man went through pain similar to that felt during the original circumstance. Again, the other members discussed what had happened, often providing alternative explanations, reassurance and emotional support (Jones 1947). This latter form of psychodrama was similar to that carried out at Northfield. Jones went on to develop this form of therapy in later work, and Moreno visited his unit at Belmont on a number of occasions (Millard 1996, p.585).

Millard, in his sympathetic review of Jones' work at Mill Hill and later, argued that the latter inaugurated the large-group psychotherapy group there (1996, p.585). This is a difficult claim to substantiate. The approach was didactic rather than psychotherapeutic, and relied on classroom tutorials. It was clearly aimed at getting across a particular moralistic point of view rather than enabling the individual to come to their own conclusions. Even if these methods could be considered as psychotherapy, Cody Marsh was using very similar techniques in 1921, and applying them to a whole hospital. He had weekly meetings of 300 male and female patients (Marsh 1933). Joshua Bierer, as intimated earlier, could also lay claim to this role in the United Kingdom (see chapter 2). The pioneers of work with young people, such as Aichhorn, Homer Lane and David Wills, also anticipated him in environments that were much more clearly self-determining. Bion and Rickman's joint effort took place a little later in 1943, but was psychodynamic rather than educational. However, what Jones did succeed in doing, and what was not achieved in Birmingham, was involving all the clinical staff in the approach. Together, they clearly established an atmosphere of creativity, activity and optimism that engendered a similar energy in the soldiers who were patients there. Maxwell Jones subsequently became a well-respected and charismatic figure in the future development of therapeutic communities and social psychiatry (for fuller details see Millard 1996).

No interaction between the two originating sites of the therapeutic-community movement has previously been reported, and it is generally assumed that there was a form of parallel independent discovery occurring. However, this is not strictly accurate. First, we have seen that Slater took ideas stemming from Rickman at Wharncliffe back to Mill Hill (*see* chapter 4). He clearly intended that such an approach be repeated. Second, Bridger also visited, as described in chapter 6, although he did not find the methods to his taste. Mildred Creak was also with Maxwell Jones before she went to Birmingham, and alluded to this in one of the discussions on group therapy. She stressed how he brought all the nurses into the community from the start, comparing this with Northfield, where they appeared to be more peripheral. She also emphasised the rigidity of his arrangements, which caused difficulties which she didn't elaborate on, although she felt the results justified his technique (Discussion Group 7, 1945, pp.3–4). It is likely that there was more crossover, but Jones never acknowledged publicly the existence of the Northfield Experiments. The rivalry that existed amongst the practitioners at Hollymoor appears to have affected Mill Hill as well.

PLOUGHING THE LONE FURROW: FOULKES' INITIAL GROUP WORK AT NORTHFIELD

Foulkes' first year of work at Northfield was under the aegis of Lt. Col. Rosie, whose faint-hearted support allowed him to work with his patients in groups in his own time. In those early days the therapy was clearly aimed at improving the individual's health. The caustic observations that others made about his telling the patients to 'imagine he was wearing a white coat' refer to this time (e.g. Bridger 1990a).

Some of these early groups were written up briefly by Foulkes and later Martin James. The first, recorded on 13 June 1943, had seven members and lasted two hours. The record comments on individuals rather than group dynamics. A fortnight later the subject matter was discipline and reasons for the soldiers disliking the army. It was evidently quite an emotional group, with 'many strong resentments showing up' (Foulkes 1943b). It was attended by 11 soldiers as was the next, which became more heated and enquiring. They began to ask 'What's the matter with us?' and curse their experience of the army. Notes on the other meetings are irregular and very sketchy. It is unclear whether the groups were held regularly after this, as only ten were recorded between June 1943 and January 1944. Foulkes' didactic tendency showed in the last group annotated, which appeared to be a question-and-answer session on the nature of neurosis. In his replies he informed the members that 'neurosis is using the power of the mind to keep ill, instead of well' (Foulkes 1943b).

Later in 1944, some of the groups Foulkes ran with Martin James were recorded in some detail. Again the sessions appear to have been held at weekends and in the therapists' own time. A number of his preoccupations recur, including selection issues, negative transferences and silences. They were evidently open meetings in the sense that different ones were attended by different people, including some American psychiatrists, Drs Lenz and Olsen. Indeed, for that particular session the men were chased up by ward staff to attend because of the visitors' presence. This pressure led one group member to complain about 'being pried upon by Americans' (Foulkes 1944c, 19 December).

Throughout there is a sense of yearning for an ideal group, one in which the therapists speak little. The therapists wished 'to let the Group produce their own material and almost ignore F[oulkes] and J[ames]. The feeling should be one of keenness and personal involvement for each member of the Group' (Foulkes 1944c, 11 November). On one occasion the silence evidently became too much and Foulkes, after having attempted to get this discussed, 'talked for a long time on individual responsibility and the evolution of society, from groups dependent on a despotic leader to self-governing groups'. Not surprisingly, subsequent individual interviews with the patients suggested 'that the point of this was not fully appreciated' (Foulkes 1944c, 28 October). One cannot teach democratic theory and expect it to be practised after a few sessions.

The notes strongly intimate the sense of struggle, experienced by most novice group therapists, against silence. This contrasted with private interviews in which the patients became 'quite fluent'. At one point the therapists tried to utilise this by encouraging the individuals to take problems to the group. Gratifyingly, one member responded and started talking as the 'result of urging at a private interview'. This suggested to them 'that a good deal of positive encouragement at private interviews towards talking at the group is necessary during the early stages of organising a Group before a Group feeling has got up' (Foulkes 1944c, 11 November). Another tactic postulated was selection; indeed, one group was dropped altogether because of its inability to escape from hostile muteness (Foulkes 1944c, 12 October). The final two reports reverberate with this conflict. Martin James tried to overcome the groups difficulties in starting by speaking spontaneously himself; but his colleague criticised this by pointing out that whilst he wished to 'warm the group up', he had actually achieved quite the opposite effect. This stemmed from an earlier discussion about when groups actually start. Evidently, James felt that one had to wait for everyone to be present, whilst his mentor felt that groups should commence punctually 'even before all are assembled if need be'. The former persisted in arguing that the absence of a start time would avoid casual conversation (Foulkes 1945b, 16 January). The outcome of all this debate was that the next recorded session started with 'a prolonged silence' (Foulkes 1945b, 2 February). They had evidently decided to tackle the enemy head on.

There was clear hostility from group members towards Foulkes. On 12 October it is noted that 'negative feelings to F. are still manifest' (Foulkes 1944c). When James had occasion to run the group on his own, his announcement that his senior colleague was on leave was greeted with cheers, and 'the relief and gaiety were quite infectious'. They rewarded him with his 'most successful Group' (Foulkes 1944c, 5 December). The imagery referring to Foulkes' perceived malevolence was redolent with magical terror: 'F. was thought to exert a sinister influence and there was general agreement that the atmosphere was improved when he was not present. His piercing glance was singled out particularly and deep material was produced about hypnosis and the power of the human eye' (Foulkes 1944c, 5 December). One of the group members related this to the drawing power of the sea, its rhythmical, rocking and soothing movements acting hypnotically on those who observe it. Another related how he could not look his father in the eye, and that guilty people evade accusatory looks. The resulting discussion made no reference to any interpretation of these punitive phantasies. There is no evidence that this negative transference was discussed at any time, despite Foulkes' earlier excitement at his 'discovery' of the group transference (Foulkes and Lewis 1944, p.178). The only comment that James could make was that he hoped 'that some of the fantasy nature of the Group in relation to F. has been explored and that it will make his situation easier later on' (Foulkes 1944c, 5 December).

Other issues raised included James' failure to prepare the group for his period of leave, and the members' subsequent punishment of Foulkes for this by failing to turn up (Foulkes 1944c, 12 October). In general, however, the men were keen to attend the groups. On one occasion 15 were present, and on another they were disappointed that they had not been reminded by the staff that the group was running (Foulkes 1944c, 4 and 11 November).

It is not clear who wrote the notes, and whether they reflected accurately Foulkes' own thinking. However, they were preserved in his papers, and at least one of them could only have been written by him as James was away. It is evident that he had to struggle for every one of his insights; he did not set out at the beginning with a complete framework as did Bion and Rickman. Each practical aspect, such as when the group should start, who should be members, how to tackle silence and the importance of informing the group about leave, had to be considered and a solution devised.

By the end of 1944, Foulkes was able to experiment with an example of a selected closed group in 'pure form' (Foulkes 1948, pp.91–102). Charles Lewsen, the physician at the hospital, had become interested in psycho-therapy, and negotiated with Foulkes to support him whilst he treated nine patients in individual therapy. The men who took part had mostly seen some form of action in northern France. Seven were suffering from anxiety states and two from hysterical disorders. Taking advantage of this situation, Foulkes did not see them individually, but only in a group. Supported by Bridger from the social therapy department, Foulkes and Lewsen were able to manage them as a team. In the second session the men identified a project that they all could work on, that of putting the hospital stage and all its equipment in order. This was suitable because of the variety of skills that it demanded. They kept together in their ward and soon distinguished themselves with their good behaviour and morale. Increasingly, they gained confidence with each other and operated as a 'self-propelling body', engaging the staff as necessary to improve their performance. They became less preoccupied with their personal problems and more involved in their work and future. All of them remained in the army, having changed their perception of it as a 'bad' object to an acceptable one. Foulkes successfully negotiated their transfer to the convalescent depot as a single unit, arguing that they would be mutually supportive.

The unreality of this does not seem to have registered with Foulkes, despite the ward sister's sceptical comments about 'Major Foulkes' precious group'. Bridger also took issue with this approach, stating that there was no reason why a closed group should not go through an intermediate stage before leaving hospital (Discussion Group 9, 1945, p.1). Foulkes' approach further led to conflict with the commanding officer for contravening army regulations. He submitted to pressure from the men to change them from the 'blues' to khaki all in one go. This, he found, was not allowed, as only 10 per cent of the men on the ward were allowed to wear khaki at once. Whilst the regulation was evidently pettifogging, this episode demonstrated Foulkes' tendency to ignore the military environment in favour of the wishes of his patients. It is clear that whilst they were cocooned in the supportive environment of Northfield they worked together particularly well; but no one prepared them for the inevitable bereavement that would follow their break-up in their subsequent careers.

Foulkes had established a routine by July 1945. Patients were collected into groups of between eight and ten on their admission to the treatment ward. Concurrently, he would carry out one or two individual interviews to get an idea of the person's history. He carried this out with the aid of a questionnaire that enquired about 'their complaints, recent history and relevant experiences, ideas of treatment and cure' in a manner similar to Paul Schilder's practice described earlier (*see* Chapter 2; Foulkes 1945a, p.7). One or two men might not be suitable for working in a group, and they would be discharged from such an approach to be replaced by other new patients. The team would at this time be 'sharing the same sleeping quarters with beds in close proximity'. They would be encouraged to discuss and agree on a joint work project on which they could start as soon as possible, usually during the second meeting (Foulkes 1945a, p.7).

By early 1945, Foulkes had become an acknowledged expert on group therapy. A memorandum he wrote for the Army Medical Department for Psychiatry distilled what he had learnt so far (Foulkes 1945a).[2] It is clear that later he moved a long way from this particular position, but the document remains significant in that it outlined one moment in his progress. At this time he still saw the advantages of group psychotherapy as being economic, emphasising the practical advantages with regards to time-saving rather than recognising its relevance in the communal environment of the army. The paper is preoccupied with the aim of achieving the perfect group. It is clear that had there been enough time he would have preferred to be developing group analysis: 'deep' individual analysis within the group setting. However, due to the rigours of war he threw himself into exploring what he then saw as a limited version. His model was the psychoanalytic session, and from this many solutions came lock, stock and barrel.

For Foulkes there was a continual conflict between the professed ideal of the group as a self-sustaining unit and the need for the therapist to assist it towards this end. This caring, if potentially inhibiting, approach was demonstrated by his advice that novices be guided gradually towards a freer style of leadership. He recommended that inexperienced psychiatrists adopt the seminar style of the ABCA groups. The doctor could be kept informed of the progress of small gatherings of patients and pass on information about their situation, including results of X-rays, blood tests or other investigations. When questions arose, the therapist could give a short lecture or demonstration on the spot, or recommend that it might form the basis for

---

2 This is a typescript manuscript apparently for circulation to all military psychiatrists. It is not known how widely it was distributed.

the next ward ABCA meeting (Foulkes 1945a, p.1). If the therapist was particularly anxious, he could hide behind a set programme of discussions, similar to that of Blair described earlier. The therapist could thus take on the role of teacher rather than exposing his uncertainty.

Foulkes argued that one of the advantages of working with a group was that it enabled the doctor to get to know his patients better than he could just seeing them alone. Symptoms and signs could be observed for their functional rather than subjective effect. The person's abilities would be seen in a more realistic setting and they could demonstrate unsuspected skills or deficits. In fact, he found that individual interviews gave little extra information, except in the case of those patients who made it clear that they would only disclose information privately. The men, as their interest in group was awoken, became more active, learnt about social adaptation and began to recognise which of their own behavioural difficulties caused difficulties for others.

As the therapist gained experience he or she could evolve towards a freer style. He or she would recognise the group's mirroring of the social dynamics of the hospital and the army, and its role as a building-block of these wider organisations. By understanding these the therapist could use them as levers to influence the therapy, as predicated by Foulkes' tutor Kurt Goldstein. Previous psychoanalytic training would enable him or her to take into account intra-personal unconscious processes. If the therapist wanted to go further along the Freudian path he or she could advise the group to talk about anything that they wished. In this situation, explanations about particular conditions would be kept to a minimum, and the members would be encouraged to discover as much as possible for themselves.

Neurotic patients were, in Foulkes' experience, reluctant participants in therapy. Groups operated similarly. It was important to stimulate the person's interest; once they were engaged the next step was to encourage them to become active participants rather than passive commentators. This nurturing process was implemented by education, explanation and discussion at every opportunity, and individual therapy where necessary. Once the resistances were overcome the group could take on a life of its own, displaying unexpected talents, ingenuity and enthusiasm. This flourishing of creativity was Foulkes' overall aim. He endeavoured to sustain it by preserving the group in which it was engendered rather than enabling the individuals to take the skills they had learnt to new situations.

This exposed the novice therapist to new threats. He or she needed to switch from being an encourager and carer in the earlier stages to handling merciless questioning once the group had achieved this sense of autonomy. This was the acid test of whether the therapist could relinquish his or her powerful and protective role of nurturer, and truly and modestly feel: 'Here we are, together, facing reality and the basic problems of human existence. I am one of you, not more, and not less.' The therapist had to give up the claim to perfection and acknowledge that he or she was 'wanting, imperfect and ignorant' (Foulkes 1945a, p.3).

The memorandum was written as a training tool. Foulkes made it clear that he could only give guidelines, and not 'condense the technique into a set of rules' (1945a, p.5). He was only passing on the experience he had gained so far. Selection was largely unnecessary except in ensuring that the members' intelligence, war experience and expected disposal was not too dissimilar. He considered that selection by trial was perfectly appropriate, and that people who prevented the group from functioning as it should could properly be excluded. This applied even if they themselves were benefiting: the needs of the group took precedence over individual requirements. An interesting sideline on this was his observation that whenever a group gave a person a poor prognosis, it was usually accurate and they were unlikely to benefit from individual treatment.

Foulkes discussed the issue of open and closed groups, declaring that either was acceptable, and outlining different combinations that were possible. He identified the difficulties with various sizes, coming to the conclusion that eight members was ideal, very much in line with present-day thinking on the small therapeutic group. Another guideline that persists is his conclusion that extending the group beyond two hours serves little purpose, and that an hour or an hour and a half was perfectly satisfactory.

The attitude, role and practice of the therapist had to be flexible. Even in free-floating discussions they would initially have to take an active role in getting things going and demonstrating what was expected. New practitioners would ask how they could start the group. With increasing insight, the therapist would shift from this active, controlling role to a more passive, receptive one. The leader could then explore how the group's perception of him or her inhibited their spontaneity. What unconscious, magical role did the leader have? This might then be reflected back to the group. Gradually, he or she would recede more and more into the background, becoming superfluous, whilst at the same time steering the group 'delicately towards a therapeutic end' (Foulkes 1945a, p.4).

By phasing the process in this manner Foulkes attempted to avoid the contradiction of being both passive and directive concurrently. When a group was unsuccessful he would intervene in a number of different ways, including individual counselling, didactic interventions and interpretation of resistances. His ambivalence was again reflected in another statement that the psychiatrist should bring 'forth the spontaneous activity' of the group.

This could be put down to his poor command of the English language, in which case his unconscious exposed his dilemma for him. It is of course only possible to provide conditions in which spontaneity can occur, and encourage it. It is not possible to make it happen. The therapist's role in this case is passive rather than active.

Despite the emphasis on the group eventually being weaned from dependency on therapists, Foulkes could not disengage himself from his prime directive, the treatment of the individual:

> But since the psychiatrist in a hospital is after all concerned with the treatment of individuals he can perhaps not help putting the individual to some extent in the limelight and engaging in a more individually-centred group therapy. (Foulkes 1945a, p.2)

He unwittingly illustrated his dilemma in describing a later episode. During his intervention in a dispute in the hospital band later in 1945, he felt it was necessary to privately encourage one soldier, whom he considered to represent a good model of behaviour (Foulkes 1948, p.103). Again, he had to actively foster what he considered to be a satisfactory outcome, rather than relying on the group process to achieve this. A little later in the year he saw the basic tasks of treatment to be restoring the man's self-confidence and ability to do some form of work, and enabling him to manage the strains of army life better. The soldier's attitude had to be corrected so that he could be open to the 'wholesome influence' of the group (Foulkes 1945c, p.2).

Broader social issues, whilst acknowledged, remained in the background (Foulkes 1945c, p.2). As noted earlier, Rickman visited Northfield on a number of occasions. In 1945 he attended a conference in which Bion presented a paper. In the discussion that followed, Rickman reported on a group therapy session he had been invited to at the hospital, in which the therapist, later identified by Harold Bridger as Foulkes, introduced the session by stating that 'you can say what you like here, for within these four walls we are not in the Army!' (Bridger 1990a; Rickman 1945). Rickman found this statement shocking, as the denial of the real military situation prejudiced the development of open and honest relationships (Rickman 1945).

It was instances like this that led to Tom Main's impassioned condemnation of many therapists at Northfield: 'they wanted to go on treating people, but it was inappropriate in war. They wanted to pursue this selfish interest of theirs when there were bloody great issues to be solved' (Main 1984).

There is a constant sense that Foulkes was prevented from seeing the overall consequences of his work by the individual orientation of his therapy. He could understand that the planets circled round the sun, but was still so firmly tied to the ground that he operated as if the earth was the centre of the universe. He was intellectually aware of the wider social systems which ebbed and flowed around him, but was unable to free himself emotionally from the doctor-patient relationship, which at this time he saw as central.

Following Rickman's visit in late August of 1945, Tom Main complained bitterly about his influence:

> Some of the group discussions here do not differ much from ABCA... This is at once an apology for Northfield and an explanation of our present state of development. The only alternative was a leader and disciples for the particular cult about which you felt such dismay, a set, in fact of Foulkes worshippers. (Main 1945)

These particular criticisms were to a large extent unfair. Foulkes himself had already acknowledged the value of ABCA groups as a training environment, and furthermore had extended the role of group therapy throughout the hospital. It is also unlikely that he was deliberately attempting to form a cult. Many people considered him to be a considerate and likeable man (Lewsen 1993). However, Main was reacting to the prolonged failure of Foulkes to understand the real role of group therapy in a military hospital. In contrast, Main complimented the work of Harold Bridger, who he felt had grasped the necessities more effectively. The groups he was involved with formed around particular tasks. Although there was no formal discussion of particular issues in Bridger groups, Main noted that:

> there is a reshuffling of interpersonal relationships and there are crises about the function and the relating deficiencies of members. Whilst these crises may be about applied skill they are also about emotional attitudes of certain group members which are discussed openly, sometimes before Bridger, occasionally with a psychiatrist, but usually alone by the group themselves. One of the immediate jobs is to explore the tensions in these groups and help the discussion of the group problem in regard to the cohesive or disruptive effect of its members, in relation to a particular function. I underline here because I believe this matter of function, like geography, allows or prevents the growth of relationships and like geography can be altered, to shelve a disruptive crisis, in an emergency, and to allow of its discussion later. (Main 1945)

Such task-orientated groups would have had the full support of Rickman. Here again is the concept of work as a means of exploration of the real world, echoing Freud's dictum that 'No other technique in the conduct of life so firmly attaches the individual to reality' (Freud 1991, p.268; first published 1930).

Main described other work being carried out. Some therapists were using the groups to emphasise the moral aspects of being a soldier during a war;

others were aiming to help individuals establish more sincere relationships. He justified the latter, despite its apparently rather idealistic nature, as being important in providing 'some of our isolated patients with a set of warm human relationships even for a short time' (Main 1945). He was concerned about what to do once positive, co-ordinated group relationships had been established. He was not happy for them to be utilised solely for the exploration of neurosis and personal difficulties, but wasn't sure how else they should be handled. What impressed him was that, despite its vagueness, the work being done had a value in 'reducing isolation and fostering social contacts in a way which allows the working out of a neurotic attitude in a socially acceptable way and further provides a sense of security and social support which often badly needs restoration' (Main 1945).

Main reflected on the fact that Bion and Rickman's work on laying bare and mastering intra-group tensions was only being implemented by Bridger. In his letter to Rickman he wrote that in his view:

> This stage is now overdue – and your visit made it plain. For instance thinking it over I wish now that the awkward, individually hostile and socially disruptive depressives I had in a group could now have had a wiser therapist than myself, one who, having raised the astonishingly quickly agreed matter of ambivalence could have proceeded to stimulation of recognition of its operation within that group instead of, as I did, merely discussing then its personal significance for them. Now I think I know better – and my next difficulty is immediate – how to handle such a discussion. (Main 1945)

It was time to bring the consequences of neurotic disorders to light within the group by demonstrating their operation 'here and now'.

WALKING THE TALK: TAKING GROUP THERAPY OUT OF THE WARD

One solution to this was to encourage Foulkes to use his talents on a roving commission around the hospital, and in the autumn of 1945 this is precisely what Main did (Main 1989, p.134). This led to the former acting as a 'troubleshooter' and peripatetic therapist.

Foulkes gave an example of how this worked (1948, pp.102–105). Having heard that there were troubles with the hospital band, he visited their rehearsal hut to find that a new pianist was having difficulties in settling in to his new role. The previous pianist, and band leader, continued to find fault in his successor's playing, despite the fact that he was soon to leave the hospital. Having surveyed this conflict for a little while, Foulkes reflected back his observations to the whole group. He started by pointing out that disparaging the new performer in front of them all was not having a good effect on their cooperation. Furthermore, however good the previous pianist had been he was not going to be present for much longer, and it would be better for him to let the band reform without his intervention. The latter, after some consideration, shrugged his shoulders and left. Foulkes then offered to help drum up more new members amongst the hospital population by asking some friends in the painting hut to make posters to put up around the hospital.

He saw this as a way of fostering links between different sections of the hospital and bringing the hospital activities to life again. This was his approach to Bridger's 'hospital-as-a-whole-with-its-mission'. Typically, he took a nurturing stance rather than confronting the neuroses.

Further discussion took place. From this it emerged that there was some anxiety that success in the band would jeopardise members' chances of leaving the army. Foulkes could reassure them on this point, because the primary task of the hospital then was to rehabilitate people for civilian life. After this the band settled down, gained new members and became very successful. He later met the displaced musician and was able to help him towards gaining insight into how his behaviour disturbed others.

Foulkes' wanderings took him frequently to the art hut (Bradbury 1990a). He would spontaneously initiate group discussions there, often taking as the theme whatever painting was being engaged in. In one instance everyone present was agreed that a particular collection was unremittingly drab and uninteresting (Foulkes 1948, pp.137–138). This provoked a normally reserved private into a serious monologue on the 'unresurrected dead', which formed the subject of one of them. Another work stimulated a debate about English women, their lack of loyalty and the men's own attitudes to other countries. This argument was engaged in heatedly by a staff sergeant who had clearly suffered at English women's hands. The whole discussion lasted about two hours.

In Foulkes' view, these illustrations demonstrated his success in such informal situations. After fitting himself into the group and their problems, he was able to make a very active, but brief, intervention that enabled them to solve the problems for themselves. He prided himself on the fact that this form of therapy created no dependency.

Most of the wards held meetings in which all the patients and staff met. Foulkes was asked by Tom Main to take over William Ward, as the psychiatrist previously in charge was ill. The morale on this unit had deteriorated because of the lack of leadership. In Main's view, it was 'in a dreadful state, and must be taken by storm' (Foulkes 1948, p.105). Foulkes was thus in a similar position to Bion some two years earlier. The contrast between their two styles is exemplified by how Foulkes tackled the task of bringing order into the chaos (Foulkes 1948, pp.105–111).

At first he merely walked about the ward, observing and talking to different men to gain some idea of the atmosphere. In one side room a gambling school was blatantly in progress. He noted the empty beds. The general indifference was exemplified by the fact that the ward meeting was attended by only a third of the patients, and the staff turned up late regularly.

Foulkes set up his office in a side room at the heart of the ward. Although he spent less than three to four hours a day there, it allowed him to demonstrate his presence and be in close contact with the main activity area. In order to establish discipline he himself attended the ward meeting meticulously on time, and commenced it whether there was a full quota of soldiers and staff or not. He made contact with all the patients, both on and off the ward, observing what they were doing and offering comments. Ad hoc individual interviews contributed to an understanding that responsibility was a two-way process. One man who had been 'Away Without Leave' requested some medication for headaches. Instead of responding to this directly, Foulkes enquired about what he was going to do to gain appropriate treatment (Foulkes 1948, p.106).

Foulkes quickly found two or three men who were willing to assist him, creating a core group very much as Bion had done in his small group work. He interviewed them individually and helped them to sort out their problems, and in return they aided him. One function they carried out was to prevent unauthorised individuals gaining access to Foulkes' office. After meeting with the sisters and other staff, they began to take an interest. The nurses started to take social histories of the patients and learn about their backgrounds. Foulkes' popularity began to grow, and he was able to establish good relationships with most of the men.

Attitudes began to change. It became a wise move not to miss the ward meeting, as decisions made there affected everyone, and by attending it was possible to find out how the system operated. The men became lively and began to take an interest in the affairs of the hospital as a whole. The 'soap' story exemplified the improvements. Foulkes heard that this article was being regularly stolen, and questioned the assembled ward about this over three successive weeks. On the first two occasions the response was an equivocal silence. On the last the reply was unanimous: it was no longer happening, and such things did not happen on William Ward.

One corporal, wanting his discharge from the army, demanded to see the personnel selection officer (PSO), and was surprised to find that only Foulkes, as the officer in command, could sanction this. The man was not happy with this and insisted on seeing the commanding officer. Happy with his apparent outmanoeuvering of Foulkes, the soldier went off, whistling, for his interview. Rowlette, forewarned, evidently gave him short shrift, because three days later the soldier 'returned to his unit without a murmur'. As a consequence, the PSO was invited to attend the meeting to explain his role (Foulkes 1948, p.107).

Another focus of resistance was a side ward of 12 to 15 patients, many of whom were amongst the most disturbed in the unit. Foulkes visited regularly, and on one occasion found the men, who should have been participating in other activities, lying about, playing cards or doing nothing at all. One particularly obstinate man, mildly unwell, refused to answer questions and ignored Foulkes altogether. He was discharged from the hospital back to his unit within 48 hours. This followed on from Foulkes' dictum, cited earlier, that the individual could be sacrificed for the sake of the whole unit; this man's truculent and insubordinate manner needed to be dealt with through army discipline rather than therapy. This man's 'gang', other residents of the side ward, surrendered without a fight, much to Foulkes' surprise, and rapidly established friendly and cooperative relationships. Foulkes emphasised that this sternness was not characteristic of his behaviour. Indeed, he went out of his way to show kindness and to be helpful (Foulkes 1948, p.108). This disclaimer certainly fitted in with his nurturing tendancy, noted earlier.

Much of this approach to the ward was very similar to Bion's, and showed how much Foulkes' practice had changed. He employed techniques that eschewed selection, breaking silences and concern over transferences. He concentrated on the here and now, and encouraged the men to face up to the realities of their situation. The 'management by wandering about' established the belief that he was concerned about the individuals, but also determined to rally the troops to face the enemy. Perhaps this was the time when the two men's practices came closest to each other.

Foulkes appears to have been equivocal as to whether this form of therapy was group analysis or not. Clearly, there was a difference between this practical, short-term work in the setting of a military hospital and the longer-term therapy of individuals on a weekly outpatient basis, and in his memorandum he emphasised that it was not (1945a, p.1). However, 20 years later he described his work, using examples from Northfield, as group analysis (1964, p.187).

THE WORD SPREADS: OTHER THERAPISTS

Foulkes illustrated the further development of small-group therapy by describing the work of one of his colleagues, George Day (1946b). This probably took place in the latter part of 1945, as it consisted of eight ex-prisoners of war. Clearly, Day was able to allow a silence to inaugurate the session, as the first question, asked directly to him, was from a corporal wanting to know about his tendency to cry easily. In response, Day asked a general question as to whether the others had a similar experience. Most did, and all quickly stirred with interest. He then enquired about other changes, and was rewarded with many examples of their social difficulties. The discussion was soon free-flowing, with the therapist taking a back seat. The men were surprised that they had gained enough confidence to talk about thoughts and behaviours that they had thought they would never share with anyone else, particularly angry thoughts about their loved ones. The sense of mutuality and sharing predominated, so that innermost concerns were shared in an atmosphere of humour, teasing and reminiscence. The role of the psychiatrist was similar to that of a conductor of an orchestra, encouraging the shyer individuals and 'preventing the extrovert from swamping the rest with his solos' (Foulkes 1946b). After exploring the sense of being cut off from other people, the men began to ask how they might overcome this. Day reflected back that they had just been doing this for the previous hour, and followed up this observation by deciding that this was the appropriate time to terminate the meeting.

This was closer to Foulkes' ideal group, though it is noticeable that the therapist still controlled it to the extent that he decided when it was to end, rather than relying on a specific predetermined time. The very powerful effect of his astute but *ex cathedra* interpretation would have been to leave the members with a continued sense of dependence on him and undermine their own hard-won sense of thinking things through for themselves. This would have been exacerbated especially by the fact that there was no chance to discuss the matter any further.

Reflecting what she had learnt from Bion, Bridger and Main, Millicent Dewar gave an account of her technique of group therapy in the *Bulletin of the Menninger Clinic* (1946). In her view, the primary role of the therapist was to concentrate on the group rather than the individuals. Her sessions, when given in combination with individual therapy, were held once a week. Where the group was the only form of therapy this would increase to two or three times. Ideally the men should have worked together from their admission. Where possible they would be informed about the nature of the group prior to the first meeting, which reduced their contact with the psychiatrist and confronted them with their task of examining their relationships from the outset. They sat in a circle, usually in one of the side rooms on the ward. The first session often started awkwardly, as the men had no idea what to expect, and the therapist had to confront an uneasy silence. They all became painfully aware of the 'here and now', real situation, and were led to face the intra-group tensions engendered by the uncertainty about their role and that of the therapist.

Because treatment had to be rapid, the average stay at that time being about three months, Dewar and Main would break this initial tension after about five minutes if the patients had been unable to. Leaving it for longer would have led to the surfacing of deeper unconscious trends, which could not have been managed in the therapeutic time available. Dewar favoured two tactics for breaking the silence. One was to 'throw in a controversial remark', and the other was to invite the group to examine the silence itself. Some form of superficial talk would ensue, which the therapist allowed to continue so that the men could get to know each other. The next session would then usually start with less overt nervousness. In further meetings the members would deepen their mutual exploration of emotional problems.

The leader's main role was to identify and elucidate central themes that affected the whole group. For instance, when the iniquities of sergeants and officers and the odiousness of discipline had formed the main topics of discussion, it would be opportune to draw attention to the underlying cause for this distaste for authority and authoritarian figures. Dewar was at pains to emphasise the relative passivity and reserve of the therapist, except when insightful comments could be effective in moving the group on. Sometimes arguments might develop which got out of hand. On these occasions the psychiatrist would have to act in a parental manner by defusing the situation with some form of explanation, reassurance or 'even a word of ridicule' (Dewar 1946, p.84). This would settle the insecurity, and the men could continue to examine their problems more calmly. In a situation in which an individual was being rounded upon by the rest, her tactic would be to get them to examine their motives for this, treating it as a group dynamic.

Dewar's style contrasted with that of Foulkes and those who followed him in a number of ways. This is best illustrated by her way of handling members who remained silent. She considered that it was best for the group as a whole to tackle such difficulties, which it usually would. If a silent member was ignored for some sessions then he might be drawn into the discussion directly, but this was thought best avoided.

A series of meetings described in some detail by Susan Davidson exemplify the format typical at the end of 1945 (Davidson 1946). Her account followed the progress of a group of six ex-prisoners of war, all non-commissioned officers, from forming to boarding out over a period of six weeks from 29 August to 5 of October.

Interestingly, the first meeting was on the same day that John Rickman made his final visit to the hospital. They were still on the admission ward, in the 'blues', and had been interviewed briefly on the previous day. The session started with an explanation that they were now a team, and that they would remain together for their stay. They were told that they were free to discuss anything that they wished to and could run the meeting how they wanted (Davidson 1946, p.92). An emaciated corporal, who was panicky and had problems mixing with people, quickly vented his frustration about the uniform. This provoked a general agreement about the members' sense of being singled out in a manner similar to that of the POW camps, where they had had to wear patches to mark their status as prisoners. The presence of guards and 'Out of Bounds' notices in the hospital reminded them further of their gruelling experiences and revived their sense of imprisonment. This was followed by a request that they be allowed to go for walks when they wished to. As it was not possible to immediately satisfy their requests they became rather tense and silent.

After Major Creak asked about the difficulties that led to them coming to the hospital they became more animated again and described the difficulties they had found in relating to others on returning home. They felt out of place and wanted to do something useful to fit in again. The second session, which Bridger attended, applied itself to this yearning. The meeting, which was brief, concentrated on identifying a group project for them to work on. As a number of them were in the building trade they decided to build a toy village and doll's house for a Child Guidance Clinic. As a result of this interest, Creak gave a talk about child psychiatric services soon after. They also wanted to make some things to take home for their families.

Three days later they were evidently progressing. Corporal J., who had been nursed in a side room, was now taking meals on the ward and was sleeping better. Their discussion centred on the dullness of the city centre on a Sunday and plans for their project. The next session, on 5 September, showed more improvement. They were now on William Ward, a proper treatment unit, and Corporal J. had left his side room to join the others. Perhaps most importantly for their morale, they were wearing the khaki again, removing the most obvious evidence of stigma. Their overall task at the hospital was clarified. As they were to be discharged from the army, they needed to consider what their civilian roles were going to be and prepare for them. This led to discourse on their lives as prisoners of war and the ways they had devised to outwit their captors. They were also interested in knowing more about Child Guidance Clinics, criticising Birmingham for only having one. This led naturally to describing the work they were doing and their future plans with regards to the toys they were building.

Four days later they reconvened. During the intervening period they had all moved to Charlotte Ward, where they and some other friends formed a small party of 13 that remained loyal to William Ward, with whom they still played football. They all did their own chores, cleaning and tidying, and happily accepted that they were now largely being left to their own devices. They discussed other cultures, Jewish, Italian and German, finding faults and virtues in each of them, and were able to refer to their prison experiences with humour and in a relaxed manner. Corporal B. was depressed. He had seen the medical specialist and there were concerns about his physical health, but it was not possible to clarify what was wrong as some blood tests had not yet been reported on. He had been advised to avoid strenuous activity, and this worried him because he wanted to join the police force after discharge from the army.

They met again on 14 September, with a trainee, Lt. (Miss) Hussy attending. A mutual friend of some of the members had joined the group, ousting a well-established individual from the task of painting. This led to conflict. The latter had begun to behave erratically and was demoted to wearing the 'blues' again, which his colleagues considered to be unfair. He continued to stay out late, making his delinquency obvious to others by getting caught easily. His friends, in particular another corporal, had tried to advise and support him. He explained that he was yet again 'on a charge' for being out late and had to leave the meeting early because of this. His behaviour caused some concern, and after he had gone they discussed his family circumstances sympathetically. The issue of disciplinary problems and the difficulties of being in the hospital by 9.30 at night were mulled over. It was surprising to them, given the large numbers of POWs in the hospital, that there were not more disciplinary problems.

After weekend leave, extended because of the Victory in Japan (VJ day) celebrations, the next session was seven days later. There had been further improvements in their health. They were asked to describe what had happened that led them to be admitted to hospital. Their prison experiences varied from extreme deprivation and times when they feared for their lives to relatively safe jobs working on a farm. The most difficult issue facing them on repatriation was uncertainty about what to do. They had anticipated the peace eagerly, and yet when they were released they felt that they were 'in a rut', unable to plan for the future. They felt 'cheesed off', irritable and restless. In common with other men in a similar situation, they struggled with guilty feelings about being a 'liability to the country' and working for the enemy when others were fighting, whilst at the same time wishing for sympathy with regards to the awful conditions they had experienced.

They continued to improve, becoming increasingly involved in activities throughout the hospital and not needing the support of the original group. The project was completed, and each also found time to make something, such as a toy or handbag, for members of their family. The delinquent found it difficult to modify his actions until he was elected as the ward representative to the Hospital Committee. Once given this opportunity he became very conscientious and responsible, relishing his new role and the sense that he was again a valuable member of the community.

The final occasion was on 5 October, when Major Foulkes also attended. The first part of the meeting was taken up collecting facts about their stay at Piper's Wood Selection and Training Batallion after their return to England. They then discussed the changes they would like to make at Northfield. In their view, the psychiatrists had changed with the times whilst the administration had not. They considered that Northfield should perform more along the lines of a Civil Resettlement Unit than a military establishment, and rules such as the pass out until 9.30 p.m. should be abolished. They also thought that the hospital should be more like the rest camps in the Middle East, where all ranks were suspended and everybody called each other by their first names (Davidson 1946).

This account has been given in some detail, as it captures much of the spirit of the therapeutic work done at Northfield. It was given as an example of the approach in the *Bulletin of the Menninger Clinic* in 1946, and describes how the transitional nature of work and the 'hospital-as-a-whole' was integrated with individual therapeutic needs. The support of the whole group for a particular individual who was experiencing difficulties was classic example of how the therapist, by keeping a hands-off approach, could enable effective therapy by other means.

TENSIONS ON STAGE: PSYCHODRAMA

Unfortunately, although psychodrama was apparently used quite frequently at Northfield, there are very few accounts of its practice there. As a result, this section is less detailed than those describing group therapy in general.

The first tentative consideration of Moreno's work started with Foulkes' reading of the journal *Sociometry* after some copies were loaned to him by Hargreaves in 1944 (*see* Chapter 6). One of these papers, on interpersonal relationships, outlined his psychodrama technique (Moreno 1937). However, in his notes Foulkes did not refer to this at all, but concentrated on the theoretical issues alone (1944b). Some notes written by Foulkes in June

1945 show that even then psychodrama was still considered to be in 'an experimental stage'. He made it clear that they did not intend to copy Moreno's methods, but wrote that 'while preserving our liberty to experiment with it...we prefer to refer to this method of treatment as enactive therapy.' He insisted that, even with this proviso, group psychotherapy methods remained preferable (Foulkes 1945c, pp.3–4).

This ambivalence can be seen in a slightly garbled letter to Foulkes from John Rickman, who wrote, after emphasising the nature of working with intra-group tensions:

> only when he has begun to master these aspects of group discussion (& may I say, not before then) is a psychiatrist ready to be let loose on the boards of a Psycho or Socio drama... (I might be going too far) ...if you can't interpret the global, whole, over-all (call it what you will) experience of your present G[roup]T[herapy] situation in terms of psychodrama (granted that the material is not at all abundant for the purpose) you won't make much of a fist of the psychodrama when you get it. ... A round stage and all the carpentry in England wouldn't begin to give psychodrama – like the Brass instruments which bedazzle the academic psychologists, a hell of a lot of thinking has to go on in order to prevent the apparatus getting in the way of the experiment so to speak. (Rickman 1944)

Millicent Dewar attributed the introduction of enactment therapy to Foulkes, but the first recorded description came from Martin, in May 1945 (Dewar 1994, p.8). He recounted that he had five men 'on psychodrama', one of whom had won the Military Medal. One was asked to relive his experiences in order to demonstrate what had happened to him. Two colleagues assisted him whilst the remaining pair watched. The audience became very distressed, wiping their foreheads and sweating. The following group therapy session became very tense, emotional and verbally aggressive, and the feelings remained unresolved at the end. It resulted in a couple of the men refusing to take part again. Martin found the psychodrama more artificial than the group and also somewhat less effective. Bridger held the view that it might have been better to start the discussion in the therapy group, and use the psychodrama to utilise the tension left at the end (Discussion Group 4, 3 May 1945, pp.1–2).

By the end of 1945 a 'Moreno Stage' consisting 'of a round platform in three tiers' was built and installed in the lecture theatre at the hospital. This was where the psychiatrists held their weekly clinical meetings (Foulkes 1948, p.115). In order to demonstrate the work of the co-ordination group to them Foulkes staged a sociodrama as a teaching session. The members' only directions were that they should carry out their daily business in view of everyone. They could not all sit on the same level. This led almost immediately to a Sergeant Major finding that a colleague of similar rank was seated beneath his juniors. In exasperation he expostulated to the assembled doctors 'I ask you! *Why?*', evidently feeling that his pal was insulted by such a placement. The psychiatrists started to respond and became involved in the action. The debate that followed extinguished the difference between the performers and the audience. As a result, the doctors learnt a great deal about group therapy and the social field they were working in. They also gained a better understanding of how the co-ordination group worked, and were brought closer to their patients and each other.

The members of the newspaper group also regularly enacted their difficulties on stage. Because of the gifted nature of many of them, they became their own producers, directors and performers concurrently. Their subjects would include topics taken from the hospital, or their lives in the army or at home. Sometimes they would concern the problems of running the newspaper. On one occasion, because it was felt that they were losing contact with the rest of the hospital, they enacted their business in front of one of Foulkes' therapy groups. The resulting interaction became very lively and re-established the contact between the magazine and its customers. Following this, the newspaper group was able to solve its problems more effectively and gained a lot more new ideas for its material (Foulkes 1948, p.116).

Others made tentative experiments. For instance, Stein tried out psychodrama on a group of men who stammered. But many of the psychiatrists remained inhibited about using this form of therapy, and others were downright suspicious, finding that it provided a stage for the person with histrionic tendencies, without therapeutic benefit (Discussion Group 8, 31 May 1945, p.1; Dewar 1993). Millicent Dewar remembered having one individual who was an excellent actor, but was also devious. He performed with great ability, but achieved nothing in terms of therapy for either himself or others. She found it unhelpful. At times she felt it could be dangerous, because it allowed individuals to act out their fantasies, and thus could reinforce neurotic traits (Dewar 1994, p.8). Main was highly sceptical 40 years later, paraphrasing Dorothy Parker's criticism of a play: 'Oh boy, is it psychological. But it didn't help' (Main 1984).

Moreno's influence expressed itself in other ways. By using questionnaires it was possible to establish the person's preferences and place him together with others of similar tastes. This technique was used for both establishing groups and placing people together on wards. Main recalled running a whole ward on these sociometric lines (1984).

DESCRIBING THE ELEPHANT:
DISCUSSION GROUPS

There is a famous Sufi story about three blind men who were asked to describe an elephant. One, who touched the ear, asserted that it was a large leathery mat. Another, who felt the trunk, argued vehemently that it was nothing of the sort and claimed it was a flexible hollow pipe. The third, after having examined the elephant's leg, disagreed with both, declaring that it was thick and firm like a pillar (Shah 1973). Similarly, those who initially explored group therapy at Northfield were unsure of what was going to happen, nervous about what was expected of them, and worked largely in isolation. The result was inevitably a tangle of discordant approaches. When Foulkes and Bridger started the weekly discussion groups in 1945 as part of the attempt to weld the hospital into one co-ordinated unit, they offered the psychiatrists the opportunity to share their experiences and gain a clearer overall picture of the animal they were dealing with.

These sessions were recorded in varying amounts of detail, and demonstrate the many dilemmas facing the therapists. They were possibly the first recorded peer-group seminars on group psychotherapy in the world, and certainly in the United Kingdom. The debates were archetypal, rehearsing all those that would follow. In them Foulkes was able to test his ideas against those of Bion, and explore some of the contrasts between them. Most of those attending looked on the former as the expert, and it was against some resistance that Bridger and Main represented the ideas of the latter. Rickman's visit at the end of August was a welcome support for them, and the inspiration they gained from it was evident from Main's later letter:

> All, not merely worshippers [of Foulkes], are now handling groups and this was a useful state for our own psychiatric group to be in – at one it narrowed the split between the disciples and the philistines and created a common purpose, and also it allowed heart searching to be a group affair rather than an affair of an out group of emotionally reacting sceptics wondering whether Christ was as phoney as he seemed.
>
> So your visit was timely, and believe me, useful, in the way that a bomb in a slum is useful. (1945)

The central concern was the struggle of doctors to establish their role in the groups. Should they lead from the front or allow the members to take the initiative, what should they do about disruptive individuals, should they select who was to attend, and did their presence even matter? McLean's initial scepticism about group therapy was based, he realised eventually, on his perception of it as a threat to his role as a doctor. He was 'unwilling to expose' himself and his weaknesses to a group of patients. This was because he 'had the conception that a psychiatrist must be someone who is omniscient in the psychological field, superior to the patient, who must be a psychological God' (Discussion Group 19, 8 November 1945, p.1).[3] Main pointed out that this was a consequence of his medical training (p.3). Not everyone was convinced of the benefits of group therapy anyway. Colonel Sutton remained sceptical, asking whether it made any contribution 'which could not be achieved by individual interviews' (Discussion Group 12, 8 August 1945, p.3). Bridger, in response, argued that this was a false dichotomy, rather like discussing 'the relationship of heredity and environment and any attempt to locate the exact value of either'. He emphasised that it was the conjunction of the two that was important, not their separateness (p.2).

Unlearning these traditional attitudes was difficult and painful, and made more so because the soldiers themselves were more comfortable with pills, medicines and individual interviews. In the absence of these they felt that their individual problems had not received due and proper attention. Group therapy seemed to many of them a second-best, or commonly not a treatment at all. They were often reluctant to join it, and when they did their perception was that they just seemed to get better. As a result, they rarely gave credit to the doctor for their improvement. Foulkes drew attention to how similar these experiences were for both the patients and the therapists (Discussion Group 19, 8 November 1945, p.3). However, as Main argued, it was important to remember that the group leader was an officer and a psychiatrist, and to pretend to the group that he was anything else was a 'masquerade' (Discussion Group 15, 12 September 1945, p.9). The task was to work with the real 'here and now' situation, sharing the enigmas and contradictions with the men. Foulkes had come to similar conclusions, rejecting his earlier practice of exhorting the men to imagine that he was a doctor in a white coat. By this time it was his opinion was that one had to be 'honest about the whole thing. I told the group what my position is, whether they approve or not I involve my own difficulties with those of the group'. However, he couldn't desist from adding the patronising postscript 'It is important to show them the way out where conflicts may be reconciled' (Discussion Group 8, 31 May 1945, p.2).

After this initial reluctance had been overcome, debate centred around the question of what the group leader was supposed to do. A new draft of junior doctors explored this issue with Foulkes in November (Discussion

3   This and following references refer to a series of records of meetings of the psychiatrists at North-field throughout 1945. They are typescript reports, and many have misprints, sometimes trans-forming the meaning of what is being stated. They are also evidently not complete accounts, but summaries of the main points being made.

Group 18, 1 November 1945). One of them, Kaufman, enquired how to start a group and on what principles selection criteria should be based. These were subjects that had figured frequently in previous discussions.

Foulkes consistently reiterated the importance of selection, and tried a number of experiments with it. There was general agreement that people with learning difficulties did not do well alongside those of more ability, and tended to hinder the discussion process. This was because, amongst other things, they did not have the language to verbalise their feelings, would repeat the same thing over and over again, and found it difficult to understand what was being discussed. The idea of special groups for these people was mooted but never executed (Discussion Group 18, 1 November 1945, pp.1–2). Depressed men also appear to have presented difficulties. Often they were silent, and therapists felt that they had to take a more active role. Foulkes avoided having a group of them together, and Millicent Dewar also did not like to work with them (Discussion Group 11, 2 August 1945, p.4). Exploring these issues, Main did hold a group that consisted entirely of depressed individuals. He found that they became hostile towards each other, and as a result he handled the situation poorly. He was not able to examine with them their aggression as it related to the group (Discussion Group 14, 5 September 1945, p.5). Men described as psychopaths were also unwelcome, as they had little ability to concern themselves with the needs of others (Discussion Group 12, 8 August 1945, p.2). Cassells insisted on more subtle criteria. He excluded people on the grounds of having no insight, and tried to put together people who had some understanding of each other's problems (Discussion Groups 14, 5 September 1945, pp.1, 5; 15, 12 September 1945, p.7).

Mildred Creak described the effect of poor selection in one group:

> One topic after another was brought up and dropped and we ended up with a subject that no one was interested in. That was a reflection of a rather ill chosen group, dull intelligence, quite schizoid people who didn't contribute much anyway and the other five were rather quiet and shy (Discussion Group 11, 2 August 1945, p.5).

During his exploration of these issues Foulkes was at pains to emphasise that selection for treatment differed from selection for the group. To identify that a man may benefit from group therapy was not the same as placing him in a particular group. Foulkes lamented the fact that patients were assigned on a rota basis to the psychiatrists, as this prevented him from experimenting further with specific groups for particular disorders, such as men who stammered. His practice was to select those men with a good prognosis in the army. These were soldiers who were reasonably cooperative, had a 'fairly good approach', needed treatment and wished for it. He found that these made up about a quarter of his case load (Discussion Group 5, 10 May 1945, p.1). He refined this procedure by testing out the individuals in the group. Those he considered unsatisfactory he rejected early on (Discussion Groups 5, 10 May 1945, p.1; 11, 2 August 1945, p.7; 12, 8 August 1945, p.1). Bridger, emphasising the range of groups within the hospital, suggested that men might benefit from different ones depending on their needs. The social club could benefit shy, inhibited men. The closed group may be too advanced for the beginner in group therapy, who could gain experience initially through social activities rather than jumping in at the deep end (Discussion Group 5, 10 May 1945, p.2).

Kaufman's next question concerned how to start the group (Discussion Group 18, 1 November 1945, p.1). This had perplexed the doctors from the very first session, when they had 'felt at a loss to know what to do to start off and what happened when one gets an impasse' (Discussion Group 1, 12 April 1945). Perhaps more than any other issue, this went to the heart of the differences between Foulkes' approach and that of Bion's advocates. Foulkes nurtured his groups from the beginning by giving explanations, leading the discussion and generally encouraging the members. Noticeably, he continued this practice in the discussion groups themselves, frequently starting them off with an opening question or statement. As we have seen, Dewar was happy to wait for the group members to initiate the discussion themselves. In this she reflected the practice of Main and Bridger. Lt. Magnus visited her group and commented that she interfered very little in comparison to other therapists and that the group got on very well as a result (Discussion Group 11, 2 August 1945, p.1).

Mute group members threw into relief the anxiety of the therapist. When it occurred Martin James would think to himself 'God, here is a silence', and would start worrying about it. Although rationally he knew that silences were not necessarily negative, he recognised that he tended to project his own distress and assume that they were (Discussion Group 6, 17 May 1945, p.2). The therapists looked around for methods by which they might terminate them. Mildred Creak felt compelled to ensure that everyone in her group had a good time, and described this as her 'hostess reaction' (Discussion Group 11, 2 August 1945, p.4). Copying Foulkes, James asked what the members were discussing before the group commenced (Discussion Group 6, 17 May 1945, p.2). However, Foulkes himself warned against techniques, or 'tricks'. He acknowledged that some silences were creative and positive, but emphasised that most were hostile, containing the implicit demand that the therapist act in some way. At times he felt that this was appropriate, and would respond. He argued that 'I would rather give them something on the whole than strain the group' (Discussion Group 6,

17 May 1945, p.2). On another occasion he reported that his present group was 'uphill work' and that he felt that he had to talk more (Discussion Group 11, 2 August 1945, p.4). This contrasted vividly with Bion's later reflections. In his first group at the Tavistock in 1948 he experienced the group members becoming silent and focusing on him, expecting him to do something. As a consequence he felt uneasy, and his intervention was to report this back to them (Bion 1961, p.30). This approach of taking the 'here and now' emotional experience as material to be examined from the start, rather than avoided, contrasted with Foulkes' more conciliatory technique. The latter himself was keen to stress the importance of the present, as it contained both the past or future (Discussion Group 4, 26 April 1945, p.3). However, he found it difficult to act on this perception. In the sixth session he replied to Dewar's question about the nature of indifference as a resistance to therapy by stating:

> That is one of the worst forms. Take this seminar for instance. Very few have turned out and this is not the first time. There is something very serious about the situation and it isn't very good. If a patient doesn't worry at all and doesn't come to a group session, then it serious. If he is most negative but makes a positive effort in coming it is good, even if he says nothing... (Discussion Group 6, 17 May 1945, p.1)

Foulkes then subverted the impact of this challenging observation about the 'here and now' experience of the group by first presenting value judgements on people's behaviour, and then diverting the attention of those present to theory and other situations. Had he taken the Bion route he might have commented on his reaction to the situation and left it for the other members to reflect on.

Kaufman's line of questioning was taken up by de Maré, who sought to establish the separate domains of group and individual therapy. This was another regular controversy that had begun in April. Then the subject matter had concerned a patient who had monopolised a group session so much that the other members didn't speak. A range of suggestions were put forward, without any evident conclusion being reached (Discussion Group 2, 19 April 1945). Later, a loquacious sergeant in another group felt it incumbent on him to make sure that there was no silence in his group. Davidson felt he had to be checked (Discussion Group 11, 2 August 1945, p.2). On another occasion a soldier upset his colleagues during discussions which were held outside of the established therapy sessions (Discussion Group 8, 31 May 1945, p.2). More problematic situations arose when the tensions grew to such an extent that members felt that they had to leave their group. On one occasion it was the ward sister who was being criticised, and on another it was a bandsman (Discussion Groups 10, 19 July 1945, p.1; 2, 8 August

1945, p.1). In answer, Foulkes tended to reiterate his point about selection, and his approach of rejecting a number of individuals during the course of therapy (Discussion Group 12, 8 August 1945, p.1). As has been referred to earlier, his view was that once a group had decided a man was a bad bet for therapy, it was likely that this person would not succeed in any other form of treatment. This was confirmed by Cassells' experience with one man who tended to disrupt an otherwise effective group. The man requested that he be allowed to leave, and once this was granted Cassells took him on in individual therapy. Although he was more cooperative it was not therapeutically successful (Discussion Group 12, 8 August 1945, pp.1–2). Essex tried another tactic, which was to take one man out of a group in which he had become the butt of others' hostility and place him in another. The same thing happened again, repeating a long-established pattern (Discussion Group 12, 8 August 1945, pp.1–2). There was always the option of commanding an offender to carry out orders. Sutton employed this approach for someone who was refusing to wear the 'blues', pointing out that if this continued disciplinary action could be taken (Discussion Group 10, 19 July 1945, p.3). Bridger preferred to share the problem with the person's comrades, and found that commonly they would look at ways of reintegrating him (Discussion Group 12, 8 August 1945, p.1). Main advocated a similar process, giving as an illustration the example of the patient in Davidson's group quoted earlier in this chapter, in which his companions took on responsibility for trying to resolve the problems (Discussion Group 15, 12 September 1945, p.7).

This question extended to whether individual problems could be discussed in a group setting (Discussion Group 3, 26 April 1945, p.3). The earlier debates tended to search for techniques with which this could be done. Thoms' tactic was to announce generally to the group: 'There is a man who has so and so. I don't know if he would care to talk about it' (Discussion Group 4, 3 May 1945, p.4). Other doctors recounted episodes in which men had felt more able to talk about particular issues in the group than in individual therapy, and argued that such issues could lead on to a general discussion. One man said in a private interview that he had shot his friend, but wouldn't talk about it in the group. Yet he was able to discuss it openly in the very next session (Discussion Group 4, 3 May 1945, p.4).

The debate about the relative activity and passivity of the psychiatrist continued throughout. In April, Magnus wanted to know 'How can we help them and explain it to them?' (Discussion Group 3, 26 April 1945, p.2). In August, Mclean asked 'I want to know what I am intended to do with the group, what I am going to advise?' (Discussion Group 11, 2 August 1945, p.6). Earlier on, the former felt that he wanted 'to tell [himself] to do more'

(Discussion Group 11, 2 August 1945, p.2). In Sutton's opinion, the doctor had to 'have certain ideas of what he is expecting in that discussion, and what he is aiming at, and then he finds his role' (Discussion Group 11, 2 August 1945, p.2). This yearning for structure was most clearly demonstrated in a session when Foulkes, Main and Bridger were absent. The resultant insecurity led to Sutton, as the senior officer present, taking charge and speaking more than in any other group that he attended. He always found it difficult to tolerate silence and always had to 'edge in' on meetings, feeling impelled to organise the process (Bridger 1990b). However, his activity failed to prevent a general air of despondency ensuing. The psychiatrists felt that groups were being used less, that social therapy might mean that psychiatry was unnecessary, and indeed that the meeting itself seemed to be a lot of 'hot air'. To counteract this sense of gloom it was suggested that the meeting required a chairman 'to keep people to the point', ignoring the fact that Sutton was already attempting to do this (Discussion Group 16, 19 September 1945). Markillie contrasted the 'body of security' that built up in the subsequent session, when Foulkes was present, with the anxiety engendered in the previous one. However, nobody articulated the sense of dependency that existed, despite the fact that the main subject of discussion, apprenticeships in group therapy, further expressed their unconscious wish for parental guidance (Discussion Group 17, 11 October 1945).

Describing his own methods, McLardy stated that after selecting his patients through individual assessment he then tried to direct the discussion towards issues he had previously identified with them. Tom Main argued in reply that though this approach was an important step, it did not fulfil the preliminary aim, which was for the members to gain a sense of comradeship, common allegiance, fellowship, and responsibility towards each other and the external world (Discussion Group 15, 12 September 1945, p.7) It was only once this had been achieved that they could begin to examine their interrelationships.

Throughout the discussions, Foulkes encouraged doctors to abandon a directive and organised role, avoiding rules of behaviour, techniques and attempts to tackle symptoms rather than causes. This led inevitably to the question of what skills the psychiatrist needed to be a group therapist. Magnus raised this question in April, emphasising the problems the men had addressing and being addressed by officers. He concluded that the problem lay in their lack of confidence. In answer, Bridger recounted a talk with Bion, in which he had referred to his own non-medical status. They had agreed that it was not necessary to be a doctor, because the group's task was to handle its own tensions. The caring, responsible and active role of the doctor could actually be a handicap. The task of the therapist was to deal with his or her own frustrations and be able to tolerate the stress of the group while they set about their purpose, which was primarily to face the problem of neurosis and return to health (Discussion Group 3, 26 April 1945, p.2). When Magnus continued to articulate his lack of confidence, Foulkes elaborated further, pointing out that he could take this issue to the group members themselves: 'Discuss it with them at their own level – it is therapy and you will learn too. After all to many patients confidence may be a concrete thing that they feel they have lost.' Bridger added that discussing what is meant by confidence would be valuable (Discussion Group 3, 26 April 1945, pp.2–4). Six months later, Main's reply to Mclean's concerns about losing his status as a doctor ran along very similar lines. He recognised that the patients were also uncertain about their new roles, and so should be supported by discussing the issues openly (Discussion Group 19, 8 November 1945, p.3). Similarly, Bridger in the very first discussion suggested that the appropriate thing to do when starting the group was to ask the members what they felt about talking in such a group (Discussion Group 1, 12 April 1945). Of course, one of the issues that faced doctors with this loss of control was the fear that things would get out of hand. Martin recounted the events that took place in one group in which he was involved when the members became angry and aggressive towards each other. The group ended on a note of tension, unlike the WOSB group, in which 'you seal things off to avoid anxiety'. Foulkes was very uncertain whether this unresolved stress was a good thing (Discussion Group 4, 3 May 1945, p.2). A number of accounts emphasise the fact that tensions could run very high.

Another illustration of the different approaches is provided in a dialogue between Martin and Main. Martin argued that it was important to get group members to do things for themselves and overcome their fear of participation. If the man is able to speak

> he begins to be aware of the social implications. He is doing something positive and something social. It is very important that a man should speak in a group as that is the only way in which one can see what is happening in the group. (Discussion Group 13, 29 August 1945, p.2)

Main retorted that he had 'said the right thing the wrong way round', implying that the important thing was to create the environment and understanding in which the person felt able to speak, rather than concentrate on the individual's personal activity in isolation. If the person experienced being part of a safe, supportive and creative process he would become involved (Discussion Group 13, 29 August 1945, p.2). It wasn't what the therapist could do for the individual, but what could be done to help the group understand the forces in the social field. Rickman's earlier visit had been disturbing because his notions reinforced this move away from the treatment of individual symptoms of illness to the gaining of insight into the interpersonal relationships of the neurotic group tensions (Discussion Group 14, 5 September 1945, p.1).

Bridger took the same line when he reframed the debate about activity and passivity, emphasising that the key issue was participation (Discussion Group 11, 2 August 1945, p.3). This led to further debate about when and how to intervene. Main emphasised that just letting a man join groups willy-nilly did not lead to group therapy. It was a staged process in which the person had to sense that they belonged before embarking on any further steps. In the instance of a group discussing someone who was not present, he declared that the group leader should intervene to ensure that the displaced anxieties were manifest in the group, not projected outside of it (Discussion Group 15, 12 September 1945, p.8). Bridger elaborated on this by denying the separation between individual and social therapy. He contended that both were carried out within the overall social field and the forces operating within it. Individual therapy could only be carried out if it was not divorced from the environmental setting, taking place as a stage in the individual's passage to recovery (Discussion Group 13, 29 August 1945, p.6). He was evidently unhappy with the psychiatrists' estrangement from the overall process of the hospital:

> Let us get back to the total field situation and get back to what Major Foulkes described as treating cross infection [the contagion of feelings and attitudes amongst the soldiers] positively and let us also be very frank. This group therapy discussion is attended by Psychiatrists interested in Group Therapy. This week everyone was supposed to attend. You see the result here today. It is no different from when it was voluntary. This is to my mind significant because dynamically it corresponds with the effort of the social therapy group in dealing with the whole hospital. I feel that the Psychiatric group must examine its own attitude. The treating of a hospital as a unit and the purpose for which this group meets are topologically similar. All this is highly significant and relevant to the problem. For cross infection to be positive, groups and in particular the psychiatric group, need to be positive. (Discussion Group 7, 24 May 1945, p.4)

One can imagine how the doctors felt 'got at', similarly to the soldiers in Bion's training wing 30 months earlier. Foulkes immediately defused the tension by adding his own questions, and the discussion veered onto safer issues such as the gradings of other staff.

Most of the groups discussed technique in as dispassionate a manner as possible. Foulkes was looked on as the fount of information about this and for much of the time attempts to examine the doctor's own state of mind were ignored. However, as many of them became more confident, there were sporadic attempts to reflect on the impact that the therapy had on themselves and how their emotions influenced the patients. In September, Mclean recognised that 'Group treatment has affected the psychiatrist as much as the patient' (Discussion Group 16, 19 September 1945, p.2). James outlined the therapeutic effect that they had on him: 'I was feeling none too good just prior to a group session, and yet no sooner had we settled down, than it was one of the best we had ever had' (Discussion Group 6, 17 May 1945, p.1). In response, Foulkes underlined how responsive the group was to its therapists (p.2). At times, some of the therapists were able to recognise the parallels between their own feelings and those of the patients. Day realised that both he and the group had similar positive feelings about the end of the war and the fact that most of them would soon be released from the army. But this form of insight was unusual, and Essex's question about what form of treatment was useful for the psychiatrist was ignored when he put it to the discussion group, as was Mclean's contentious idea that the psychiatrist was just as dependent on the patient as vice versa (Discussion Groups 16, 19 September 1945, p.2; 19, 8 November 1945, p.1). This led to Main and Bridger having to reiterate the idea that there was little difference between the men and the officers who were treating them. Foulkes identified that the patients had the same emotional difficulties as the doctors in facing the group idea and Main took this further by suggesting that the traditional roles of doctor and patients should be discussed openly as part of therapy (Discussion Group 19, 8 November 1945, p.3).

Tom Main attempted to use his own experience of arriving at the hospital to illustrate how other visitors experienced their reception:

> There is a social technique of hostility, isolating a visitor is to make him do the talking. I noticed this was the way this hospital received me. I was a stranger so I was a bar to any conversation between people. There was silence and I had to work my passage and the person was put to test. There is a gathering of the forces and he either runs out or comes in. There is a hostile kind of listening which can be turned to an interesting kind of listening. (Discussion Group 13, 29 August 1945, pp.2–3)

A week later he emphasised the importance of the session which had discussed its own tensions:

> Last week we had a very interesting discussion and it was interesting because we ourselves discussed our own tensions as a group. We discussed the effects of visitors, the real situation, the rationalisation. We did attempt to discuss technique. We were handling the discussion as if

the group itself was a social organism. (Discussion Group 14, 5 September 1945, p.1)

As stated earlier, the groups tended to resort to the search for technical solutions to emotional problems. Whilst much of this was sterile, some basic issues were debated. A general conclusion was reached that for a specific therapy group eight was about the right number of patients (Discussion Groups 5, 10 May 1945, p.2; 10, 19 July 1945, p.1). The length of the sessions varied. Bridger found that some of the ward and committee meetings lasted for up to three hours (Discussion Group 10, 19 July 1945, p.1). The frequency also varied, ranging from once to three times a week. The debate about whether groups should remain consistent, with a set membership, or whether they should be more open, allowing for a fluctuating membership, led Bridger to emphasise yet again that this was dichotomising unnecessarily. The ideal was a 'continuous project', with the group adapting to the needs of its membership (Discussion Group 9, 21 June 1945, p.1). This sense of dynamism was central to his observations. He recognised that how you approached the group changed as the membership matured (Discussion Group 11, 2 August 1945, pp.1–3).

Theoretical considerations were referred to from time to time. Psychoanalytic ideas were brought up almost exclusively by Foulkes, who talked of interpretation, transference, group transference and resistances (Discussion Groups 4, 3 May 1945, p.3; 6, 17 May 1945, p.1; 7, 24 May 1945, p.2; 9, 21 June 1945, p.1; 11, 2 August 1945, p.5). However, these references appear to have made little impact, as other members rarely used the terminology at all. 'Lewinfiltration' also figured, rather more overtly, with many people talking about the social field, particularly Bridger. Moreno's spontaneity figured briefly, being mentioned by Foulkes on a couple of occasions (Discussion Groups 6, 17 May 1945, p.1; 8, 31 May 1945, p.2). In general, however, there was little use of jargon, and there is the genuine sense of issues being explored very directly without preconceived ideas by most of those present.

Given the amount of time spent on how groups should be run, there was relatively little debate about their nature or advantages. Demonstrating the variety of group approaches present in the hospital, Thoms held the view early on in the discussions that the task was to ensure that the patient realised that he was not in a mental hospital, to discuss with him the causes of his illness and to gain insight into his disorder (Discussion Group 4, 3 May 1945, p.1). This hangover from more didactic approaches did not linger long amongst those who attended the discussions regularly. Captain Day suggested that the advantages of working with a group lay in the fact that one saw the individual's problems against the background of the social setting. This ability to be more objective benefited the psychiatrist as well as the patient (Discussion Group 1, 12 April 1945). This view was shared by Collins six months later when he stated: 'I can judge patients much better in the space of half an hour by watching their reactions and noting their silences in a group than I can in half an hour [individual] interview. (Discussion Group 14, 5 September 1945, p.2).

Much to people's surprise, group therapy was not a time-saving exercise (Discussion Group 5, 10 May 1945, p.1). Its benefits lay elsewhere. It provided camaraderie, and the sharing of experiences gave the men a 'fellow feeling of sympathy' (Discussion Groups 6, 17 May 1945, p.1; 14, 5 September 1945, p.2). Going closer to the heart of the matter, Foulkes identified groups as the 'ideal medicine for that aspect of neurosis that is social' (Discussion Group 12, 8 August 1945, p.3). However, the social adaptation offered by the groups, in some doctors' opinions, didn't appear to resolve the personal difficulties that people had. Mclean saw patients who were 'adapted to the hospital but still undoubtedly have their own personal problems' (Discussion Group 11, 2 August 1945, p.6). This question vexed de Maré, who took it a stage further, arguing that it was possible to adjust people to all sorts of groups, including those with Nazi sympathies. An argument could be made by psychiatrists that if the individual didn't fit in with the social group around them they were a psychopath (Discussion Group 14, 5 September 1945, p.3). It is not clear from Main's reply that he understood the question that de Maré was posing; but Rickman's answer would have plainly been that the healthy therapeutic group is one that is exploring and open to new information, not one that has fixed and rigid conclusions.

The question of whether groups affected people at a deeper level continued to cause uncertainty. Davidson finished one discussion group with this issue, explaining that she was 'content if... [she could] get... [her] patients to get any insight at all' (Discussion Group 14, 5 September 1945, p.7).

As one might expect, Main tended to reiterate Bion's views. He stated on one occasion:

> The fundamental difference in group treatment is the basis of the examination of tensions within groups and the attempt to resolve them. If the social disturbance can be resolved, if the man can be given social insight by the group, why he is hostile to a group or overanxious to please, if they can be discussed in relation to the group and the man improve his performance as a group member, he will have achieved a chance to be happy in society. His adjustment to life is better and

frustrations would be fewer. (Discussion Group 14, 5 September 1945, p.2)

In another meeting Main emphasised that the purpose was not just to get the individual well within himself, but also to get him healthy with regards to the society he was living in (Discussion Group 15, 12 September 1945, p.5).

There was some debate about the difference between a group and a crowd, and during this Markillie almost paraphrased Le Bon. He argued that where panic occurs a 'mob and a rabble have features in common. You get infection to such a degree that the outskirts of a rabble have no idea of the precipitating cause' (Discussion Group 20, 15 November 1945, pp.3–4). The soldiers arriving at the hospital were in a similar state of mind. For them to recover they needed first to feel that they belonged somewhere, thus replacing the comradeship that they had lost. They achieved this by joining the more organised structure of a group, which Main defined as 'a living organism with a structured emotional framework, a body of people all of whom have some kind of allegiance to each other' (Discussion Group 14, 5 September 1945, p.5).

The concept that the group was a microcosm of the social situation that it was in was constantly reiterated by Bridger and Main. They acknowledged that there was a tension between the military requirements of the army and the clinical needs of therapy, but argued that there was a chain of groups through which the individual might pass from the requirements of treatment to re-establishing himself as a functioning citizen (Discussion Group 10, 19 July 1945, p.2). Each stage reflected the activities of the system around it. For instance, the incident in which a sister left the therapeutic group was significant in that it demonstrated difficulties within the ward as a whole (p.1). The doctor was not just a clinician, but also, as an officer, a representative of the military hierarchy (Discussion Group 8, 31 May 1945, p.2). This meant that these issues had to be brought out into the open before they could be resolved. The staff had to treat the hospital as a quasi-military unit in order for therapy to be effective (Discussion Group 7, 24 May 1945, p.3). Their wider role in the army was emphasised by the stream of visitors that came. These ranged from officers, doctors and ex-prisoners of war visiting prior to setting up the Civil Resettlement Units to American and Canadian staff learning about British military psychiatry. The staff at the hospital had to learn how to make them feel welcome, let them join therapy groups, and understand what was significant about the process of what was happening there. Trying not to perceive them as a source of irritation and interruption was often particularly difficult.

RESHAPING THE DOMAIN: GROUP
THERAPY AT NORTHFIELD

Like Maghull in the First World War, Northfield trained a generation of psychiatrists in a new treatment for neurosis. Whilst the total numbers trained were many fewer, at least ten continued working in the field, and their impact has been profound. Foulkes went on to set up the Institute of Group Analysis. Bion's influence is more nebulous, most directly expressed in the work of the Tavistock Institute. De Maré, E.J. Anthony and Joshua Bierer are amongst the other names who made a subsequent impact. The literature on the field is huge and continues to accumulate. Unlike the previous war, detailed records of how the practice developed give a vivid picture of many of the dissensions and agreements amongst the pioneers.

Bion and Rickman drew together concepts from Lewin's field theory, their military experience and psychoanalysis. This, combined with their clarity about the therapeutic objective, gave them a clear vision of how to achieve it. Foulkes, on the other hand, had to fight for every insight. His understanding of the purpose of group therapy evolved as he gained experience. He moved from conducting individual therapy in a group setting to a position that was not far removed from that of his predecessors at Northfield. However, he had to contend continually with his tendency to avoid confrontation and his reparative, protective nature. This led to misunderstandings, particularly with Tom Main, who was himself struggling to understand the full implications of Bion's approach. In many ways, he similarly had to learn everything for himself, in contrast to his friend, Bridger, who grasped intuitively the underlying concepts of working with the 'here and now' realities of group situations. Perhaps the fact that he wasn't a doctor made it easier. Bridger also seems to have taken Foulkes in his stride. However, it is interesting to observe the behaviour of the latter in the group discussions. Frequently, he adds to Bridger's observations, and not infrequently diverts their impact. He appears to have consciously wanted he and Bridger to be allies, and yet unconsciously wanted to undermine him at the same time. The rest of the psychiatric staff tended to remain the shadow of these three, and indeed in their absence the discussion group drifted like a rudderless ship. A number of people, particularly Millicent Dewar and Ronald Markillie, have subsequently commented on the tensions amongst the psychiatrists (Dewar 1993; Markillie 1993). It is evident that they were reacting to the dissensions between these three as well as the inherent conflicts with the administration.

It is perhaps inevitable that this concatenation of ideas and protagonists should have carried with it such discomfort. Apart from Bridger, each went off after the war to found and rule their own domain, Main at the Cassell,

Bion with his particular brand of psychoanalysis, and Foulkes in the Institute of Group Analysis. Bierer continued to plough his own furrow at the Marlborough Day Hospital, whilst Bradbury left the world of therapy altogether to finish up as a Professor of Art. The cauldron of intellectual debate at Northfield was highly creative at the same time and also potentially destructive. In retrospect it is evident that the intra-group tensions of the psychiatrists themselves were never resolved.

Perhaps Moreno's most important contribution was his emphasis on the value of spontaneity. This commonplace word was used frequently throughout the discussions and related writings, and only when its conceptual value is recognised does its relevance becomes apparent (e.g. Foulkes 1948, p.116; Main 1984).[4] Enactive therapy attempted to capitalise on serendipity, as did much of Bridger's work. Bradbury remembered him squatting on the stage in the Great Hall confronting a large group of men who had illegally spent the previous night in the pub. Instead of lecturing them, he merely waited for their response and allowed the session to develop from this (Bradbury 1990a). He built the 'here and now' into drama and extracted the psychological essence from the event, making it explicit. Some years later, Bridger emphasised the importance of process in enabling the release of creativity, rather than relying on outcome as a measure of success (1990b). The latter approach is inhibitive, and restricts the possibilities to those which can be forseen; the former, on the other hand, allows for new, unpredictable achievements.

The great task of the group therapies and the social therapy department was to create an environment in which trust could develop and the men could achieve a sense of belonging and self-worth. Once this had been achieved they were able to re-examine their lives and begin to break loose from the chains of neurosis. Integral to this process was the enabling of those spontaneous moments, when new ideas and insights could rupture old set patterns of thought and action, and open up fresh worlds of opportunity.

---

4   The discussion at the beginning of Discussion Group 8, 31 May 1945, emphasised the problems of inhibition and started to look at how to counter them.

CHAPTER 8

'The Sum of Our Gifts':[1]

Overview and Future

It is an advance on a different front. (Tom Main in Discussion Group 15, 12 September 1945, p.2)

MAN OR MANKIND: THE OVERALL TASK

In 1940, during the invasion of France, Antoine de Saint-Exupéry pondered on why he continued to contribute to the futile defence of his country. He was flying reconnaissance flights in an unarmed aeroplane over occupied territory, with the daily expectation of death and in the face of imminent defeat. The task was to all intents and purposes pointless. He came to the conclusion that his only strength lay in the community of mankind, not as a system that reduced every individual to conformity, but one that celebrated variety. It was not himself, but the universal family of humanity that was worth fighting for (de Saint-Exupéry 1995, p.127–129).

This paradoxical, poetic airman had come to conclusions similar to those reached by the protagonists of this book. Like Foulkes, he had to struggle towards these conclusions. War evokes such soul-searching, and it is perhaps unsurprising that such speculation inevitably impacts on psychiatry, with its close alliance to philosophy and psychology. It was not just the exigency of neurosis in soldiers that forced the development of psychotherapy in the two World Wars, it was also the consequences of a conscript army. The recruitment of men and women whose ambitions lay outside of the field of arms introduced new ideologies into the traditional military sphere. Inevitably, this provoked conflicts. Few people wish to kill others, and, whilst the majority avoided such direct involvement, the overall product of their work was to maximise the slaughter of the enemy.[2]

---

1   From de Saint-Exupéry 1995, p.127.
2   The findings of S.L.A. Marshall in the American army that no more than 25% of front line troops actually fire at the enemy with whatever weapon they are provided with provides ample evidence

Doctors were torn by a variety of dilemmas: the problem, for male doctors, of reconciling their masculinity with their 'feminine' role, the conflict between their prime directive of preserving life and their senior role, and their relative safety compared with most of their patients. There would always be a group for whom further physical assaults on those whom they were treating was an anathema. Rest, even enforced chemically, could be perceived as beneficial, but the more radical procedures such as surgery, convulsive treatment, applying electric shocks or other physically invasive therapies were repugnant. It is noticeable that the most ardent advocates of such procedures were also those who had the most negative views of those whom they were treating. The possibility of talking to their patients, demonstrating their own humanity and 'befriending' them, would have appealed to the more sensitive practitioners. The spread of didactic therapies, educating the soldiers about their disorders, exemplifies the success of one solution to this. It preserved the professional's status, whilst satisfying his or her wish to respect the individual's humanity.

However, this was not enough. The difference between the work of Bion and Rickman, and that of Foulkes, is that the task was seen from entirely different angles. For the latter, the ideal aim was individual treatment, evolving to achieve the perfect group, which would almost incidentally provide good soldiers, especially if they were kept together. The army and its rigours tended to get in the way of this. Foulkes continued to emphasise the individual over humanity, despite his protestations to the contrary.

For the former two, the overall task was to win the war by providing effective soldiers in a variety of roles. The army was a group environment and consequently group approaches were the most effect method to realise this. The military environment was the actuality which had to be accepted and understood. Saint-Exupéry's dilemma was whether he should continue to carry out an increasingly absurd task. He concluded that to subsume his own wishes to the discipline of the greater whole was the only way he could remain true to mankind and himself. Bion and Rickman agreed wholeheartedly.

Winning battles or winning wars: Successes and failures

A fundamental enquiry about the Northfield Experiments is whether or not they were successful. This then begs a further question: what are the relevant measures of this?

of this. Even those who were under direct attack and in danger of being wiped out would fail to defend themselves (Marshall 1947, pp.50–63).

The first potential measure, which directly addresses the issues raised by Rickman and Bion, is the number of soldiers returned to effective service. In common with most research in psychiatry at this time, there is no relevant evidence available. Crude outcome figures would have been of little or no help because of the numerous confounding variables and lack of controls.[3] Reports from men who were present at the time are too few to be strictly helpful, though it is noticeable that the more critical ones tend to come from the later years, when the hospital had reverted to being a poorly-staffed traditional unit.

More positive evidence comes from the Civil Resettlement Units that were set up to help ex-prisoners of war readjust to life after war. These were directly modelled on the work at Northfield, and, as we have seen, many of their staff spent time there, absorbing the approach more or less successfully. At their peak there were 20 such units operating, each capable of dealing with 240 men at a time (Curle 1947, p.42). They were described, in a manner similar to that of Bridger on the social therapy centre at Northfield, as transitional communities. The plan was to 'assist the passage of individuals' from their role as ex-captives to one of functioning citizens.

The Civil Resettlement Units were run quite openly by the army, on quasi-military lines. The individual who attended them volunteered to do so, and there was no coercion. This ensured that those who did so took responsibility for their cooperation in the process. On its part, the CRU structure had to be entirely consistent with its aim, as any insincerity on its part would have been rapidly recognised by its clients. The organisation was run explicitly on group lines. The trauma of the prisoner of war had taken place in the context of a body of people relating to their captors, and his difficulties on returning concerned his relationships with the social community around him.

The milieu aimed to encourage initiative, spontaneity and the ventilation of personal problems, and to replace external military discipline with inner self-control. More than half the staff were women, in order to help the men

---

3   Some evidence of outcomes was given in the quarterly records of Dennis Carroll in September 1944. He was able to report that, in August of that year, 91% of discharges from the hospital went back to duty. Seven hundred cases came from Normandy, of whom 96% returned to duty, including 75% who were fit for overseas duty. Three months later the picture was not so positive, with 85% of cases returning to duty, four-fifths of whom were in category C 2 (the lowest category for service). This latter figure was flattering, because the triage before admission allowed more difficult cases through and the workload was very high (Carroll 1944b and c). These figures are fairly unhelpful in deciding on the efficacy of the unit, as they do not state how long the men were able to sustain their improvement, and they do not distinguish which treatments were the most successful. The fluctuations were also sensitive to the type of case being received.

to overcome their shyness (Wilson, Doyle and Kelnar 1947). The soldier was at no time ordered to attend any particular activity, but a range of discussion groups, vocational opportunities and recreational events were available. While there, the individual passed through a series of stages. Initially, he had to learn about the unit, then orientate himself to the surrounding social and industrial organisations. Finally, he would begin to make preparations for the future. Accompanying this process was a psychological evolution that began with reducing suspiciousness of authority and improving socialisation, and ended with testing out possible life plans.

The tackling of neurotic problems by the whole unit if necessary was entirely congruent with Bion and Rickman's work, and indeed was consciously patterned on it. The report of Main, Bridger, Foulkes and others in the *Bulletin of the Menninger Clinic* provided a care model (Wilson, Doyle and Kelnar 1947).

Adam Curle and Eric Trist evaluated the outcome of this work in one city by following up 50 men who had graduated from a CRU, comparing them with 100 ex-prisoners of war who had not been through the service and 40 families who had not experienced either. Those who had taken advantage of the transitional-community experience consistently displayed evidence of a significantly better social adjustment than those who had not. There are of course a number of confounding variables in this. For instance, those who chose to undergo the course may have already been better adjusted than those who could not face the idea, and the group chosen was very small compared with the overall numbers involved. However, the findings are very suggestive of the beneficial effects of such an approach (Curle and Trist 1947). Incidentally, this was probably one of the first controlled studies carried out in social psychology in the United Kingdom.

Other potential measures of success include the dissemination of practice. In this field again, the evidence is patchy, other events confuse the picture. Looking particularly at the development of the therapeutic community, only two units can be strictly described as stemming directly from Northfield – the Cassell Hospital, where Tom Main went on to be director, and Warlingham Park, where T.P. Rees worked. The success of Maxwell Jones in promoting his model overshadowed the less well-publicised work of Main. Also, whilst the Northfield Experiments are widely referred to in psychiatric and psychotherapeutic literature as being historically significant, little is made of what specific contributions came from that source.[4]

The evidence for these men's influence in group psychotherapy relies most heavily on the work of Foulkes, and the Institute of Group Analysis. This latter has of course become widely influential, and has promulgated a rather distorted version of events in the hospital. Bion developed his theories further at the Tavistock Clinic and this work, whilst evidently being derived from his few weeks at Northfield, tended to eclipse the earlier insights. Rickman went on to write about the factor of number in groups, but his early death in 1951 prevented any further development of his thoughts in this area. In consequence his work is now largely neglected.

Despite this dearth of definitive verification of the impact of the Northfield Experiments in the psychodynamic field, there is some evidence of a more covert, even subversive, influence. First is the regular, if often inaccurate, acknowledgement of their influence in a wide range of textbooks, lectures and discussions. Present-day practitioners working in group therapy and therapeutic communities are nearly all aware of this predecessor, although they remain vague about the details. Northfield has an enormous mythic importance, with the accounts by Bion, Main, and Foulkes providing the central dogma. Some few, rare, practitioners are aware of the reports in the *Bulletin of the Menninger Clinic*, and another few have read Bridger's succinct chronicles. Some of the conceptualisations realised then, such as the emphasis on the 'here and now', have gained a familiarity that indicates a less formal route of transmission. As Ernest Jones has already been quoted as stating, more ideas have been promulgated by word of mouth than through written literature, and this is surely true of Northfield.

Northfield was of course part of a much wider series of social–psychological innovations, much of which was taken up by the Tavistock Institute of Human Relations. It is through this organisation that many of the ideas were developed and broadcast to a wider audience. Their focus, however, moved away from psychiatry and mental illness to preventative work, particularly in industry. Bridger, in particular, exemplified this shift, moving from Northfield to the Tavistock Institute, and subsequently working independently in the field of leadership training.

---

4   An ad hoc survey of textbooks revealed about twenty references to Northfield, all of which confined themselves to terse statements about how Northfield was a forerunner, but gave little or no further information.

THE ENIGMA REVISITED: BION AND RICKMAN

Part of the failure of the Northfield Experiments to influence future generations can be paid at the door of one of their most clear-sighted participants. Throughout Bion's career in the army he was dogged by a sense of resentment, feeling that he was undervalued and misunderstood. He left the WOSB board following conflict with his commanding officer, the Board President, and left Northfield in similar circumstances. It is interesting how Trist and Sutherland in particular take his part in all of this, and ignore his failings as a self-appointed leader. Perhaps this is because of their awe of him: they were much younger men who considered that they were in the presence of a genius. However, his inability to share his ideas in a manner which others could understand and his continued sense of resentment towards figures of authority, including J.R. Rees, were failings in someone who undoubtedly revolutionised group therapy. Perhaps in this self-imposed isolation lay the seeds of the riddle with which we are now left. Sutherland relates how in the first of the trial 'study' groups that led to the Leicester Conferences, he and Rickman felt themselves to be lagging behind Bion's comments about the group. The fact that two of his closest colleagues could feel so unclear about what he was doing in a group appears to have been part of his problem (Sutherland 1985, p.52). Maybe the enigma lies more in his unwillingness to share his thinking with many of his colleagues, and his disdain for their opinions, than in the nature of group theory.

One answer could have lain in the work of Rickman, who also, through his diffidence, failed to elaborate on his own thinking. His strength was in discussion. His impact on the Second Northfield Experiment was considerable. Dewar recalled the privilege of being invited to join him for a coffee evening whilst he was staying at Northfield, and Main remained convinced of his prime importance forty years later (Dewar 1993; Main 1984). Bridger believed that Rickman brought a profound anthropological sense to his understanding of societal forces and group tensions. It is unfortunate that he wrote little; but for Bridger and others of his generation 'who were fortunate enough to take part in them', his 'coffee-pot sessions' were unforgettable (Bridger 1985, pp.97–98).

What would have happened had Rickman lived longer? Unlike Bion, he did not feel the need to retreat to individual psychodynamics to further understand the group. Indeed, he was more interested in exploring other arenas of social psychology, including becoming involved in trying to keep the Peckham Experiments going after the institution of the National Health Service.

Would he have continued to develop the idea of amalgamating psychotherapy with the development of social roles? One of the challenging aspects of the Northfield Experiments was their holistic approach. The soldier was able to explore his personal dilemmas and his effect on others, and in parallel develop a sense of purposefulness through his vocational role. Treatment today tends to be much more disaggregated, with different therapies being provided in isolation from each other.

SPLIT LOYALTIES: FOULKES AND BION
AFTER FIFTY YEARS

Tensions continue to plague the relationship of the adherents of the two traditions even now. Represented by the Institute of Group Analysis and the Tavistock Clinic, they continue to debate the relative merits of each approach. The followers of Bion have been characterised as cruel, harsh and traumatising, in contrast to the friendly, caring disciples of Foulkes, A recent debate discussed the 'split' between the two (Hinshelwood 1999). During this, it became clear that the personalities of the initiators have tended to obscure their messages. The veiled antagonisms of Northfield have become openly polarised, a thesis and antithesis for which no synthesis appeared to be forthcoming.

Of course, this dichotomy would have been ridiculed by Kurt Lewin, as an example of Aristotelian thinking. To take the analogy of a painting, what has happened is that the figure and ground have been divorced. Bion's emphasis on the social context and the intra-group tensions has been contrasted with Foulkes' concentration on the individual. This oversimplification of the division lies at the heart of the conflict.

Again, it is interesting to speculate how Rickman would have viewed the present schism. The person who has most closely sustained his outlook has been Harold Bridger, who has brought a humanity to his interpretation of Bion's work which often appears to be lacking in more orthodox adherents. He has repeatedly emphasised the task orientation, the process, and the relationship of internal and external factors in group functioning.

The task is the key. This predicates the tensions in the group, or team, as well as how they might be resolved. Bion's basic assumptions become tools by which to understand the process. All groups oscillate between the wish to sustain the group for its own neurotic needs and the imperative to perform the task. By understanding the processes that encourage the former, it is possible to improve progress in the latter.

Different tasks require different solutions. For many individuals the experience of a supportive, nurturing group environment provides a transitional stage towards a more realistic setting. Others are able to develop their own practice in the stressful milieu of a two-week-long leaderless group.

Bridger consistently emphasises the real-world setting in which the group has to operate according to his training methods. An instance of this is his request to members of otherwise 'taskless' training groups, attending a course, to keep in mind the fact that they would need to report their activities to the other groups. This subtle instruction is zen-like in its apparent simplicity and actual complexity. How does a group tackle its internal tensions without an agenda, whilst having to keep in mind the necessity to relate their experience to the outside world? This requirement forces a constant interplay of figure and ground. The individual exchanges no longer occur in a vacuum; they have to be related to an external social reality.

BACK TO THE RUBBER BALL: CAN THE LESSONS BE LEARNT EVEN NOW?

It was perhaps absurd to expect the discipline of psychiatry to maintain its pre-eminence in the army once the group of individuals who had inspired that pre-eminence had been demobbed. The ordinary psychiatrist rarely has the depth and breadth of knowledge possessed by the members of the 'Tavistock Group'. Their theoretical resources ranged from industrial psychology to educational methods, and it was the melding of these that gave them their vision. As we have seen, they spread out into a variety of different fields after the war, and apart from Brigadier Rosie, none of the key players remained in the army.

Foulkes was relatively unusual in that he spent most of his military service at Northfield. Most of the other psychiatrists either had or were to have widely varying experiences in army psychiatry. Apart from those who feature significantly in this book, others like Emanuel Miller and Ronald Markillie had worked in other military hospitals. Alfred Torrie had worked in the Middle East with acute war casualties. Jack Pearce went to Italy as Adviser in Psychiatry to Allied Forces Headquarters. Ellis Stungo went to work in the Far East, having had a lot of earlier experience with physical treatments in psychiatry in civilian practice. Eric Wittkower had been involved in the early development of selection procedures, and was later to pursue his interest in psychosomatic medicine in other arenas. Lt. Col. Rosie went on to become a Brigadier and the Director of Army Psychiatry.

As a result of this flow through the hospital, the activities there were known of, not always approvingly, by a wide circle of psychiatrists and other doctors. The end of the war, however, took them out of the army, and very rapidly the knowledge and skills there evaporated. This is well illustrated by the descriptions of Northfield Military Hospital in 1947 (*see* Chapter 6). By the time of the Falklands War, memories had faded so much that it was possible for the expectation to be that there would be little or no psychological trauma. The British Soldier just wasn't like that! The subsequent high prevalence of Post Traumatic Stress Disorder in the men came as a complete surprise.

A particularly irrational outcome of the pioneering work at Northfield has been the divorce of the therapeutic-community approach from rehabilitation. One of the successes of the service provided by Northfield was the integration of the exploration of interrelationships with practical experience in work settings. Therapeutic communities since have generally tended to concentrate on the psychotherapeutic aspects, whilst rehabilitation psychiatry has taken over the vocational training. This divorce was exemplified by the comparison of three hospitals in the 1960s by Wing and Brown (1970). Of these, one was identified as a work-orientated unit, the second as a therapeutic community and the third as providing a traditional mental-hospital approach. Even today the integration of psychotherapeutic approaches with practical skills training for life remains rare in all fields of mental health. Certainly, the idea that patients with mental disorders should be approached about their future employment within the first week of treatment is not put into practice anywhere in the United Kingdom to this author's knowledge.

It is lessons such as this that make the Northfield Experiments still so vibrantly relevant today. Psychiatry has tended to concentrate on the individual almost to the exclusion of all other factors, in particular the family. It is only with the implementation of 'community care' that this process is being reversed. When a person is treated at home, it becomes less possible to ignore the circle of family and friends that he or she lives with. Therapy thus increasingly has to address the issues of the social group, the responsibilities of the patient and the wider social issues of discrimination, role and employment. Exploring with the members of that group the consequences of their interactions would appear to offer opportunities of integration and amelioration of distress that other therapies tend to ignore.

To achieve this, the therapist needs to begin to take a much wider view of his or her role. He or she needs to be able to helicopter above the immediate situation and take an overview. Present-day therapeutic endeavour is nearly always individually-orientated, and development crawls from stage to stage within one system level, usually that of the patient–doctor relationship. There is a need for a broader vision which takes into consideration technologies from completely different fields of endeavour: the team in industry, communication skills, sociology, media skills and education, to name but a few.

The Northfield Experiments demonstrated the possibility of a caring system co-ordinating in such a way that the whole organisation could work as one with the aim of enabling people who had experienced some form of disability to function effectively in society. Given the enormous benefits that could ensue from this combination of unidirectional energy, it seems strange in retrospect that this method of operating hasn't become more widespread, or even 'normal' practice. The therapeutic community was hijacked by philosophies and mutually exclusive ideals, and lost its way. Psychiatric rehabilitation somehow became separated and fossilised into large workshops and programmes in which the personal development of the individual tended to be neglected.

Perhaps the analogy of the rubber ball introduced in chapter 5 is more pertinent than at first it might appear. Pressure applied can achieve one of two results. Either the ball returns to its old shape when the pressure is released, or it splits. Can the hospital system ever be reformed, or does it need to be reinvented? One is reminded of Wilfred Trotter's view that societies need to maintain their illogical and primitive belief systems in order to survive. In other words, democratic societies as a whole tend to act as basic assumption groups, except occasionally in times of extreme need.

Antoine de Saint-Exupéry, in describing French society before the invasion, likened it to a jumbled field of stones. Everyone was concerned with their own rights and wishes. The Germans, on the other hand, took their pebbles and formed them into a uniform heap, which seemed well able to overwhelm the chaotic cultures that faced them. However, this uniformity had within it its own seeds of failure. A diverse, cohesive society, in which each person contributes his or her differing skills within an overall strategy, has the greater strength to survive in the long term. He and John Rickman clearly shared the same vision.

Appendix 1

Official Army Nomenclature of Mental Disorders

The nomenclature was finalised in 1942, and circulated in the Technical Memoranda of the Department of Army Psychiatry for use 'by all Army Psychiatrists in their reports' (War Office 1946a). That part referring to the majority of patients who would have been in Northfield is reproduced below:

B. MENTAL DISORDERS OF PSYCHOGENIC ORIGIN WITHOUT CLEARLY DEFINED ORGANIC CAUSE OR STRUCTURAL CHANGES

ANXIETY STATE

Specify: (i) duration (recent or chronic)

             (ii) severity (mild or severe)

             (iii) type: (a) unspecified

                           (b) with gross somatic dysfunction[1]

                           (c) predominantly phobic

HYSTERIA

Specify: (i) amnesic

             (ii) motor

             (iii) sensory

             (iv) visceral[2]

OBSESSIONAL STATE

Specify: (i) rumination

             (ii) thought

             (iii) impulse

PSYCHOPATHIC PERSONALITY

Specify: (i) with emotional abnormality

             (ii) with antisocial trends

             (iii) with pathological sexuality

1 Effort syndrome, neurotic dyspepsia, neurotic diarrhoea
2 Hysterical vomiting or enuresis

Appendix 2

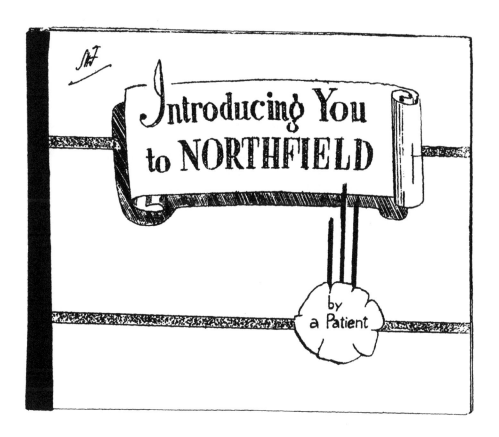

Cover of the pamphlet 'Introducing You to Northfield', given to patients during 1945 on arrival at the hospital
Reproduced by kind permission of the Wellcome Contemporary Archives Centre

Text of the Patients' Booklet: 'Introducing You to Northfield'

The following is the text of the Patients' Booklet, produced by the soldiers themselves, that was handed out to, and discussed with, the new admissions (see Chapter 5). The front page is reproduced above.

Introducing You to NORTHFIELD

by a Patient.

Editors note

This magazine has been compiled as clearly and concisely as possible to give you some idea of why you are here, and the facilities and entertainments available during your stay at this Hospital. We are going to try to solve some of your difficulties in the light of those we have experienced ourselves.

A useful map to be found on the back page which will tell you where you are at present and where you can go during your stay.

If you are in the slightest doubt about ANYTHING after reading this Magazine, the Sister will be only too pleased to help you … further information can be obtained from a Group Activities Office in the Hospital Club Corridor.

The correct address when writing is: —

Number, Rank and Name,
Military Hospital
Northfield, Birmingham
THE EDITOR

THE HOSPITAL NEWSPAPER

'The Mercury' is a newspaper published weekly on Friday mornings. This paper depends entirely on your articles so give it your best support.

INTRODUCTION

We have been sent here because our health has been impaired. There may be many reasons for this. It may be due either to the way a man is constituted or to the experience that he has been through at various times during his life; one might say quite clearly that it is due to both these causes but the degree to which each is involved differs with each of us, as individuals. It is therefore in our interest to explain to our Psychiatrist (the specialist who helps us on the road recovery), as much as we can about ourselves and to confide in him. His chief concern is to help us to overcome our present difficulties and thereby become healthy and able to take up our life and work anew. This calls for our closest co-operation in everything that is done here. Anything we tell our psychiatrist is, of course, treated as strictly confidential.

As far as treatment is concerned one might well say that everything we do here is treatment. It is for this reason that our treatment does not consist solely of bed and rest, or the usual bottle of coloured medicine. Besides interviews with our Psychiatrist, we spend much of our time in various forms of exercise and activities. We will discuss the details later in this Magazine because they differ for each of us, though it is often more helpful to work in teams the same way as they do on the 'Mercury' Staff, rather than as individuals … our special activity is selected in one of our earliest private discussions with our Psychiatrist.

You are at present in Charles Ward, which is the admission ward. You will stay in bed the morning following your arrival until your Psychiatrist has visited you. Once again, this is the admission ward so most of us spend only two or three days here before being transferred to our particular Psychiatrist's ward … a few, for various reasons, remain in Charles Ward.

When you reach your new ward you'll be expected to follow the Programme which is posted on your Ward Notice Board, which consists of a Selected Activity (explained later in this Magazine), an easy P.T. programme, which consists of walks, indoor games and swimming, Cinema Shows and one or more Group Discussions per week.

Selected Activities, Entertainment, Parties and Recreation are all 'good medicine' as well as enjoyable for their own sake, and we hope that in a very short space of time you will returned to the state of health and happiness you once knew...

MAIL...

On arrival in Charles Ward, paper and stamped envelopes can be obtained from the Sister free of charge. Mail collections from the post box in the Information Corridor (see map), are as follows: —

> 0800 hrs
> 1045 hrs
> 1300 hrs
> 1645 hrs

A list of unregistered letters is posted up on the Ward Notice Board and whilst you are in Charles Ward you'll be able to collect your letters at breaktime.

On Treatment Wards you may not get your letters until 1200 hrs because the Wards are close when we leave for our activities at 0915 hrs.

Registered letters and parcels will be listed on the Notice Board opposite the Post Office and must be collected personally.

TELEGRAMS AND TELEPHONE

Two phone boxes are available and telegrams may be sent by this means — lift receiver, dial '0' and ask for telegrams — remember, have plenty of change in your pocket! If a telegram comes for you, you'll be notified IMMEDIATELY and it can be collected from the A & D (Admission and Discharge).

LEAVE and PASSES

PASSES As soon as your Psychiatrist has seen you and if he considers you fit enough, you will be issued with a Pass Card and the standard Hospital past times are: —

Thursdays, Saturdays and Sundays — 1330 hrs until 2130 hrs.

Should your wife, parents or relations come to see you on a 'non-pass' day and you wish to accompany them outside the Hospital, apply to your Psychiatrist with the necessary evidence and if you are fit enough he will recommend it. It is advisable

to apply at least one day before they arrive. If,
however, your people arrive unexpectedly, see your
psychiatrist and he will do what he can to help you.

Late passes are only granted under very special
circumstances and then only with the Commanding
Officer's permission. Write out your reason as
clearly as possible, attach it to a Pass Form
(obtained from the Wardmaster) then consult your
Psychiatrist on the matter.

48 HOURS Leave can be granted on urgent family or
business grounds is that recommended by your
Psychiatrist, in this case you go on leave in blues
and do not have to follow the procedure has laid
down for ordinary leave.

PRIVILEGE LEAVE AND DISEMBARKATION LEAVE

Provided you are due for leave, you can, during your
stay at this Hospital, be granted one of the
following leaves:

URGENT COMPASSIONATE LEAVE

Apply IMMEDIATELY to the Military
Social Worker (Richard Ward) and in
such urgent cases a special programme
will help you to get home quickly!

(a) Hospital Privilege Leave – 7 full days arriving
    from B.L.A.
(b) Disembarkation Leave if you have arrived from
    the Middle or Far East – governed by length of
    overseas service, i.e. Two years or less, 14
    days; Two to four years, 21 days; or Four years
    and longer, 28 days.
(c) Privilege Leave (9 days).

Procedure for going on Leave

Leave procedure is a little complicated owing to the
many units under our care and the return to England
of so many men from various theatres of operations,
this procedure is very necessary, we assure you, and
if you follow the procedure carefully it turns out
easier than it at first seems.

1 Apply to your Psychiatrist for permission, stating whether it is Privilege, Disembarkation or Compassionate.

2 Collect your Leave Proforma from the Wardmaster and your Psychiatrist will complete it.

3 Return the Proforma to the Wardmaster who will get the O.C. of your Division to sanction it.

4 Go to the General Office and the Leave Clerk will check up dates and fix up details. He will present the Leave Proforma to the Registrar, who, with the C.O.s authority, grants leave and completes the form with his signature.

5 Take the Proforma to: -

PAY OFFICE - From here you will collect your ration allowance and pay for the leave period. Credits CANNOT be paid - they must be obtained by sending your Part II to your Regimental Paymaster (in a registered envelope), stating that you require your credits...

PACK STORE - Collect your kit and change into khaki.

LINEN STORE - Hand in the WHOLE of the kit originally issued to you and they will give you a Clearance Chit.

SISTER i/c WARD - Report the fact that you are going on leave and hand in your crockery - plate etc., and knife, fork and spoon.

WARDMASTER - Who then know you are going on leave and that you will remain on the 'bed strength' of the Hospital.

GENERAL OFFICE - Return the completed certificate and collect your Leave Voucher and Ration Card.

On leaving the Hospital report to the Guard Room and hand in the Linen Store Clearance Chit, Sister's Clearance Chit, A.B. 42 and your Leave Certificate.

ENTERTAINMENTS!

In this Hospital you will find many entertainments.
A programme is produced weekly and can be seen on
the Ward Notice Board of all wards. A rough idea of
this entertainment is as follows:

            Monday - Film Show
            Tuesday - Stage Show (or Whist Drive)
            Wednesday - Film or Stage Show
            Thursday - Badminton
            Friday - Patients' Dance
            Saturday - Badminton.

LIBRARY A library, sponsored by the Red Cross, will
be found in Bond Street - there is a wide selection
of books and these may be borrowed between the hours
of 1300 and 1400 on Mondays, Tuesdays, Wednesdays
and Fridays. Clearance Chits will be issued from
0830 and 0930 hrs EACH morning.

SWIMMING Watch your weekly programme - this takes
the place of P.T. and Games.

ICE SKATING This is held in the Birmingham Ice Rink
on each Thursday and tickets may be obtained (free)
from the Group Activities Officer.

BADMINTON Instruction and facilities for playing
Badminton are available to those interested, in the
Gym on Thursdays and Saturdays.

THE HOSPITAL CLUB

This Club is open at the times stated on your Ward
Notice Board.

The Club is looked after and run by a group known
as Hospital Stewards - this is a full-time activity
for those interested in this kind of work. The Club
is a great boon to the rest of us here and this work
enables the Club Rooms to be ready for any programme
suggested, as well as seeing that the games and
tables are always kept in good order.

Facilities are available for writing, Table
Tennis, Snooker, Billiards, Darts, Cards, etc.

The Social Activities Room may be booked for Ward
Socials, Whist Drives, Tombola (Housey-Housey),
Gramophone Concerts and Dancing Lessons, etc. During
the day the room may be used for our friends and

relations if we should like to talk to them in private.

CRICKET AND FOOTBALL Matches can be arranged by Wards whenever required - this is up to you and your Wardmaster. Matches with local teams take place regularly.

TENNIS At the time of this Magazine going to press, the Tennis Court is in the process of having a new top dressing. It will soon be available for play. Racquets can be obtained from the Entertainments Office.

DO YOU WANT TO GO TO A PARTY?

The parties offered to us by the people of Birmingham are very good, and by saying very good we can assure you of an excellent time. Your Ward Committee representative will post a list on your Notice Board to which you must append your name. Coach or bus will take you and bring you back from the party - and whatever or wherever it is we are sure you will have a grand time. Remember, first names on the list receive first consideration, so make sure yours is the FIRST!

We ask one thing of you - if you put your name down for a party, be sure to turn up on time - latecomers cause great inconvenience to the rest of their comrades as well as to our hosts and hostesses, who take up so much of their own time in giving us such grand times - try one, you'll like it!

PAY PARADE is in the Gym on Thursdays at 1045 hrs. Bed patients will be paid later in the day.

SELECTED ACTIVITY

A Card will be issued to you as soon as your Psychiatrist considers you fit enough - this will be carried at all times and will act as a pass when leaving the Hospital grounds.

It would take far too long and be beyond the scope of this booklet, to describe in detail all the Selected Activities. There is a list on the Pass

Card but this only covers a part of a very wide field … one need know little or nothing about an activity to take part in it, and we have found this a great opportunity to 'have a go' at something which many of us have wanted to do. Instructors are there to help us, and to see that we have a chance to develop any ideas that we do have.

Those of us who work in Groups have what is called a full time activity – these are activities which require teams to carry out the job in hand. In these circumstances we have an opportunity of tapping the resources of Birmingham, as well as those of the hospital – the 'Mercury' is an example.

If the activity that has been chosen, after discussion between the Psychiatrist and yourself is not one of those to be found on the pass card, then you may rest assured that a means will be found for you to carry it out. The Social Therapy Officer's will give you their fullest assistance in this … for example, it is possible to work on a farm or even teach at a local school. Your activity can be changed at any time by having a talk with your Psychiatrist about it.

PAY

In Hospital our basic rate of pay is 14/- per week for all men below the rank of sergeant, 17/6 Sergeants and 21/- W.O.s. Extra money will only be granted for 48 hrs and longer periods of leave or in EXTREME cases of hardship.

A form, called a Hospital Remittance Form can be obtained from the Pay Office and credits can be sent to relatives. To find out how much you have in Credit go to the Pay Office in Bond Street between the hours of 0830 – 0930 (except Sundays) and ask them to send a P.1483 (Statement of Accounts) to your Paymaster this will be returned in due course and then you can send a Hospital Remittance Form. The time this form takes to come through varies, depending on where you have come from … from England and BLA it takes anything from 8-14 days, so don't worry if it doesn't come through before. The Pay Office and the Paymaster work as quickly as possible but they can't work miracles so please be patient whilst waiting, they are doing their utmost.

ALL QUESTIONS REGARDING PAY WILL DEALT WITH AT THE
PAY OFFICE 0830 hrs - 0900 hrs (except Sundays)

MEAL TIMES

BREAKFAST...............	0730 - 0745 hrs
DINNER..................	1230 - 1240 hrs
TEA (Mondays to Fridays) 1630 - 1700 hrs	
TEA (Sats and Suns)...... 1600 - 1630 hrs	

NAAFI

MORNINGS	STAFF WEEKDAYS	09.40 - 10.00 hrs
	PATIENTS "	10.05 - 11.00 hrs
	ALL SUNDAYS	10.30 - 11.20 hrs
LUNCHTIME	ALL DAILY	13.00 - 14.00 hrs
	PATIENTS DAILY	17.30 - 21.00 hrs
EVENINGS	SATURDAY	18.00 - 21.00 hrs
	STAFF DAILY	17.30 - 21.00 hrs
	EX. FRIDAY	17.30 - 20.30 hrs
	SATURDAY	18.00 - 21.00 hrs

GENERAL

VISITS Relations and friends may come to visit us on
Mondays Wednesdays and Fridays from 14.00 - 18.00
hrs. Should any of our relations have to travel long
distances it is possible, with permission from the
Sister i/c Ward and the Orderly Medical Officer, for
them to visit us at other times.

BARBERS This is to be found by going up the stairs
on the left of the stage in SHOP the Gymnasium.
Opening hours are from 0900 hrs patients (staff 0800
hrs) until 1200 hrs. Afternoons from 1400 - 1700
hrs.

CHURCH TIMES Roman Catholic's may attend Mass at
1745 hrs in the room opposite the Hospital Club
Entrance. Mass is also held at St Brigid's Church at
0930 hrs.

   C of E Service is held in the Hospital Chapel at
0930.

   A Sabbath morning Service is held for the Jewish
Faith in the Singers' Hill Synagogue every Saturday

at 0900. Facilities are provided for those wishing to attend.

<u>TAILOR AND SHOE REPAIRS</u> Consult your Sister and she will do her best to help you in this matter…

WELFARE AND FAMILY PROBLEMS

Throughout our stay in Hospital you can consult the Military Social Worker's who have an office on Richard Ward. They are two ATS Officers who will help you at any time and they have done magnificent work for us all. To give you an idea, here are some of the things they can do for us:

1 If we have friends or relatives coming to visit us and they want to stay overnight nearby, arrange an interview with one of the Welfare Officers and she will furnish you with an address at which your people can stay at

2 If you are urgently in need of money for compassionate reasons, a certain amount can be granted from the Benevolent Fund.

3 If you have any problems affecting your family that you wish to settle, go and see the Welfare Officer as soon as you can.

WARD MEETINGS

Your Ward holds a weekly meeting which is attended by all members of the Ward, the Psychiatrist and your Ward Sister. All matters affecting the Ward are discussed - if you feel you have a grouse or a complaint mention this to your Ward Representative who will bring it up at the next Ward meeting. Ward Committee members are elected, one of whom acts as chairman of the meeting. All Ward Representatives attend the meeting of the Ward Committees (see below).

COMMITTEE MEETINGS

(I) <u>Meeting of Ward Committees</u> - held on Fridays at 0915 hrs in the Hospital Club.

The representatives of your Ward meet all the representatives of other Wards to discuss suggestions and interchange ideas brought forward at the meetings above. Minutes of these

meetings are available for your own ward
meetings so that information can be passed
directly back to the ward members.

(2) <u>Entertainments Sub Committee</u> - held on Tuesdays
at 0915 hrs in the Hospital Club.

One of your Ward representatives attend this
meeting where all matters affecting Hospital
entertainment are discussed.

Things TO REMEMBER...

<u>NO SMOKING</u> is allowed in the Gym, Dining Hall, or
Corridors of this Hospital.

<u>THE NOTICE BOARD</u> in your Ward should be consulted
twice daily - morning and afternoon.

<u>HOSPITAL NOTICES</u> on the Notice Board by the door
leading to the NAAFI should be read daily because
items of some importance to YOU appear from time to
time.

<u>ROLL CALL</u> is held in every ward at 2130 hrs - should
you miss this report to the guard room as soon as
possible.

<u>HOSPITAL BLUES</u> will be worn at all times except
under special circumstances.

<u>BOOTS OR SHOES</u> will be worn at all times except on
P.T. parades when plimsolls will be worn.

<u>STRAIGHT TALK</u> Drinking and staying out late is 'bad
medicine'. Lay off and you'll get well all the
quicker. Do your share by giving co-operative
behaviour and you will be helping your treatment and
the Hospital which is helping you. We must warn you
that if you are put on a charge, and it is
substantiated, you will forfeit your pass, until
your Psychiatrist recommends the C.O. to return it.

AUTHOR'S NOTE

With thanks to the Wellcome Contemporary Medical Archives for the
possibility of reproducing the above (Anon, (undated), *Introducing You to
Northfield*, by a Patient. PP/SHF/1.11.1, Foulkes Archives, Wellcome
Contemporary Medical Archives). The format is similar to the original which
was typed. The punctuation, and spelling, are as in the original.

References

Abrahams, S. (1944) *Letter to J. Rickman*. Rickman Papers, Archives of the British Psycho-Analytic Society, CRR/F19/01.

Adair, J. (1984) *The Skills of Leadership*. Aldershot: Wildwood House.

Adam, R. (1949) *Foreword* in H. Harris (1949) pp. vii–viii.

Adrian, E.D. and Yealland, L.R. (1917) 'The treatment of some common war neuroses.' *Lancet 1*, 867–872.

Ahrenfeldt, R.H. (1958) *Psychiatry in the British Army in the Second World War*. London: Routledge and Kegan Paul.

Ahrenfeldt, R.H. (1968) 'The Army Psychiatric Service' in A.S. MacNalty and W.F. Mellor (eds) *Medical Services in War, History of the Second World War*. London: HMSO.

Aichhorn, A. (1936) *Wayward Youth*. London: Putnam.

Anderson, C. (1942) 'Chronic head cases.' *Lancet 2*, 1–4.

Anderson, C., Jeffrey, M. and Pai, M.N. (1944) 'Psychiatric casualties from the Normandy beach-head: first thoughts on 100 cases.' *Lancet 2*, 218–221.

Anderson, M.B. (1944) *Matron's Quarterly Report Nursing Staff, 18/12/44*. Public Record Office, WO 222/846.

Anon (undated) *Introducing You to Northfield, by a Patient*. S.H. Foulkes Papers, Wellcome Institute for the History of Medicine: CMAC: PP/SHF/1.11.1.

Anthony, E.J. (1983) 'The group-analytic circle and its ambient network.' In M. Pines (ed) (1983). Ch. 3, 29–53.

Appel, J.W. and Beebe, G.W. (1946) 'Preventative psychiatry: an epidemiological approach.' *Journal of the American Medical Association 131*, 1469–1475.

Armson, M.W. (1943) Letter to John Rickman, 28/2/43, Rickman Papers, Archives of the British Psycho-Analytic Society, MRB/F01/01.

Babington, A. (1986) *For the Sake of Example: Capital Courts Martial: 1914–1920*. London: Paladin.

Backus, P.L. and Mansell, G.S. (1944) 'Investigation and treatment of enuresis in the army: preliminary report on 277 cases.' *British Medical Journal 2*, 462–465.

Baker, D. and Tegner, W.S. (1945) 'Effort syndrome at an army physical development centre.' *Journal of the Royal Army Medical Corps 84*, 232–234.

Bartemeier, L.H., Kubie, L.S., Menninger, K.A., Romano, J. and Whitehorn, J.C. (1946) 'Combat exhaustion.' *Journal of Nervous and Mental Diseases 104*, 358–389, 489–525.

Baruch, L. (1998) *Correspondence and interview*. Unpublished.

Bavin, M.G. (1947) 'A contribution towards the understanding of the repatriated prisoner of war.' *British Journal of Psychiatric Social Work*, 29–35.

Baynes, J.C.M. (1972) *The Soldier in Modern Society*. London: Eyre Methuen.

Baynes, J.C.M. (1987) *Morale: A Study of Men and Courage*. London: Leo Cooper.

Beccle, H.C. (1942) 'War psychoses: their nature and treatment.' *Medical Press And Circular* 208, 136–139.

Bellamy, W.A. (1945) 'Battle exhaustion.' *Medical Press And Circular 214*, 155–156.

Bennet, E.A. (1941) 'Anxiety states in war.' *Medical Press And Circular 205*, 128–130.

Berrios, G.E. and Freeman, H. (eds) (1991) *150 Years of British Psychiatry: 1841–1991.* London: Gaskell.

Bidwell, S. (1979) *The Chindit War: The Campaign in Burma 1944.* London: Hodder and Stoughton.

Bierer, J. (1942) 'Group psychotherapy.' *British Medical Journal 1*, 214–216.

Bierer, J. (1944) Quarterly Report for the Recreational Therapy Department for the Quarter ending 18 December 1944. Northfield Military Hospital, Public Record Office, WO 222/846.

Bierer, J. (1948) 'Modern social and group therapy.' In N.G. Harris (ed) *Modern Trends in Psychological Medicine.* London: Butterworth.

Bierer, J. and Haldane, F.P. (1941) 'A self-governed patients' social club in a public mental hospital.' *Journal of Mental Science 87*, 419–426.

Bion, F. (1982) Introduction to W.R. Bion (1986).

Bion, W.R. (1940) The 'War of Nerves': Civilian Reaction, Morale and Prophylaxis, Chapter 10, 180–200, in E. Miller.

Bion, W.R. (1946) 'The leaderless group project.' *Bulletin of the Menninger Clinic 10*, 77–81.

Bion, W.R. (1948) Paper on Advances in Group and Individual Therapy, in J.C. Flugel (ed).

Bion, W.R. (1961) *Experiences in Groups and Other Papers.* London: Tavistock.

Bion, W.R. (1986) *The Long Week-end 1897–1919: Part of a Life.* London: Free Association Books.

Bion, W.R. and Rickman, J. (1943) 'Intra-group tensions in therapy.' *Lancet 2*, 678–681.

Birmingham Asylums Committee, (1915) Letter from Board of Control, and minutes of a special meeting of the Asylums and Committee for the Care of the Mentally Defective. 5 February, City of Birmingham Central Library Archives.

Birmingham Asylums Committee, (1920) Report of the Asylums Committee for the Care of the Mentally Defective. City of Birmingham, City of Birmingham Central Library Archives.

Birmingham City Council, (1942) Report of the Proceedings of the Birmingham City Council. Mental Hospitals Committee's Report, 11 December 1942.

Blair, D. (1943) 'Group psychotherapy for war neuroses.' *Lancet 1*, 204–205.

Bléandonu, G. (1994) *Wilfred Bion: His Life and Works 1897–1979.* London: Free Association Books.

Bleckwenn, W.J. (1930a) 'Production of sleep and rest in psychotic cases.' *Archives of Neurology and Psychiatry 24*, 365–372.

Bleckwenn, W.J. (1930b) 'Narcosis as therapy in neuropsychiatric conditions.' *Journal of the American Medical Association 95*, 1168–1171.

Bleuler, E. (1902) 'Dementia praecox.' *The Journal of Mental Pathology 111*, 113–120.

Bloch, S. and Crouch, E. (1985) *Therapeutic Factors in Group Psychotherapy.* Oxford: Oxford Medical Publications.

Braceland, F.J. (1947) 'Psychiatric lessons from World War II.' *American Journal of Psychiatry 103*, 587–593.

Bradbury, L. (1990a) Interview with the author and D. Clarke.

Bradbury, L. (1990b) Letter to the author 22/6/90.

Bradbury, L. (1990c) Letter to the author 30/6/90.

Bridgeland, M. (1971) *Pioneer Work with Maladjusted Children*. London: Staples Press.

Bridger, H. (1946) 'The Northfield Experiment.' *Bulletin of the Menninger Clinic 10*, 3, 71–76.

Bridger, H. (1985) 'Northfield revisited.' In M. Pines (ed) *Bion and Psychotherapy*. London: Routledge and Kegan Paul.

Bridger, H. (1990a) 'The discovery of the therapeutic community: the northfield experiments.' In E.L. Trist and H.A. Murray (eds) *The Social Engagement of Social Science 1: The Socio-Psychological Perspective*. London: Free Association Books.

Bridger, H. (1990b) Interview with the author (unpublished).

British Medical Journal (1939) 'Neuroses in war time: memorandum for the medical profession.' *2*, 1199–1201.

British Medical Journal (1942) 'Editorial: applied psychology in the army.' *2*, 74–75.

British Medical Journal (1945) 'Editorial: Progress in the Psychiatry of War.' *1*, 913–914.

British Medical Journal (1947) 'Psychology and psychiatry in the services.' *1*, 892–893.

Brooke, E. (1946) 'Battle exhaustion: Review of 500 cases from Western Europe.' *British Medical Journal 2*, 491–493.

Brown, J.F. (1936) *Psychology and the Social Order*. London: McGraw Hill.

Burroughs, P. (1985) 'Crime and punishment in the British army: 1815–70.' *English Historical Review 100*, 545–71.

Burrow, T. (1927a) 'The social basis of consciousness: A study in organic psychology.' *International Library of Psychology, Philosophy and Scientific Method*. London: Kegan Paul, Trench and Trubner.

Burrow, T. (1927b) 'The problem of the transference.' *British Journal of Medical Psychology 7*, 193–202.

Burrow, T. (1927c) 'The group method of analysis.' *Psychoanalytic Review 14*, 268–280.

Burrow, T. (1928a) 'The basis of group-analysis or the analysis of the reactions of normal and neurotic individuals.' *British Journal of Medical Psychology 8*, 198–206.

Burrow, T. (1928b) 'Biological foundations and mental methods.' *British Journal of Medical Psychology 8*, 49–63.

Calder, A. (1994) *The People's War: Britain 1939–1945*. London: Pimlico.

Cameron, K. (1940) 'Occupation therapy for war neuroses.' *Lancet 2*, 659–660.

Cantlie, N. (1948) 'Forward psychiatry: Address given to a conference in 1944 on the same subject.' *Journal of the Royal Army Medical Corps 91*, 3, 93–95.

Carroll, D. (1944a, b, c) Commanding Officer's Quarterly Reports on Northfield Military Hospital, a) 25/6/44, b) 25/9/44, c) 18/12/44. Public Records Office, WO 222/846 XC23303.

Cartoon of John Rickman (1942) 'The Freudian: Rickman Rorsached' artist unknown (signed XX, dated 28/9/42). Papers of John Dalziel Wyndham Pearse, Wellcome Institute for the History of Medicine: CMAC: GC/192/18.

Casson, F.R.C. (1945) *Letter to J. Rickman,* 2/7/45. Rickman Papers, Archives of the British Psycho-Analytic Society. CRR/F20/22.

Cerletti, U. and Bini, L. (1938) 'Un nuovo metodi di shock terapia bollettino della.' *Acadamia di Medica di Roma 64,* 136–138.

Clayton, J. (1991) Ex-Pathology Laboratory Technician. Interview with author (unpublished).

Cochrane, A.L. (1946) 'Notes on the psychology of prisoners of war.' *British Medical Journal 1,* 282–284.

Collie, G.F. (1943) 'Returned prisoners of war: A suggested scheme for rehabilitation.' *Fortnightly 153,* 407–411.

Cook, G.T. and Sargant, W. (1942) 'Neurosis simulating organic disorder.' *British Medical Journal 1,* 31–32.

Cooper, J.E., Kendell, R.E., Gurland, B.J., Sharpe, L., Copeland, J.R. and Simon, R. (1972) 'Psychiatric diagnosis in New York and London.' *Maudsley Monograph 20.* London: Oxford University Press.

Cope, V.Z. (ed) (1952) 'Psychological medicine.' In *History of the Second World War; Medicine and Pathology.* London: HMSO.

Corbin, R.C.H. (1990) Letter to author (unpublished).

Corsini, R.J. (1957) *Methods of Group Psychotherapy.* New York: McGraw Hill.

Cottrell, A. (undated, c. 1945) RAMC. London: Hutchinson.

Craigie, H.B. (1942) Letter: 'Physical treatment of acute war neurosis.' *British Medical Journal 1,* 675.

Craigie, H.B. (1944) 'Two years of military psychiatry in the Middle East.' *British Medical Journal 2,* 105–109.

Crew, F.A.E. (1953) *The Army Medical Services, Administration 1.* London: HMSO.

Crew, F.A.E. (1955) 'The army psychiatric service.' In *The Army Medical Services, Administration 2,* 467–497. London: HMSO.

Culpin, M. (1940a) 'A week-end with the war neuroses.' *Lancet 2,* 257–9.

Culpin, M. (1940b) 'Mode of onset of the neurosis of war.' In E. Millar (ed) *The Neuroses of War.* London: Macmillan.

Cunningham Dax, E. (1945) Letter to L. Bradbury (unpublished).

Cunningham Dax, E. (1998) Letter to the author (unpublished).

Curle, A. (1947) 'Transitional communities and social reconnection: a follow-up study of the civil resettlement of british prisoners of war. Part I.' *Human Relations, 1,* 42–68.

Curle, A. and Trist, E. (1947) 'Transitional communities and social reconnection: a follow-up study of the civil resettlement of british prisoners of war. Part II.' *Human Relations 1,* 240–288.

Curran, D. (1941) Letter to John Rickman, 13/6/41, . Rickman Papers, Archive of the British Psycho-Analytic Society CRR/F16/17.

Curran, D. and Guttman, E. (1946) *Psychological Medicine.* Edinburgh: Livingstone.

Daily Mirror (1915) Advertisement for Phospherine, 8/12/15 p.15.

Da Costa, J.M. (1871) 'On irritable heart'. *American Journal of Medical Science 61,* 17–52.

Danson, J.G. (1942) 'The effort syndrome.' *Medical Press and Circular 208,* 185–188.

Darwin, C.R. (1871) *The Descent of Man.* London: John Murray.

Davidson, S. (1946) Notes on a Group of Ex-Prisoners of War, *Bulletin of the Menninger Clinic 10*, 90–100.

de Maré, P.B. (1972) *Perspectives in Group Psychotherapy: A Theoretical Background.* London: George Allen and Unwin.

de Maré, P.B. (1983) 'Michael Foulkes and the Northfield Experiment.' In M. Pines (ed) *The Evolution of Group Analysis.* London: Routledge and Kegan Paul.

de Maré, P.B. (1985) 'Major Bion.' In M. Pines (ed) *Bion and Group Psychotherapy.* London: Routledge and Kegan Paul.

de Maré, P.B. (1993) Interview with the author (unpublished)

de Maré, P.B. (1994) Interview with A.Wilson (unpublished).

de Saint-Exupéry, A. (1995) *Flight to Arras.* Harmondsworth: Penguin.

Debenham, G., Sargant, W., Hill, D. and Slater, E. (1941) 'Treatment of war neurosis.' *Lancet 1*, 107–109.

Dewar, M. (1946) 'The technique of group therapy.' *Bulletin of the Menninger Clinic 10*, 82–84.

Dewar, M. (1993) Interview with author (unpublished).

Dewar, M. (1994) Interview with A. Wilson (unpublished).

Dicks, H.V. (1970) *Fifty Years of the Tavistock Clinic.* London: Routledge and Kegan Paul.

Directorate of Army Psychiatry (1944) *The Prisoner of War Comes Home.* Technical Memorandum No. 13. In War Office (1946).

Discussion Groups 1–21 (1945) Discussions on Group Therapy, 12 April 1945 – 20 December 1945, Northfield Military Hospital. S.H. Foulkes Papers, Welcome Institute for the History of Medicine: CMAC: PP/SHF/C.3/8.

Dixon, N.E. (1979) *On the Psychology of Military Incompetence.* London: Futura.

Douglas–Wilson, I. (1943) 'Minor psychological disturbances in the services.' *Journal of the Royal Army Medical Corps 81*, 283–288.

Douglas–Wilson, I. (1944) 'Somatic manifestations of psychoneurosis.' *British Medical Journal 1*, 413–415.

Duke-Elder, P.M. and Wittkower, E. (1946) 'Psychological reactions in soldiers to the loss of vision of one eye, and their treatment.' *British Medical Journal 1*, 155–158.

Edkins, J.R.P. (1948) 'Further developments in abreaction.' In N.G. Harris (ed) *Modern Trends in Psychological Medicine.* London: Butterworth.

Elias, N. (1969) 'Sociology and psychiatry.' In S.H. Foulkes and G. Stewart Prince (eds) *Psychiatry in a Changing Society.* London: Tavistock.

Elliot-Smith, G. and Pear, T.H. (1918) *Shell Shock and its Lessons.* Manchester: Manchester University Press.

Ellis, J. (1990) *The Sharp End: The Fighting Man in World War II.* London: Pimlico.

Euripides (1976) *The Bacchae.* Harmondsworth: Penguin Classics.

Fairbairn, W.R.D. (1940) 'Schizoid factors in the personality.' In W.R.D. Fairbairn *Psychoanalytic Studies of the Personality.* London: Tavistock.

Fairbairn, W.R.D. (1941) 'A revised psychopathology of the psychoses and psychoneuroses.' *International Journal of Psycho-Analysis 22*, parts 3 and 4.

Fairbairn, W.R.D. (1943) 'The repression and return of bad objects.' *British Journal of Medical Psychology 19*, parts 3 and 4.

Fairbairn, W.R.D. (1946) 'Object-relations and dynamic structure.' *International Journal of Psycho-Analysis 27*, parts 1 and 2.

Fairbairn, W.R.D. (1952) *Psychoanalytic Studies of the Personality.* London: Tavistock.

Fenton, T.W. (1990) Personal communications.

Fidler, R.F. (1946) 'A psychiatrist's observations in the BLA.' *Journal of the Royal Army Medical Corps 85*, 186–191.

Flugel, J.C. (ed) (1948) 'Proceedings of the International Conference on Medical Psychotherapy.' *International Congress on Mental Health 3*, London, 11–14 August 1948. London: H.K. Lewis.

Foulkes, E. (ed) (1990) *S.H. Foulkes: Selected Papers: Psychoanalysis and Group Analysis.* London: Karnac Books.

Foulkes, S.H. (as S.H. Fuchs) (1936) 'Sum Stand der heutigen Biologie. Dargestellt an Kurt Goldstein: Der Aufbau des Organismus.' *Imago 22*, 210–241.

Foulkes, S.H. (1937) 'On introjection.' *International Journal of Psycho-Analysis 18*, 269–293.

Foulkes, S.H. (as S.H. Fuchs) (1938) Review of N. Elias, *Über den Prozess der Zivilisation. 1: Wandlungen des Verhaltens in den Weltichen des Abendlandes,* In *International Journal of Psychoanalysis 19*, 263–265.

Foulkes, S.H. (1942) Review of N. Elias, *Über den Prozess der Zivilisation. 1, Wandlungen des Verhaltens in den Weltichen des Abendlandes.* In *International Journal of Psychoanalysis 23*, 94–95.

Foulkes, S.H. (1943a) *Notice of transfer to Northfield Military Hospital,* S.H. Foulkes Archives, Wellcome Institute for the History of Medicine: CMAC: PP/SH/1/11.1.

Foulkes, S.H. (1943b) *Notes on patients and groups at Northfield,* S.H. Foulkes Papers, Wellcome Institute for the History of Medicine: CMAC: PP/SH/C.3/2.

Foulkes, S.H. (1944a) Syllabus for lectures March/April 1944, S.H. Foulkes Papers, Wellcome Institute for the History of Medicine: CMAC: PP/SH/1/C.3/11.

Foulkes, S.H. (1944b) *Sociometry: Seminar Notes.* S.H. Foulkes Papers, Wellcome Institute for the History of Medicine: CMAC: PP/SH/C.3/11.

Foulkes, S.H. (1944c) *Notes on Group Therapy,* S.H. Foulkes Papers, Wellcome Institute for the History of Medicine: CMAC: PP/SHF/C.3/2.

Foulkes, S.H. (1945a) *A Memorandum on Group Therapy,* A.M.D.11, B.M., 33/02/2, PP/SHF/1.11.1, S.H. Foulkes Papers, Wellcome Institute for the History of Medicine: CMAC: PP/SHF/C.3/11.

Foulkes, S.H. (1945b) *Notes on Group Therapy,* S.H. Foulkes Papers, Wellcome Institute for the History of Medicine: CMAC: PP/SHF/C.3/2.

Foulkes, S.H. (1945c) *Address to the American Visitors,* 6/6/45 S.H. Foulkes Papers, Wellcome Institute for the History of Medicine: CMAC: PP/SHF/C.3/9.

Foulkes, S.H. (1945d) *Major Foulkes' Communiqués,* 1–4, S.H. Foulkes Papers, Wellcome Institute for the History of Medicine: CMAC: PP/SHF/C.3/11.

Foulkes, S.H. (1946a) 'On group analysis.' *International Journal of Psychoanalysis 27*, 46–51.

Foulkes, S.H. (1946b) 'Group analysis in a military neurosis centre.' *Lancet 1*, 303–306.

Foulkes, S.H. (1946c) 'Principles and Practice of Group Therapy.' *Bulletin of the Menninger Clinic 10*, 3, 85–89.

Foulkes, S.H. (1948) *Introduction to Group-Analytic Psychotherapy: Studies in the Social Integration of Individuals and Groups*. London: Heinemann.

Foulkes, S.H. (1955) *The Position of Group Analysis Today, with Special Reference to the Role of Group-Analytic Society*. Address to the Group-Analytic Society, 31/1/55. Reprinted in Foulkes (1990), 145–150.

Foulkes, S.H. (1964) *Therapeutic Group Analysis*. London: George Allen and Unwin.

Foulkes, S.H. and Lewis, E. (1944) 'Group analysis: A study in the treatment of groups on psycho-analytic lines.' *Journal of Medical Psychology 20*, 1.

Foulkes, S.H. and Stewart Prince, G. (eds) (1969) *Psychiatry in a Changing Society*. London: Tavistock.

Fox, J. (ed) (1987) *The Essential Moreno: Writings on Group Method, and Spontaneity by J.L. Moreno, M.D.* New York: Springer Publishing Company.

Franklin, M.E. (ed) (1943a) *Q Camp: An Experiment in Group Living with Maladjusted and Anti-Social Young Men*. London: Planned Environment Therapy Trust.

Franklin, M.E. (1943b) 'Introductory, including notes on the origin and inception of the work.' In M.E. Franklin (ed) *Q Camp: An Experiment in Group Living with Maladjusted and Anti-Social Young Men*. London: Planned Environment Therapy Trust.

Franklin, M.E. (1943c) 'Summary of methods used.' In M.E. Franklin (ed) *Q Camp: An Experiment in Group Living with Maladjusted and Anti-Social Young Men*. London: Planned Environment Therapy Trust.

Franklin, M.E. (1966) Preface to reprint of M.E. Franklin (ed) *Q Camp: An Experiment in Group Living with Maladjusted and Anti-Social Young Men*. London: Planned Environment Therapy Trust.

Fraser, D. (1983) *And We Shall Shock Them: The British Army in the Second World War*. London: Hodder and Stoughton.

Freeman, H. and Berrios, G.E. (eds) (1996) *150 Years of British Psychiatry, Vol 2: The Aftermath*. London: Athlone.

Freeman, T. (1989) Letter to the author (unpublished).

French, J.R.P. (1941) 'The disruption and cohesion of groups.' *Journal of Abnormal Social Psychology 36*, 362–377.

Freud, S. (1911) 'Formulations Regarding the Two Principles of Mental Functioning.' In S. Freud *On Metapsychology*. London: Penguin.

Freud, S. (1922) *Introductory Lectures on Psycho-Analysis*. London: George Allen and Unwin.

Freud, S. (1923) 'The Ego and the Id.' In S. Freud *The Ego and the Id and Other Works, Vol 19: The Standard Edition of the Complete Psychological Works of Sigmund Freud*. London: Hogarth.

Freud, S. (1930) 'Civilisation and its Discontents.' In S. Freud *On Metapsychology*. London: Penguin.

Freud, S. (1939) Civilization, War and Death: Selections from three works by Freud, (ed. J. Rickman) publisher unknown; noted in G. Gorer and J. Rickman (1949) under publication.

Freud, S. (1940a) *Totem and Taboo*. London: Harmondsworth.

Freud, S. (1940b) *Group Psychology and Analysis of the Ego*. London: Hogarth Press.

Freud, S. (1961) *The Ego and the Id and Other Works, Vol 19: The Standard Edition of the Complete Psychological Works of Sigmund Freud*. London: Hogarth.

Freud, S. (1991) Civilisation, Society and Religion, Vol 12: The Penguin Freud Library. London: Penguin.

Freud, S. (1991) On Metapsychology, Vol 11: The Penguin Freud Library. London: Penguin.

Friedlander, K. (1947) *The Psycho-Analytical Approach to Juvenile Delinquency. Theory: Case-Studies: Treatment.* London: Routledge and Kegan Paul.

Garrett, R. (1981) *POW: The Uncivil Face of War.* Newton Abbott: David and Charles.

Gaskin, I. and Gaskin, S. (1990) Interview with author (unpublished).

Gill, G.V. and Bell, D.R. (1981) 'The health of former prisoners of war of the Japanese.' *The Practitioner 225,* 531–538.

Gilman, S.W. (1947) 'Methods of officer selection in the army.' *Journal of Mental Science 93,* 101–111.

Glover, E. (1944) *The Diagnosis and Treatment of Delinquency: Being a Clinical Report on the work of the Institute during the Five Years 1937 to 1941.* London: Institute of Scientific Treatment of Delinquency.

Goldstein, K. (1939) *The Organism: A Holistic Approach to Biology.* New York: American Book Company.

Goldstein, K. (1940) *Human Nature in the Light of Psychopathology.* Harvard: Harvard University Press.

Good, R. (1941) 'Convulsion therapy in war psychoneurotics.' *Journal of Mental Science 87,* 409–418.

Good, R. (1942) 'Malingering.' *British Medical Journal 2,* 359–362.

Greenberg, I.A. (1974) *Psychodrama: Theory and Therapy.* New York: Behavioural Publications.

Gregg, A. (1947) 'Lessons to learn: Psychiatry in World War II.' *American Journal of Psychiatry 104,* 217–220.

Griesinger, (1867) *Mental Pathology and Therapeutics (1861).* London: The New Sydenham Society.

Grosskurth, P. (1986) *Melanie Klein – Her World and her Work.* London: Hodder and Stoughton.

Guttman, E. and Thomas, E.L. (1946) A Report on the Re-Adjustment in Civil Life of Soldiers discharged from the Army on account of Neurosis. Report on the Public Health, Medical Subjects (Ministry of Health), *93.* London: HMSO.

HMSO (1923) 'The History of the Great War: Medical Services – Diseases of the War,' *2, Neurasthenia and War Neuroses.* London: HMSO.

Haas, H.E. (1989) Interview with author (unpublished).

Hadfield, J.A. (1940) 'Treatment by suggestion and hypnoanalysis.' In E. Miller (1940).

Hadfield, J.A. (1942) 'War neurosis: A year in a neuropathic hospital.' *British Medical Journal 1,* 281–285 and 320–323.

Haldane, F.P. and Rowley, J.L. (1946) 'Psychiatry at the Corps Exhaustion Centre.' *Lancet 2,* 599–601.

Harding, G.D. (1947) Daily Orders Part One, 15 April 1947. (Copy in possession of author).

Hargreaves, G.R. (1944) *Letter to S.H. Foulkes 27/10/44.* S.H. Foulkes Papers, Wellcome Institute for the History of Medicine: CMAC: PP/SHF/C.316.

Hargreaves, G.R. (1945) *Letter to S.H. Foulkes* 30/8/45. S.H. Foulkes Papers, Wellcome Institute for the History of Medicine: CMAC: PP/SHF/C.316.

Harris, H. (1949) *The Group Approach to Leadership Testing.* London: Routledge and Kegan Paul.

Harris, N.G. (ed) (1948) *Modern Trends in Psychological Medicine.* London: Butterworth.

Harrison, T.M. (1995) Interviews with ex-prisoners of war from the Far East.

Harrison, T.M. (1997) 'Battlefields, social fields and Northfield.' *Therapeutic Communities 17, 3.*

Harrison, T.M. and Clarke, D. (1992) 'The Northfield Experiments.' *British Journal of Psychiatry 160,* 698–708.

Harrisson, T. (1976) *Living Through the Blitz.* London: Collins.

Healy, D. (1993) *Images of Trauma: From Hysteria to Post-Traumatic Stress Disorder.* London: Faber and Faber.

Hearnshaw, L.S. (1964) *A Short History of British Psychology: 1840–1940.* London: Methuen.

Henderson, D. and Gillespie, R.D. (1950) *A Text-Book of Psychiatry for Students and Practitioners,* 7th edition. London: Oxford University Press.

Henry, W. (1970) *Surgeon Henry's Trifles: Events of a Military Life.* Edited by P. Hayward. London: Chatto and Windus.

Heppenstall, R. (1953) *The Lesser Infortune.* London: Jonathan Cape.

Hewitt, L. (1989) Interview with the author (unpublished).

Hill, I.G.W. and Dewar, H.A. (1945) 'Effort syndrome.' *Lancet 2,* 161–164.

Hinshelwood, R.D. (1999) 'How Foulkesian was Bion?' Annual Foulkes Lecture read to the Group Analytic Society, May 1999, also to be published in *Group Analysis* (in press).

Hogben, L. and Johnstone, M.M. (1947) 'Relation of morbidity to age in the army population.' *British Journal of Social Medicine 1,* 149–181.

Hollymoor Hospital (1956) *Booklet.* Birmingham: Publisher unknown.

Hollymoor Hospital Records (1920–1939) *Admission and Discharge Register.* City of Birmingham Central Library Archives.

Hollymoor Hospital Records (1939–1942) *Admission and Discharge Register.* City of Birmingham Central Library Archives.

Holmes, R. (1987) *Firing Line.* Harmondsworth: Penguin.

Homer, (1964) *The Iliad.* Harmondsworth: Penguin.

Horsley, J.S. (1936) 'Narco-analysis.' *Journal of Mental Science 82,* 416–420.

Hubert, W.H. de B. (1941) 'Acute nervous illness in active warfare.' *Lancet 1,* 306–308.

Hughes, J.M. (1989) *Reshaping the Psycho-Analytic Domain.* Berkeley: University of California Press.

Hunter, H.D. (1946) 'The work of a corps psychiatrist in the Italian campaign.' *Journal of the Royal Army Medical Corps 86,* 127–130.

Industrial, M.O. (1943) 'The Neurotic Ex-Soldier.' *Lancet 1,* p.477.

Interview: Mr A. (1990) Interview with ex-patient (unpublished).

Interview: Mr B. (1990) Interview with ex-patient (unpublished).

Interview: Mrs B. (1990) Interview with hospital visitor (unpublished).

Interview: Mr C. (1990) Interview with ex-patient (unpublished).
Interview: Mrs C. (1994) Interview with hospital visitor (unpublished).
Interview: Mr D. (1990) Interview with ex-patient (unpublished).
Interview: Mrs D. (1994) Interview with hospital visitor (unpublished).
Interview: Mr E. (1990) Interview with ex-patient (unpublished).
Interview: Mrs E. (1998) Interview with ex-patient (unpublished).
Interview: Mr F. (1992) Interview with ex-patient (unpublished).
Interview: Mr G. (1995) Interview with ex-staff (unpublished).
Interview: Mr H. (1994) Interview with ex-patient (unpublished).
Interview: Mr I. (1996) Interview with ex-patient (unpublished).
Interview: Mr J. (1995) Interview with ex-Far Eastern Prisoner of War (unpublished).
Interview: Mr K. (1994) Interview with ex-patient (unpublished).
Interviews: Mr L. (1998) Interview with ex-patient (unpublished).
Interview: Mr M. (1994) Interview with ex-patient (unpublished).
Interview: Mr N. (1994) Interview with ex-patient (unpublished).
Interview: Mr O. (1995) Interview with ex-patient (unpublished).
Interview: Mrs O. (1995) Interview with ex-member of staff (unpublished).
Interview: Mr P. (1993) Interview with ex-member of staff (unpublished).
Interview: Mr Q. (1990) Interview with ex-member of staff (unpublished).
Interview: Mrs R. (1998) Interview with hospital visitor (unpublished).
Isaacs, S. (1943) 'The Nature and Function of Phantasy.' In P. King and R. Steiner (eds) *The Freud-Klein Controversies 1941–1945*. London: Tavistock/Routledge.
James, G.W.B. (1944) 'Operational Strain: Experiences with the Middle East Force.' In H.L. Tidy (ed) (1947) *Inter-Allied Conferences on War Medicine 1942–1945*. London: Staples Press.
James, G.W.B. (1952) 'Psychiatry in the Middle East Force, 1940–1943.' In V.Z. Cope *Psychological Medicine*. London: HMSO.
Jeffrey, M. and Bradford, E.J.G. (1946) 'Neurosis in escaped prisoners of war.' *British Journal of Medical Psychology 20*, 422–435.
Jones, E. (1936) The Future of Psycho-analysis, *International Journal of Psychoanalysis 17*, 269–277.
Jones, E. (1951) *Free Associations*. London: Hogarth Press.
Jones, M. (1942) 'Group psychotherapy.' *British Medical Journal*, 276–278.
Jones, M. (1944) 'Group treatment, with particular reference to group projection methods.' *American Journal of Psychiatry 101*, 292–299.
Jones, M. (1946) 'Rehabilitation of forces neurosis patients to civilian life.' *British Medical Journal 1*, 533–535.
Jones, M. (1947) 'Emotional catharsis and re-education in the neuroses with the help of group methods.' *British Journal of Medical Psychology 21*, 104–110.
Jones, M. and Lewis, A. (1941) 'Effort syndrome.' *Lancet 1*, 813–818.
Jones, W.L. (1942) 'Psychogenic illness in regimental practice.' *British Medical Journal 2*, 338–340.
Journal of the Royal Army Medical Corps (1942a) 'Editorial: The military implications of psychiatry.' *78*, 138–140.

Journal of the Royal Army Medical Corps (1945) 'Editorial: Psychiatry.' *84*, 81–82.

Journal of the Royal Army Medical Corps (1951) 'At random: psychiatric wastages.' *90*, 389–391.

Keegan, J. (1978) *The Face of Battle.* Harmondsworth: Penguin.

Keen, W.W., Weir Mitchell, S. and Morehouse, G.R. (1864) 'On malingering, especially in regard to simulation of diseases of the nervous system.' *American Journal of Medical Sciences 48*, 367–94.

Kennedy, A. (1941) 'Hysteria in War Conditions.' *Medical Press and Circular 205*, 135–140.

Kenton, C. (1946) 'Contribution to discussion on forward psychiatry in the army.' *Proceedings of the Royal Society of Medicine 39*, 137–140.

Kersley, G.D. (1942) 'Occupational therapy.' *Journal of the Royal Army Medical Corps 78*, 236–239.

King, P. (1989) 'The history of psychoanalysis during the Second World War.' *The International Review of Psychoanalysis 16*, 1, 15–33.

King, P. (1994) Interview with the author (unpublished).

King, P. and Steiner, R. (1991) *The Freud-Klein Controversies 1941–1945.* London: Tavistock/Routledge.

Kirman, B.H. (1946) 'Mental disorder in released prisoners of war.' *Journal of Mental Science 92*, 808–813.

Kläsi, S. (1922) 'Über die therapeutische Anwendung des Danerschlafes mittels Somnifens bei Schizophrenen.' *Zeitschrift für der Gesichte Neurologie und Psychiatrie 74*, p.557.

Klein, M. (1927) 'Criminal tendencies in normal children.' In M. Klein *Contributions to Psycho-Analysis: 1921–1945.* London: International Psycho-Analytical Library, Hogarth Press.

Klein, M. (1932) *The Psycho-Analysis of Children.* London: Hogarth Press. (6th edition, 1959).

Klein, M. (1933) 'The early development of conscience in the child.' In M. Klein *Contributions to Psycho-Analysis: 1921–1945.* London: International Psycho-Analytical Library, Hogarth Press.

Klein, M. (1934) 'A contribution to the psychogenesis of manic-depressive states.' In M. Klein *Contributions to Psycho-Analysis: 1921–1845.* London: International Psycho-Analytical Library, Hogarth Press.

Klein, M. (1940) 'Mourning: Its relation to manic-depressive states.' In M. Klein *Contributions to Psycho-Analysis: 1921–1945.* London: International Psycho-Analytical Library, Hogarth Press.

Klein, M. (1965) *Contributions to Psycho-Analysis: 1921–1945.* London: International Psycho-Analytical Library, Hogarth Press.

Lambert, C. and Linford Rees, W. (1944) 'Intravenous barbiturates in the treatment of hysteria.' *British Medical Journal 2*, 70–73.

Lancet (1942) 'Editorial: Choosing the fighter.' *1*, 231–232.

Lancet (1943) 'Editorial: The neurotic ex-soldier.' *1*, 177–178.

Lancet (1948) 'Editorial.' *1*, 524–525.

Langdon-Davies, J. (1938) *Air Raid. The Technique of Silent Approach: High Explosive: Panic.* London: Routledge.

Laudenheimer, R. (1940) 'Predisposition in neuroses of war.' *Medical Press And Circular 204,* 43–45.

Lawrence, C. (1985) 'Moderns and Ancients: The "New Cardiology" in Britain 1880–1930.' *Medical History Supplement No 5,* 1–33.

Lawrence, E.S. (1970) *The Origins and Growth of Modern Education.* Harmondsworth: Penguin Books.

Lazzell, E.W. (1921) 'The Group Treatment of Dementia Praecox.' *Psychoanalytic Review 8,* 168–179.

Le Bon, G. (1952) *The Crowd.* London: Benn.

Leigh, A.D. (1941) 'Neurosis: As viewed by a regimental medical officer.' *Lancet 1,* 394–396.

L'Etang, H.J.C.J. (1951) 'A criticism of military psychiatry in the Second World War.' *Journal of the Royal Army Medical Corps 97,* 236–244 and 316–327.

Lewin, K. (1935a) *A Dynamic Theory of Personality.* New York: McGraw Hill.

Lewin, K. (1935b) *The Conflict between Aristotolean and Galilean Modes of Thought in Contemporary Psychology.* In K. Lewin (1935a)

Lewis, A. (1940) 'Note on the Maudsley in war time,' addendum to E. M. Creak, 'Child Psychiatry at the Maudsley Clinic.' *American Journal of Psychiatry 97,* 399–400.

Lewis, A. (1941) Letter to J.R. Rees. In R.H. Ahrenfeldt (1958) *Psychiatry in the British Army in the Second World War.* London: Routledge and Kegan Paul.

Lewis, A. (1943) 'Social effects of neurosis.' *Lancet 1,* 167–170.

Lewis, A. and Slater, E. (1942) 'Neurosis in soldiers: A follow up study.' *Lancet 1,* 496–498.

Lewis, A. and Slater, E. (1952) 'Psychiatry in the emergency medical service, ' In V.Z. Cope *Psychological Medicine.* London: HMSO.

Lewsen, C. (1993), Interview with the author (unpublished).

Liddell Hart, B.H. (1973) *History of the Second World War.* London: Pan.

Lindemann, E. (1932) 'Psychological changes in normal and abnormal individuals under the influence of sodium amytal.' *American Journal of Psychiatry 88,* 1083–1092.

Logan, W.R. (1941) 'Psychical illness among the services in Singapore.' *Journal of Mental Science 87,* 241–255.

Lovegrove, P. (1953) *Not Least in the Crusade: A Short History of the Royal Army Medical Corps.* Aldershot: Gale and Polden.

MacCarthy, A. (1980) *A Doctor's War.* London: Magnum/Methuen.

McDougall, W. (1920) *The Group Mind.* New York: G.P. Putnam.

MacKeith, S.A. (1942) Photograph and description of PULHEMS conference, (unpublished) donated to author by Dr. S.A. MacKeith.

MacKeith, S.A. (1944) *Memorandum to Allied Forces Headquarters* (unpublished) donated to author by Dr S.A. MacKeith.

MacKeith, S.A. (1945) Notes for a Lecture to Northern Command, York, 3/3/45, (unpublished) donated to author by Dr S.A. MacKeith.

MacKeith, S.A. (1946a) 'Lasting Lessons of Overseas Psychiatry.' *Journal of Mental Science 92,* 542–550.

MacKeith, S.A. (1946b) Principles of Psychiatry in an Expeditionary Force (Notes for a lecture April, 12th 1946); (unpublished) donated to author by Dr S.A. MacKeith.

MacKeith, S.A. (1994) Interview with the author (unpublished).

Mackenzie, S.P. (1992) *Politics and Military Morale: Current Affairs and Citizenship Education in the British Army 1914–1950*. Oxford: Clarendon Press.

Mackintosh, J.M. (1940) *War and the Doctor: Essays on the Immediate Treatment of War Wounds*. Edinburgh: Oliver and Boyd.

McLaughlin, F.L. and Millar, W.M. (1941) 'Employment of Air Raid Noises in Psychotherapy.' *British Medical Journal 2*, 158–159.

Macleod, A.W., Wittkower, E.D. and Margolin, S.G. (1954) 'Basic Concepts of Psychosomatic Medicine.' In E.D. Wittkower and R.A. Cleghorn *Recent Developments in Psychosomatic Medicine*. London: Pitman.

Main, T.F. (1945) *Letter to J.Rickman*, 7/9/45, Rickman Papers, Archives of the British Psycho-Analytic Society. CRR/F20/35.

Main, T.F. (1946a) 'The hospital as a therapeutic institution.' *Bulletin of the Menninger Clinic 10*, 77–80.

Main, T.F. (1946b) 'In: Discussion: Forward Psychiatry in the Army.' *Proceedings of the Royal Society of Medicine 39*, 140–142.

Main, T.F. (1948) 'Rehabilitation and the individual.' In N.G. Harris (ed) *Modern Trends in Psychological Medicine*. London: Butterworth.

Main, T.F. (1977) 'The concept of the therapeutic community: Variations and viscissitudes.' *Group Analysis 10*, 2–16.

Main, T.F. (1984) Interview with the author (unpublished).

Main, T.F. (1989) *The Ailment and Other Psychoanalytic Essays*. London: Free Association Books.

Markillie, R. (1993) Interview with the author (unpublished).

Marsh, L.C. (1933) 'An experiment in the group treatment of patients at the Worcester State Hospital.' *Mental Hygiene 17*, 396–416.

Marshall, S.L.A. (1947) *Men Against Fire*. New York: William Morrow.

Meduna, L. (1938) 'General discussion of the cardiazol therapy.' *American Journal of Psychiatry 94*, 40–50.

Meduna, L. and Friedman, E. (1939) 'The convulsive-irritative therapy of the psychoses.' *Journal of the American Medical Association 112*, 501–509.

Menninger, K. (1946) 'Editorial.' *Bulletin of the Menninger Clinic 10*, p.65.

Menninger, K. (1948) *Psychiatry in a Troubled World*. New York: Macmillan.

Menninger, W.C. (1947) 'Psychiatric experience in the war, 1941–1946.' *American Journal of Psychiatry 103*, 577–86.

Merskey, H. (1991) 'Shell-shock.' In G.E. Berrios and H. Freeman *150 Years of British Psychiatry: 1841–1991*. London: Gaskell.

Millard, D.W. (1996) 'Maxwell Jones and the therapeutic community.' In H. Freeman and G.E. Berrios (eds) *150 Years of British Psychiatry: 1841–1991*. London: Gaskell.

Miller, E. (ed) (1940) *The Neuroses of War*. London: Macmillan.

Miller, E. (1945) 'Psychiatric casualties among officers and men from Normandy: Distribution of aetiological factors.' *Lancet 1*, 364–366.

Mills, Sergeant, (1945) Appendix E, Occupational Therapy at Reallocation Centre (All Arms) C.M.F. In J.D.W. Pearce. Report on Military Psychiatric Services in Italy, Public Records Office: WO 222/1312.

Minski, L. (1941) 'Emergency medical service: The organisation of a neurological clinic.' *Medical Press 205*, 131–133.

Minski, L. (1944) 'War neurosis.' *Medical Press And Circular 212*, 100–103.

Minski, L. (1947) 'Modern treatment in psychological medicine.' *British Medical Journal 1*, 880–884.

Mitchell, P.R. (1945) 'Major difficulties experienced in the establishment of 600 and 1,200 bed general hospitals in Normandy.' *Journal of the Royal Army Medical Corps 85*, 228–233.

Moll, A.E. (1954) 'Psychosomatic disease due to battle stress.' In E.D. Wittkower and R.A. Cleghorn (eds) *Recent Developments in Psyhosomatic Medicine.* London: Pitman.

Moniz, E. and Lima A. (1936) 'Premiers essais de psycho-chirurgie: Technique at résultats.' *Lisboa Médicina 13*, 152–161.

Montague, C.E. (1929) *Disenchantment.* London: Chatto and Windus.

Montessori, M. (1912) *The Montessori Method: Scientific Pedagogy as Applied to Child Education.* London: Heineman.

Montgomery, B.L. (1946) 'Morale in battle.' *British Medical Journal 2*, 702–4.

Moran, H.M. (1946) *In My Fashion.* London: Peter Davies.

Moreno, J.L. (1937) 'Inter-personal therapy and the psychopathology of inter-personal relations.' *Sociometry 1*, 9–76.

Moreno, J.L. (1940) 'Mental catharsis and the psychodrama.' *Sociometry 3*, 209–244.

Moreno, J.L. (ed) (1945) *Group Psychotherapy: A Symposium.* New York: Beacon House.

Moreno, J.L. (1953) *Who Shall Survive?* New York: Beacon House.

Morris, J.N. (1945) 'Report on the health of 401 Chindits.' *Journal of the Royal Army Medical Corps 85*, 123–132.

Morselli, H. (1883) *Suicide: An Essay on Comparative Moral Statistics.* London: Kegan Paul, Trench and Co.

Mott, F.W. (1917) 'A microscopic examination of the brains of two men dead of commotio-cerebri (shellshock) without visible external injury.' *British Medical Journal 2*, 612–615.

Mulinder, E.K. (1945) 'Psychotic battle casualties.' *British Medical Journal 1*, p.733.

Murray, H. (1990) 'The transformation of selection procedures.' In E. Trist and H. Murray (eds) *The Social Engagement of Social Science, 1: The Socio-Psychological Perspective.* London: Free Association Books.

Murray, K.A.G. (undated) Reflections on Public Service Selection: The Civil Service Selection Board (CSSB), The Police, The Kirk – and Others, (ca 1950–1980). (Unpublished).

Myers, C.S. (1916) 'Contributions to the study of shell shock II: Being an account of certain cases treated by hypnosis.' *Lancet 1*, 65–69.

Myers, C.S. (1940) *Shell Shock in France: 1914–1918.* Cambridge: Cambridge University Press.

Neustatter, W.L. (1945) 'What is a "Black-Out"? A Study of Fifty Cases.' *Journal of the Royal Army Medical Corps 85*, 139–142.

Newman, P.H. (1944) The prisoner of war mentality: Its effect after repatriation.' *British Medical Journal 1*, 8–10.

Nostrand, F.H. van, (1945) 'Handling of neuropsychiatric cases in the Canadian army.' In H.L. Tidy.

Onslow, P. (1869) 'The philosophy of recruiting.' *Contemporary Review 12*, 549.

Owen, W. (1973) *War Poems and Others*. London: Chatto and Windus.

Palmer, H.A. (1945a) 'Abreactive Techniques: Ether.' *Journal of the Royal Army Medical Corps 84*, 86–7.

Palmer, H.A. (1945b) 'Military Psychiatric Casualties: Experience with 12,000 cases.' *Lancet 2*, 454–457 and 492–494.

Palmer, H.A. (1946) 'Contribution to discussion on forward psychiatry in the army.' *Proceedings of the Royal Society of Medicine 39*, p.137.

Palmer, H.A. (1948) 'Recent technique of physical treatment and its results.' In N.G. Harris *Modern Trends in Psychological Medicine*. London: Butterworth.

Parfitt, D.N. (1946) 'A comparison of prolonged narcosis and convulsion therapy in mental disorder.' *Journal of Mental Science 92*, 128–137.

Parliamentary Papers (1868) Royal Commission on courts martial and punishment, No. 4414, *12*, p.139.

Partridge, F. (1981) *Memories*. London: Phoenix Paperback.

Patrick, M. and Howells, R. (1990) 'Barbiturate assisted interviews in modern clinical practice.' *Psychological Medicine 20*, 763–765.

Payne, S.M. (1957) Foreword. J. Rickman, (1957).

Pearce, J.D.W. (1945a) Report on Military Psychiatric Services in Italy, with appendices on Special Training Barracks, Occupational Therapy at Reallocation Center (All Arms) CMF, and some statistics. Public Record Office, WO 222/1312.

Pearce, J.D.W. (1945b) 'Clinical aspects of psychiatric problems in the army.' *Practitioner 154*, 33–38.

Pearse, I.H. and Crocker, L.H. (1943) *The Peckham Experiment. A Study in the Living Structure of Society*. London: Allen and Unwin.

Pearse, I.H. (1944) *Letter to J. Rickman*, 27/11/1944, Box 3, Folder 2. Rickman Papers, Archives of the British Psycho-Analytic Society.

Peters, T. and Austin, N. (1985) *A Passion for Excellence*. Glasgow: Collins.

Pines, M. (ed) (1983a) *The Evolution of Group Analysis*. London: Routledge and Kegan Paul.

Pines, M. (1983b) 'The contribution of S.H. Foulkes to group therapy.' In M. Pines (ed) *The Evolution of Group Analysis*. London: Routledge and Kegan Paul.

Pines, M. (ed) (1985) *Bion and Group Psychotherapy*. London: Routledge and Kegan Paul.

Pines, M. (ed) (1991) 'The development of the psychodynamic movement.' In G.E. Berrios and H. Freeman (eds) *150 Years of British Psychiatry: 1841–1991*. London: Gaskell.

Pozner, H. (1950) 'Some aspects of post-war army psychiatry.' *Journal of the Royal Army Medical Corps 94*, 38–47.

Pozner, H. (1961) 'Common sense and military psychiatry.' *Journal of the Royal Army Medical Corps 107*, 155–164.

Pratt, J.H. (1907) 'The class method of treating consumption in the homes of the poor.' *Journal of the American Medical Association 49*, 755–759.

Privy Council Office (1947) *Report of an Expert Committee on the Work of Psychologists and Psychiatrists in the Services.* London: HMSO.

Psyche (1943) Magazine produced by patients at Northfield. Issues 1, 4, 9, In S.H. Foulkes Papers, Wellcome Institute for the History of Medicine: CMAC: PP/SHF/C.3/25.

Raven, J.C. (1942) 'Testing the mental ability of adults.' *Lancet 1*, 115 –117.

Rayner, E. (1991) *The Independent Mind in British Psychoanalysis.* London: Free Association Books.

Rees, J.R. (1943) 'Three years of military psychiatry in the United Kingdom.' *British Medical Journal 1*, 1–6.

Rees, J.R. (1945) *The Shaping of Psychiatry by War.* London: Chapman and Hall.

Rees, J.R. (1949) *Modern Practice in Psychological Medicine: 1949.* London: Butterworth.

Rees, J.R. (1958) *Foreword* in R.H. Ahrenfeldt (1958)

Rees, J.R. (1966) *Reflections: A Personal History and an Account of the Growth of the World Federation for Mental Health.* United States Committee of The World Federation for Mental Health.

Rees, T.P. (1943) Commentary on J. Bierer (1943) 'A new form of group psychotherapy.' *Proceedings of the Royal Society of Medicine 33*, 209.

Reeve, E.G. (1971) *Validation of Selection Boards and Procedures as exemplified in a study of the War Office Selection Boards.* London: Academic Press.

Research and Training Centre (1944) Part 2 – The Method of Leaderless Groups, from R.T.C. Memorandum No 5, 'The Work of the Military Testing Officer at a War Office Selection Board (OCTUs) Reg RTC/Inf/2 S.H. Foulkes Papers, Wellcome Institute for the History of Medicine: CMAC: PP/SH/1.11.1.

Richardson, F.M. (1978) *Fighting Spirit: Psychological Factors in War.* London: Leo Cooper.

Rickman, J. (1914–1916) Scrapbook on WWI, Rickman Papers, Archives of the British Psycho-Analytic Society. Box 2, Folder 1.

Rickman, J.R. (1934) 'Discussion: A symposium on the psychology of peace and war.' *British Journal of Medical Psychology 14*, 228–291.

Rickman, J.R. (1935) A Study of Quaker Beliefs, The Lister Memorial Lecture given to The Quaker Medical Society. (unpublished).

Rickman, J. (1937) 'On "Unbearable" ideas and impulses.' *American Journal of Psychology 50*, 248–253.

Rickman, J. (1938a) *Uniformity or Diversity in Groups.* Paper based on two public lectures which were delivered in March 1938, sponsored by the Institute of Psycho-Analysis. (unpublished).

Rickman, J. (1938b) 'Need for belief in God.' In J. Rickman *Selected Contributions to Psycho-Analysis.* London: Hogarth Press and the Institute of Psycho-Analysis.

Rickman, J. (1938c) 'Panic and air-raid precautions.' *Lancet 1*, 1291–1295.

Rickman, J. (1938d) 'A discursive review, of "Air Raid. The Technique of Silent Approach; High Explosive; Panic."' John Langdon Davies, *British Journal of Medical Psychology 17*, 361–373.

Rickman, J. (1939a) *Notes on the meeting of the British Psychological Society.* May 26th, Rickman Papers, Archives of the British Psycho-Analytic Society. CRR/F14/01.

Rickman, J. (1939b) 'War wounds and air raid casualties: The mental aspects of ARP.' *British Medical Journal 2,* 457–458.

Rickman, J. (1939c) *Haymeads Memorandum.* Rickman Papers, Archives of the British Psycho-Analytic Society, CRR/F14/07.

Rickman, J. (1939d) *Lecture Notes on: The Individual and the Group.* Given in May. Rickman Papers, Archives of the British Psycho-Analytic Society. Box 4, Folder 2.

Rickman, J. (1940a) 'On the nature of ugliness and the creative impulse.' (Marginalia Psychoanalytica. II). *International Journal of Psycho-Analysis 21,* 294–313.

Rickman, J. (1940b) *'Mental Rest and Mental Pain',* a lecture to nurses in charge of neurotic patients. Rickman Papers, Archives of the British Psycho-Analytic Society. Box 1, Folder 3.

Rickman, J. (1941) 'A case of hysteria – Theory and practice in the Two Wars.' *Lancet 1,* 785–786.

Rickman, J. (1943a) *Paper on Group Therapy,* draft of W.R. Bion and J. Rickman (1943). Rickman Papers, Archives of the British Psycho-Analytic Society.

Rickman, J. (1943b) The Influence of the 'Social Field' on Behaviour in the Interview Situation, unpublished collection of papers, edited by P. King.

Rickman, J. (1943c) 'The Psychiatric Interview in the Social Setting of a War Office Selection Board.' unpublished collection of papers, edited by P. King.

Rickman, J. (1944) *Letter to S.H. Foulkes* 29/12/44, S.H. Foulkes Papers, Wellcome Institute for the History of Medicine: CMAC: PP/SHF/C.3/6.

Rickman, J. (1945) Contribution to the Discussion of Dr. W.R. Bion's paper on *'Intra-Group Tensions in Therapy: Their Study a task of the Group'* given to the Medical Section of the British Psychological Society, 19 Dec 1945. Rickman Papers, Archives of the British Psycho-Analytic Society.

Rickman, J. (1944/50) Letters and memoranda concerning the future of the Peckham Experiments. Rickman Papers, Archives of the British Psycho-Analytic Society.

Rickman, J. (1950) The factor of number in individual- and group-dynamics. *Journal of Mental Science, 96,* 770–773.

Rickman, J. (1951) 'Number and the human sciences, psycho-analysis and culture.' reprinted in J. Rickman (1957), 218–233.

Rickman, J. (1957) Selected Contributions to Psycho-Analysis. Scott, W.C.M. (ed) London: Hogarth Press and The Institute of Psycho-Analysis.

Rivers, W.H.R. (1920a) *Instinct and Unconscious: A Contribution to a Biological Theory of the Psycho-Neuroses.* Cambridge: Cambridge University Press.

Rivers, W.H.R. (1920b) 'Report to the Air Medical Investigation Committee.' In J. Rickman 'War wounds and air raid casualities: The mental aspects of ARP.' *British Medical Journal 2,* 457–458.

Rivers, W.H.R. and Head, H. (1908) 'A human experiment in nerve division.' *Brain 31,* 323–450.

Roberts, W.W. and Moore, J.N.P. (1947) 'Mental illness among army officers: A survey of admissions to a military psychiatric hospital.' *British Journal of Social Medicine 1,* 135–47.

Robinson, J.T. (1948) 'Group therapy and its application in the British Army today.' *Journal of the Royal Army Medical Corps 91*, 66–79.

Rosie, R.J. (1952) 'Psychiatry in the Army.' In V.Z. Cope *Psychological Medicine*. London: HMSO.

Ross, T.A. (1939) 'Psychological Casualties in War (letters).' *British Medical Journal 2*, pp.925 and 1110.

Rycroft, C. (1972) *A Critical Dictionary of Psychoanalysis*. Harmondsworth: Penguin Books.

Sakel, M. (1959) 'The discovery and development of insulin therapy.' In M. Sakel *Schizophrenia*. London: Peter Owen.

Salmon, T.W. (ed) (1929) In the American Expeditionary Force, Section II of Vol 10, *Neuropsychiatry*, History of the Medical Department of the United States Army in the World War. Washington: US Government Printing Office.

Sargant, W. (1942) 'Physical treatment of acute war neuroses: Some clinical observations.' *British Medical Journal 2*, 574–576.

Sargant, W. and Craske, N. (1942) 'Modified insulin therapy in war neuroses.' *Lancet 2*, 212–214.

Sargant, W. and Slater, E. (1940) 'Acute war neurosis.' *Lancet 2*, 1–2.

Sargant, W. and Slater, E. (1941) 'Amnesic syndromes in war.' *Proceedings of the Royal Society of Medicine 34*, 757–764.

Sargant, W. and Slater, E. (1944) *An Introduction to Physical Methods of Treatment in Psychiatry*. Edinburgh: Livingstone.

Sargant, W. and Stewart, C.M. (1947) 'Chronic battle neurosis treated with leucotomy.' *British Medical Journal 2*, 866–69.

Scannell, V. (1983) *The Tiger and the Rose*. London: Robson Books.

Scannell, V. (1992) 'Compulsory Mourning.' *Ambit*, 2–4

Schilder, P. (1938) *Psychotherapy*. London: Kegan Paul, Trench and Trubner.

Schilder, P. (1939) 'Results and problems of group psychotherapy in severe neuroses.' *Mental Hygiene 23*, 87–98.

Schneider, K. (1959) *Klinische Psychopathologie*. New York: Grune and Stratton.

Scott, W.C.M. (1941) 'The soldier's defence and the public's attitude.' *Lancet 2*, 271–272.

Scull, A. (1991) 'Psychiatry and its historians.' *History of Psychiatry 2*, 239–250.

Scull, A. (1996) *Focal Sepsis and Psychosis: the Career of Thomas Chivers Graves, B.Sc., M.D., F.R.C.S., M.R.C.V.S., (1883–1964)*. In H. Freeman and G.E. Berrios (eds) *150 Years of British Psychiatry, 2: The Aftermath*. London: Athlone.

Segal, H. (1973) *Introduction to the Work of Melanie Klein*. London: Hogarth Press and the Institute of Psycho-Analysis.

Segal, H. (1989) *Klein*. London: Karnac Books.

Shah, I. (1973) *The Tales of the Dervishes*. St. Albans: Granada.

Sharman, S. (1951) 'The army psychiatrist and military law.' *Journal of the Royal Medical Corps 97*, 1–14.

Shephard, B. (1996) 'The early treatment of mental disorders': R.G. Rows and Maghull 1914–1918. In H. Freeman and G. Berrios (eds) *150 Years of British Psychiatry, 2: The Aftermath*. London: Athlone.

Showalter, E. (1987) *The Female Malady: Women, Madness and English Culture, 1830–1980*. London: Virago Press.

Sim, M. (1945) 'The NCO as a psychiatric casualty: A study of 627 cases admitted to a psychiatric hospital.' *Journal of the Royal Army Medical Corps 85*, 184–186.

Sim, M. (1946) 'A comparative study of disease incidence in admissions to a base psychiatric hospital in the Middle East.' *Journal of Mental Science 92*, 118–127.

Slater, E. (1941a) *Report on Visit to Wharncliffe Emergency Hospital*, 13 and 14 January 1941, Rickman Papers, Archives of the British Psycho-Analytic Society. MRB/FO3/9.

Slater, E. (1941b) *Letter to John Rickman*, Rickman Papers, Archives of the British Psycho-Analytic Society. MRB/FO3/12.

Slater, E. (1941c) 'War neurosies: General symptomatology and constitutional factors.' *Medical Press and Circular 205*, 133–135.

Slater, E. (1943) 'The neurotic constitution: A statistical study of two thousand neurotic soldiers.' *Journal of Neurology and Psychiatry 6*, 1–16.

Slavson, S.R. (1940) 'Group therapy.' *Mental Hygiene 24*, 36–49.

Slavson, S.R. (1943) *An Introduction to Group Therapy*. New York: Commonwealth Fund.

Slavson, S.R. (1946) 'Group psychotherapy.' In E.A. Spiegel (ed) *Progress in Neurology and Psychiatry: An Annual Review, Vol I*. New York: Grune and Stratton.

Slavson, S.R. and Scheidlinger, S. (1948) 'Group psychotherapy.' In E.A. Speigel (ed) *Progress in Neurology and Psychiatry: An Annual Review, Vol. III*. New York: Grune and Stratton.

Slim, W.J. Field Marshall Lord, (1956) *Defeat Into Victory*. London: Cassell.

Slobodin, R. (1978) *W.H.R. Rivers*. New York: Columbia University Press.

Snowden, E.N. (1939) 'Prevention of war psycho-neurosis in soldiers.' *Lancet 2*, 1130–1132.

Stalker, H.A. (1941) 'Rejection of psychiatrically unfit recruits.' *Lancet 1*, 535–536.

Stalker, H.A. (1944) 'Psychiatric states in 130 ex-service patients.' *Journal of Mental Science 90*, 727–738.

Stone, M. (1985) 'Shell shock and the psychologists.' In W.F. Bynum, R. Porter and M. Shepherd *The Anatomy of Madness, Vol. II*. London: Tavistock.

Stouffer, S.A., Lumsdaine, A.A., Lumsdaine, M.H., Williams, R.M., Smith, M.B., Janis, I.L., Star, S.A. and Cottrell, L.S. (1965) *The American Soldier, Vol. 2. Combat and its Aftermath*. Princeton: Wiley.

Strecker, E.A. and Appel, K.E. (1945) *Psychiatry in Modern Warfare*. New York: Macmillan.

Stungo, E. (1938) 'Psychological investigation by means of evipan sodium.' *Medical Press and Circular 197*, 382–386.

Stungo, E. (1946) 'Psychiatric casualties in Burma, 1945.' *Journal of Mental Science 92*, 585–594.

Sullivan, H.S. (1955) *Conceptions of Modern Psychiatry*. London: Tavistock. First published 1933.

Sutherland, J.D. (1941) 'A survey of one hundred cases of war neuroses.' *British Medical Journal 2*, 365–370.

Sutherland, J.D. (1985) 'Bion revisited: Group dynamics and group psychotherapy.' In M. Pines (ed) *Bion and Group Psychotherapy*. London: Routledge and Kegan Paul.

Sutherland, J.D. (1989) *Fairbairn's Journey into the Interior*. London: Free Association Books.

Sutherland, J.D. and Fitzpatrick, G.A. (1945) 'Some approaches to group problems in the British Army.' *Sociometry 8*, 443–455.

Swank, R.L. and Marchand, W.E. (1946) 'Combat neuroses: Development of combat exhaustion.' *Archives of Neurology and Psychiatry 55*, 236–247.

Symonds, C.P. (1941) 'Presidential address: The neurological approach to mental disorder.' *Proceedings of the Royal Society of Medicine 34*, 289–302.

Symonds, C.P. (1943) 'Anxiety neurosis in combatants.' *Lancet 2*, 785–789.

Tayleur Stockings, G.T. (1944) 'A study of acute neurotic depression as seen in military psychiatry and its differential diagnosis from the depressive psychoses.' *Journal of Mental Science 90*, 772–776.

Tayleur Stockings, G.T. (1945) 'The syndrome of hyster-encephalopathy in military psychiatric casualties.' *Journal of Mental Science 91*, 104–109.

Taylor, A.J.P. (1970) *English History: 1914–1945*. Harmondsworth: Penguin.

Tennant, C., Goulston, K. and Dent, O. (1986) 'Clinical psychiatric illness in prisoners of war of the Japanese: Forty years after release.' *Psychological Medicine 16*, 833–839.

Thorner, H.A. (1946) 'The treatment of psychoneurosis in the British Army.' *International Journal of Psycho-Analysis 27*, 52–59.

Titmuss, R. (1950) *Problems of Social Policy, History of the Second World War.* London: HMSO.

Tooth, G.C. and Newton, M.P. (1961) Leucotomy in England and Wales 1942 – 1954: *Reports on Public Health and Medical Subjects, 104*. London: HMSO.

Torrie, A. (1944) 'Psychosomatic casualties in the Middle East.' *Lancet 1*, 139–143.

Torrie, A. (1945) 'The return of Odysseus: The problem of marital infidelity for the repatriate.' *British Medical Journal 2*, 192–3.

Tredgold, R.F. (1942) 'Invalidism from the army due to mental disabilities. The aetiological significance of military conditions.' *Journal of Mental Science 88*, 444–448.

Tredgold, R.F. (1944) 'The importance of failure of concentration in the acute war neurosis syndrome.' *Journal of the Royal Army Medical Corps 82*, 177–182.

Tredgold, R.F., Kelly, G., Hefferman, H.N. and Leigh, P.R.W. (1946) 'Serious psychiatric disability among British officers in India.' *Lancet 2*, 257–261.

Trimble, M.R. (1981) *Post-Traumatic Neurosis from Railway Spine to the Whiplash.* London: John Wiley.

Trist, E. (1985) 'Working with Bion in the 1940s: The group decade.' In M. Pines (ed) *Bion and Group Psychotherapy.* London: Routledge and Kegan Paul.

Trist, E.L. and Murray, H.A. (eds) (1990a) *The Social Engagement of Social Science, 1: The Socio-Psychological Perspective.* London: Free Associations Books.

Trist, E.L. and Murray, H.A. (1990b) 'Historical Overview: The Foundation and Development of the Tavistock Institute.' In E.L. Trist and H.A. Murray (eds).

Trotter, W. (1919) *Instincts of the Herd in Peace and War.* London: Fisher Unwin.

Vernon, P.E. and Parry, J.B. (1949) *Personnel Selection in the British Forces.* London: University of London Press.

Vinden, F.H. (1977) 'The introduction of war office selection boards in the British Army: A personal recollection.' In B. Bond and I. Roy (eds) *War and Society 2*, London: Croom Helm.

Walker, E.R.C. (1944) 'Impressions of a repatriated medical officer.' *Lancet 1*, 514–515.

Waller, D. (1991) *Becoming a Profession: The History of Art Therapy in Britain: 1940–1980*. London: Tavistock/Routledge.

Warner, P. (1977) *The Fields of War: A Young Cavalryman's Crimea Campaign*. London: John Murray.

Ward, M. (1971) *The Blessed Trade*. London: Michael Joseph.

War Office (1922) Report of the War Office Committee of Enquiry into 'Shell Shock.' London: HMSO.

War Office (1942) Battle School Training and Battle Inoculation: Technical Memorandum No. 1, pps. 5 – 10, in War Office, (1946a).

War Office (1943–4a) Reports on the Work of the Medical Division Military (P) Hospital: Northfield. London: Public Record Office, WO 222/846.

War Office (1943–4b) War Diaries, Northfield Military (P) Hospital. London: Public Record Office, WO 177/133.

War Office (1943a) Nomenclature of Mental Diseases: Technical Memorandum 10., in War Office, (1946a).

War Office (1943b) TM 30–410, Handbook on the British Army, reprinted 1975 (eds) C. Ellis and P. Chamberlain. London: Military Book Society.

War Office (1944) Royal Army Medical Corps, Training Pamphlet No. 3.

War Office (1946a) Directorate of Army Psychiatry: Technical Memoranda, War Office (A.M.D. 11).

War Office (1946b) The General Service Intake Selection Procedure, Technical Memorandum 8, in War Office (1946a).

War Office (1947) Personnel Selection in the British Army: 8th International Management Congress Papers. Directorate for the Selection of Personnel.

War Office (1948) Statistical Report on the Health of the Army: 1943–45. London: HMSO.

Warren, A.J. (1943) *Letter to J. Rickman*, 29 April, Rickman Papers, Archives of the British Psycho-Analytic Society. MRB/F01/07.

Wender, L. (1936) 'The dynamics of group psychotherapy and its application, ' *Journal of Nervous and Mental Disease 84*, 54–60.

Wheeler, W. (1951) *The Letters of Private Wheeler: 1809–1828*. London: Michael Joseph.

Whiles, W.H. (1945) 'A study of neurosis among repatriated prisoners of war.' *British Medical Journal 2*, 697–698.

White, A.C.T. (1963) *The Story of Army Education: 1643–1963*. London: Harrap.

Whiteley, J.S. and Gordon, J. (1979) *Group Approaches in Psychiatry*. London: Routledge and Kegan Paul.

Wilde, J.F. (1942) 'Narco-analysis in the treatment of war neuroses.' *British Medical Journal 2*, 4–7.

Wilde, J.F. and Morgan, C.J. (1943) 'Occupational therapy for psychoneurotics in hospital.' *Journal of the Royal Army Medical Corps 81*, 24–31.

Wills, W.D. (1941) *The Hawkspur Experiment*. London: George Allen and Unwin.

Wills, W.D. (1943a) 'Internal government of the camp: Its growth and changes.' In M.E. Franklin (ed) *Q Camp: An Experiment in Group Living with Maladjusted and Anti-Social Young Men*. London: Planned Environment Therapy Trust.

Wills, W.D. (1943b) 'Summary of data derived from members' case records and after-histories.' In M.E. Franklin (ed) Q Camp: An Experiment in Group Living with Maladjusted and Anti-Social Young Men. London: Planned Environment Therapy Trust.

Wills, W.D. (1964) Homer Lane: A Biography. London: George Allen and Unwin.

Wilson, A.T.M. (1942) 'Suppose You Were a Nazi Agent: Fifth Column Work for Amateurs.' Technical Memorandum 2, in War Office (1946a).

Wilson, A.T.M., Doyle, M. and Kelnar, J. (1947) 'Group techniques in a transitional community.' Lancet 1, 735–8.

Wilson, N.S. (1948) Education in the Forces: 1939–1946: A Civilian Contribution. London: The Year Book of Education.

Windholz, G. and Witherspoon, L.H. (1993) 'Sleep as a cure for schizophrenia: A historical episode.' History of Psychiatry 4, 38–93.

Wing, J.K. and Brown, G.W. (1970) Institutionalism and Schizophrenia: A Comparative Study of Three Mental Hospitals 1960–1968. Cambridge: Cambridge University Press.

Winnicott, D.W. (1971) Playing and Reality. London: Tavistock.

Wishart, J.W. (1944) Experiences as a Psychiatrist with BNAF and CMF, January 1943 to January 1944 (with special reference to work in the forward areas). Typewritten personal account in the possession of S.H. Foulkes, Royal Army Medical Corps Muniment Collection, Wellcome Institute for the History of Medicine: CMAC: RAMC 466/49.

Wittkower, E.D. (1945) 'The war disabled: Their emotional, social and occupational situation.' British Journal of Medicine 1, 587–590.

Wittkower, E.D. (1947) 'Rehabilitation of the limbless: A joint surgical and psychologic study.' Occupational Medicine 3, 20–44.

Wittkower, E.D. (1949) 'Psychosomatic medicine.' In J.R. Rees (eds) Modern Practice in Psychological Medicine: 1949. London: Butterworth.

Wittkower, E.D. and Cleghorn, R.A. (1954) Recent Developments in Psychosomatic Medicine. London: Pitman.

Wittkower, E.D. and Davenport, R.C. (1946) 'The War-Blinded: Their Emotional, Social and Occupational Situation,' Psychosomatic Medicine 8, 121–137.

Wittkower, E.D. and Lebeaux, L. (1943) 'The Special Transfer Scheme: An Experiment in Military Psychiatric Vocational Re-Employment,' The Medical Press and Circular 209, 366–368.

Wittkower, E.D., Rodger, T.F. and Wilson, A.T.M. (1941) 'Effort Syndrome,' Lancet 531–535.

Wood, P. (1941a) 'Da Costa's Syndrome (or Effort Syndrome),' British Medical Journal 1, 767–772, 805–811 and 845–51.

Wood, P. (1941b) 'Contribution to the Discussion on the Psychiatric Aspects of Effort Syndrome,' Proceedings of the Royal Society of Medicine 34, 543–549.

Wright, M.B. (1939) 'Psychological Emergencies in War Time,' British Medical Journal 2, 576–578.

Xenophon (1951) The Persian Expedition. Harmondsworth: Penguin Classics.

Subject Index

(Page references in italic refer to illustrations)

Author Index